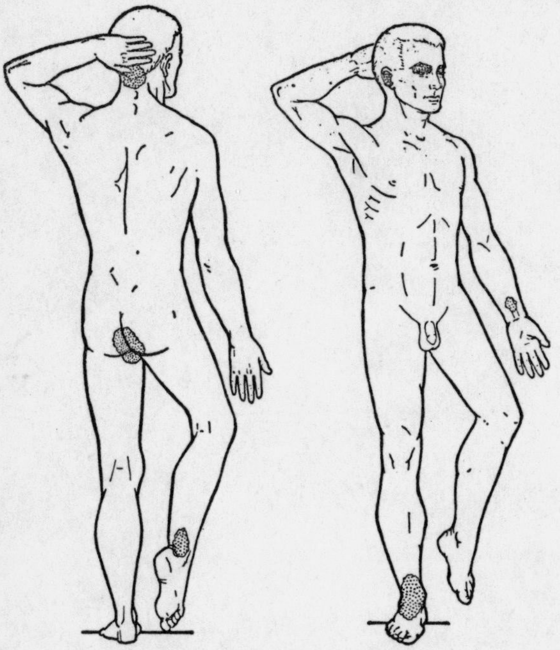

NEURODERMATITIS

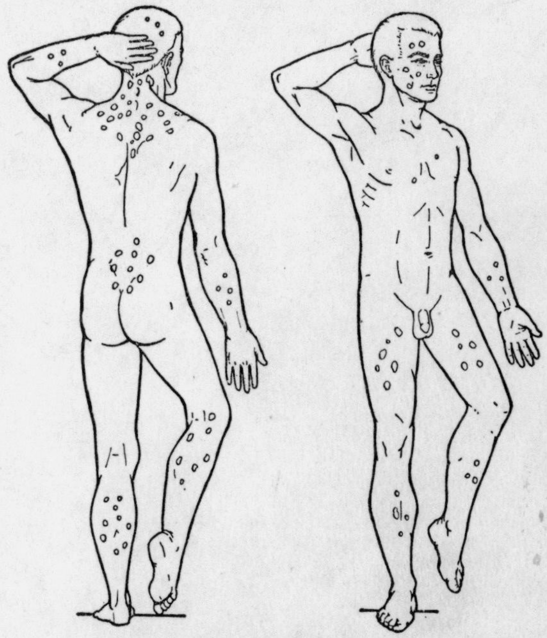

NEUROTIC EXCORIATIONS

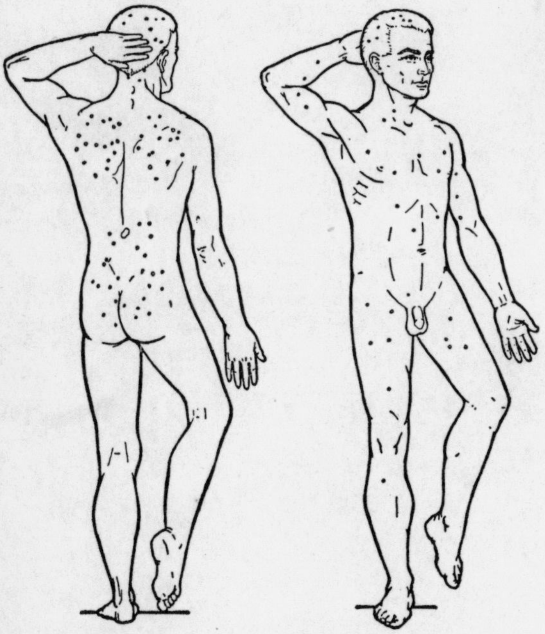

DERMATITIS HERPETIFORMIS

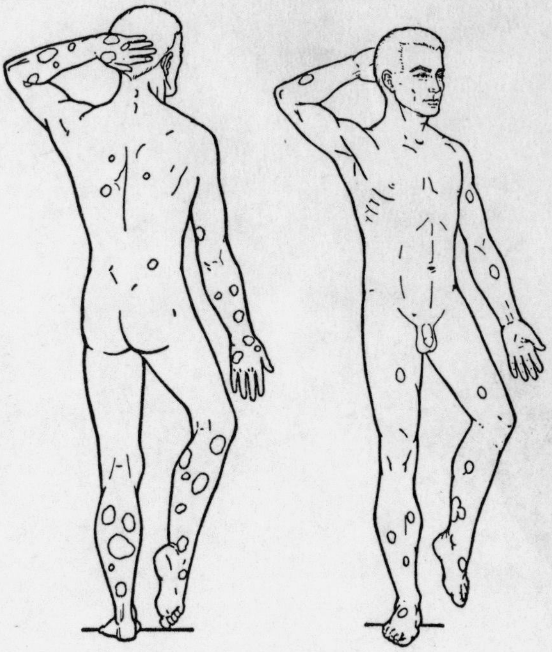

NUMMULAR ECZEMA

MANUAL OF SKIN DISEASES

MANUAL OF

SKIN DISEASES

GORDON C. SAUER, M.D.

Assistant Clinical Professor of Medicine (Dermatology) and Chief of the Section of Dermatology, University of Kansas School of Medicine; Attending Physician, General Hospital, Kansas City, Mo.; Consultant, U. S. Army Hospital, Fort Leavenworth, Kansas

151 Illustrations and 28 Color Plates

J. B. LIPPINCOTT COMPANY

Philadelphia Montreal

Second Printing

Distributed in Great Britain by
Pitman Medical Publishing Co., Limited, London

Library of Congress Catalog Card No. 59-11576
Printed in the United States of America

Dedicated to

My Family

Foreword

There has been a great need for a concise, factual book on diseases of the skin. There are many fine texts upon this subject for the specialists. However, they are so large and comprehensive that the student and the general practitioner find themselves lost in the subject matter that they wish to investigate. Since most of the physicians are not going to be specialists in dermatology, they want a book that offers practical, brief and reliable information for the diagnosis and the treatment of skin diseases.

This is such a book. Dr. Sauer approaches it from almost a personal angle, as though he were sitting by the student or the general practitioner and explaining to him the nature of the skin disease. He talks in a conversational tone about the patient's trouble. He outlines the plan of the treatment on the first visit, and upon the second and the third visits he modifies his treatment with the modification of the disease.

The illustrations, both the line drawings and the color photographs, are excellent. In many instances, the general practitioner or the student can open the book and find a color photograph of the disease which he can match with the patient's so that he can make a diagnosis and treat the patient accordingly.

The book does not go extensively into bibliographies or into lengthy discussions of the disease. This is an emergency textbook of dermatology that the general practitioner may use in treating the vast majority of his cases. If the patient has a very complicated dermatologic condition the doctor will send him to a specialist instead of trying to treat him himself.

The book is well written, concise and factual, which is high praise in itself.

Charles C. Dennie, M.D.

Emeritus Professor of Dermatology
University of Kansas
School of Medicine

Preface

The motivation for this book was a question asked of me by a senior medical student: "Where can I find a good 50-page book on dermatology?" This book is written as an answer to those students and practitioners who have asked that same general question. This book is not 50 pages long, but it is one of the shortest and most concise books published on diseases of the skin.

Approximately 15 per cent of all patients who walk into the general practitioner's office do so for care of some skin disease or skin lesion. It may be for such a simple treatment as the removal of a wart, for the treatment of athlete's feet or for something as complicated as severe cystic acne. There have been so many recent advances in the various fields of medicine that the medical school instructor can expect his students to learn and retain only a small percentage of the material that is taught them. I believe that the courses in all phases of medicine, and particularly the courses of the various specialties, should be made as simple, basic and concise as possible. If the student retains only a small percentage of what is presented to him, he will be able to handle an amazing number of his walk-in patients. I am presenting in this book only the material that medical students and general practitioners must know for the diagnosis and the treatment of patients with the common skin diseases. In condensing the material many generalities are stated, and the reader must remember that there are exceptions to every rule. The inclusion of these exceptions would defeat the intended purpose of this book. More complicated diagnostic procedures or treatments for interesting or problem cases are merely frosting on the cake. This information can be obtained by the interested student from any of several more comprehensive dermatologic texts.

This book consists of two distinct but complementary parts.

The first part contains the chapters devoted to the diagnosis and the management of the important common skin diseases. The chapter on a dermatologic formulary has been especially marked for easy reference. In discussing the common skin diseases, a short introductory sentence is followed by a listing of the salient points of each disease in outline form. All diseases of the skin have primary lesions, secondary lesions, a rather specific distribution, a general course which includes the prognosis and the recurrence rate of the disease, varying subjective complaints and a known or unknown cause. Where indicated, a statement follows concerning seasonal incidence, age groups affected, family and sex incidence, contagiousness or infectiousness, relationship to employment and laboratory findings. The discussion ends with a paragraph on differential diagnosis and treatment. Treatment, to be effective, has to be thought of as a chain of events. The therapy outlined on the first visit is usually different from that given on subsequent visits or for cases that are very severe. The treatment is discussed with these variations in mind. The first part of the book concludes with a chapter on basic equipment necessary for managing dermatologic patients.

The second part consists of a very complete dictionary-index to the entire field of dermatology, defining the majority of rare diseases and the unusual dermatologic terms. The inclusion of this dictionary-index has a twofold purpose. First, it enables me to present a concise first section on *common* skin diseases unencumbered by the inclusion of the rare diseases. Second, the dictionary-index provides a rather complete coverage of all of dermatology for the more interested student. In reality, two books are contained in one.

Dermatologic nomenclature has always been a bugaboo for the new student. I heartily agree with many dermatologists that we should simplify the terminology, and that has been attempted in this text. Some of the changes are mine, but many have been suggested by others. However, after a diligent effort to simplify the names of skin diseases, one is left with the appalling fact that some of the complicated terms defy change. One of the main reasons for this is that all of our field, the skin, is visible to the naked eye. As a result, any minor alteration from normal has been scrutinized by countless physicians through the years and given countless names. The liver or heart counterpart of folliculitis ulerythematosa reticulata (ulerythema acneiforme, atrophoderma reticulatum symmetricum faciei, atrophodermie vermiculée) is yet to be discovered.

What I am presenting in this book is not specialty dermatology but general practice dermatology. Some of my medical educator friends say that only internal medicine, pediatrics and obstetrics should be taught to medical students. They state that the specialized fields of medicine should be taught only at the internship, residency or postgraduate level. That idea misses the very important fact that cases from all of the so-called specialty fields wander in to the general practitioner's office. The general practitioner must have some *basic* knowledge of the varied aspects of all of medicine so that he can properly take care of his general everyday practice. This basic knowledge must be taught in the undergraduate years. The purpose of this book is to complement such teaching.

GORDON C. SAUER, M.D.
425 East 63rd Street
Kansas City 10, Missouri

Acknowledgments

For the most realistic presentation of skin diseases, color photography is essential. However, the cost of color reproduction is so great that it is almost impossible to enjoy the advantages of color plates and still keep the price of a book within the range where it will have the broadest appeal. The problem has been solved for this book through the generosity of the following companies which have underwritten the cost of the color plates credited to them.

- Burroughs Wellcome & Company, Inc.
- Dome Chemicals, Inc.
- Duke Laboratories, Inc.
- Geigy Pharmaceuticals
- Roche Laboratories
- Sandoz Pharmaceuticals
- Smith, Kline and French Laboratories
- E. R. Squibb and Sons
- Texas Pharmacal Company

The following pharmaceutical companies have contributed color plates from their own publications.

- Geigy Pharmaceuticals
- Smith, Kline and French Laboratories
- Upjohn Company

Anyone dealing with medical photography is fully aware of the difficulty in obtaining good illustrative cases and equally good pictures of these cases. Many hundreds of black and white, 35 mm. color, and 3¼″ x 4¼″ color pictures were taken by me and others to provide an adequate collection from which to select the illustrations for this book.

I am greatly indebted to the photographers of two institutions for their many excellent pictures. Dr. David Ruhe's Department of Audio-Visual Education at the University of Kansas School of Medicine, Kansas City, Kans., provided photographers Burton Johnson, William McGrew, Barton LaVine, Ben McIntyre, Tom Warford and Don Smith. At the Kansas City General Hospital, Kansas City, Mo., Roger Odneil was the photographer. These two institutions are credited under their photographs by the respective abbreviations, K.U.M.C. and K.C.G.H. The co-operation and the ability of these photographers is greatly appreciated. The group at the University of Kansas also had the tedious job of making black-and-white prints from my personal 35-mm. color slides.

The physician whose cases were photographed or who furnished illustration material is gratefully acknowledged under the respective picture.

The excellent line drawings were very ably prepared by Jo Ann Clifford of the University of Kansas School of Medicine, Department of Audio-Visual Education. I am grateful for her patience and for her ability to portray my rough sketches and thoughts.

A grant from the Developmental Fund of the Department of Medicine by Dr. E. Grey Dimond, Professor of Medicine, University of Kansas School of Medicine, provided additional money for illustrative work. A similar grant for additional photographic work at General Hospital was made from the Staff Fund of the Kansas City General Hospital.

The book and I profited by my association with J. Brooks Stewart, Medical Editor, Stanley A. Gillet, Production Editor, and Dr. Walter Kahoe, Director of the Medical Department of the J. B. Lippincott Company.

The material in any book comes from many sources. The majority of information in this book comes from my clinical experience in private practice and at university and hospital clinics I have directed. Various excellent textbooks have been consulted, especially the following:

Sutton, R. L., Jr.: Diseases of the Skin. St. Louis, C. V. Mosby Company, 1956. This is the modern monumental encyclopedia of all of dermatology. In addition to the help received from this excellent text, I desire to acknowledge the stimulation and the advice that I have had personally from Dr. Sutton. Additional textbooks and references are listed throughout the book as they pertain to special subjects.

I felt the need of constructive criticism of the material from a physician who had an interest in dermatology but was not a dermatologist. These requirements were happily satisfied by Dr. Lawrence Field, Resident in Internal Medicine at Kansas City General Hospital, and I am greatly indebted to him for his interest, time and advice. In addition, Dr. Field spent many hours proofreading copy.

Further thanks go to: Dr. Frank Dwyer, who read and criticized the book from the dermatologist's viewpoint; Mr. Charles Hayden, Pharmacist, who gave advice regarding the Formulary; and, finally, my secretary, Mrs. Alberta Morrell, who typed and retyped the many drafts necessary to complete this book. My thanks are profound.

G. C. S.

Contents

List of Plates

Structure of the Skin*

CHAPTER 1

THE SKIN is a barrier between the internal organs and the external environment. It is uniquely subjected to noxious external agents and is also a sensitive reflection of internal disease. An understanding of the cause and the effect of this complex interplay in the skin begins with a thorough understanding of the basic structure of this organ.

LAYERS OF THE SKIN

The skin is divided into 3 layers. From inside out they are the subcutaneous tissue, the dermis and the epidermis (Fig. 1).

Subcutaneous Tissue. This layer serves as a receptacle for the formation and the storage of fat and it supports the blood vessels and the nerves that pass from the tissues beneath to the corium above. The deeper hair follicles and the sweat glands originate in this layer.

Dermis (Corium). This layer is made up of connective tissue, cellular elements and ground substance. It has a rich blood and nerve supply. The sebaceous glands and the shorter hair follicles originate in the corium.

The *connective tissue* consists of collagen fibers, elastic fibers and reticular fibers. All of these, but most importantly the collagen fibers, contribute to the support and the elasticity of the skin.

The *cellular elements* of the corium consist of fibrocytes, histiocytes, mastocytes and migratory blood cells.

The *ground substance* is not easily seen but is of tremendous physiologic importance since it contains proteins, electrolytes, tissue fluid and hyaluronic acid.

Epidermis. This is the most superficial of the 3 layers of the skin and averages in thickness about the width of the mark of a sharp pencil. There are two distinct types of cells in the epidermis, the keratin-forming cells and the melanin-forming cells. These latter cells synthesize melanin, the principal pigment of the epidermis. The keratin-forming cells are found in the basal layer and give rise to all the other cells of the stratified epidermis.

The epidermis is divided into 5 layers from within outward (Fig. 2).

1. Basal layer
2. Prickle layer
3. Granular layer
4. Lucid layer

} Living epidermis

5. Horny layer—Dead end-product

The *basal layer* of cells lie next to the corium and contain both the keratin-forming and the melanin-forming cells. The keratin-forming cells can be thought of as stem cells which are capable of progressive differentiation into the cell forms higher up in the epidermis.

* For a more detailed and excellently written account of this introductory material consult the first hundred pages of Pillsbury, D. M., Shelley, W. B., and Kligman, A. M.: Dermatology, Philadelphia, Saunders, 1956.

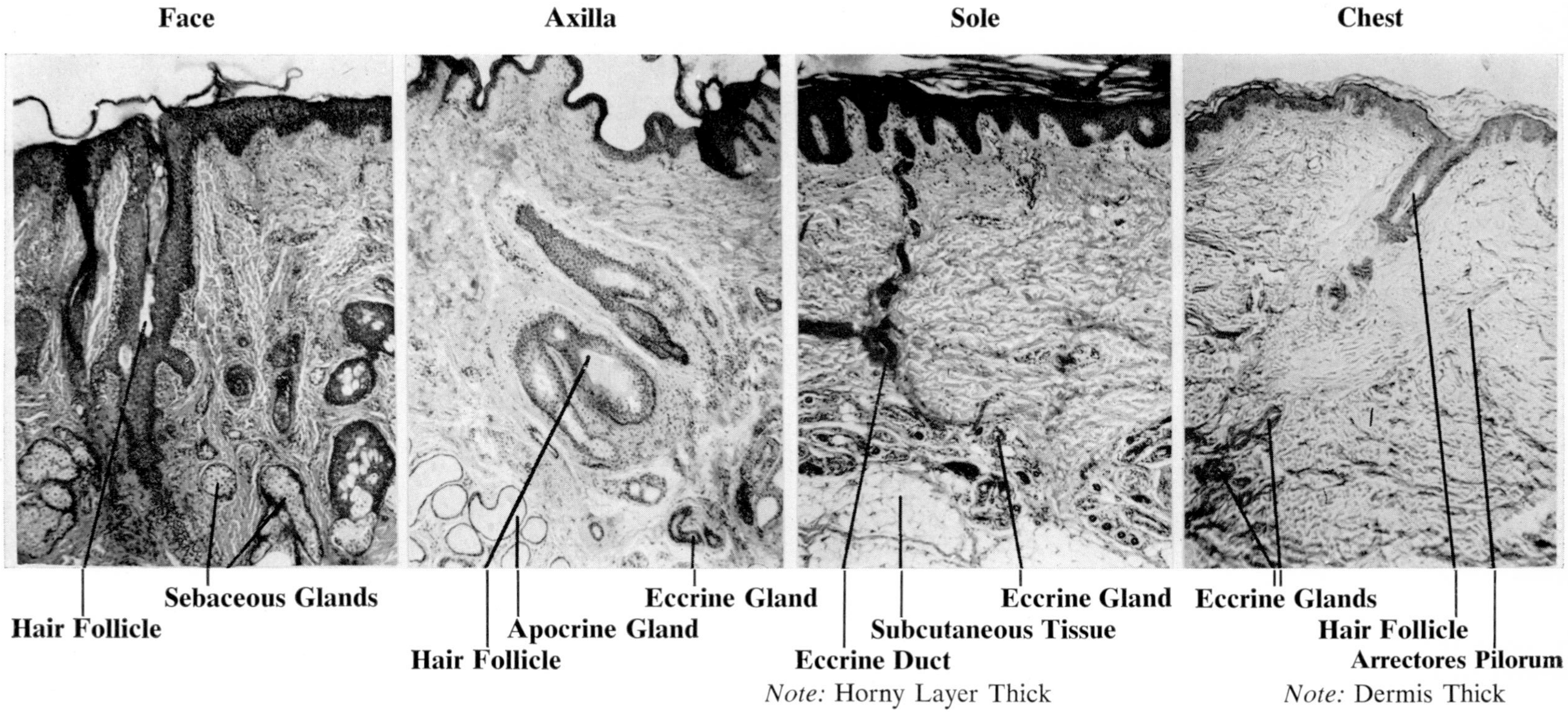

Fig. 1. Histology of the skin.

Microscopic sections from 4 different areas of the body. Note the variations in the histologic features, such as the thickness of the horny layer, the presence or absence of the 3 types of glands and the hair follicles, etc. These photographs were taken at the same magnification.
(*Dr. David Gibson*)

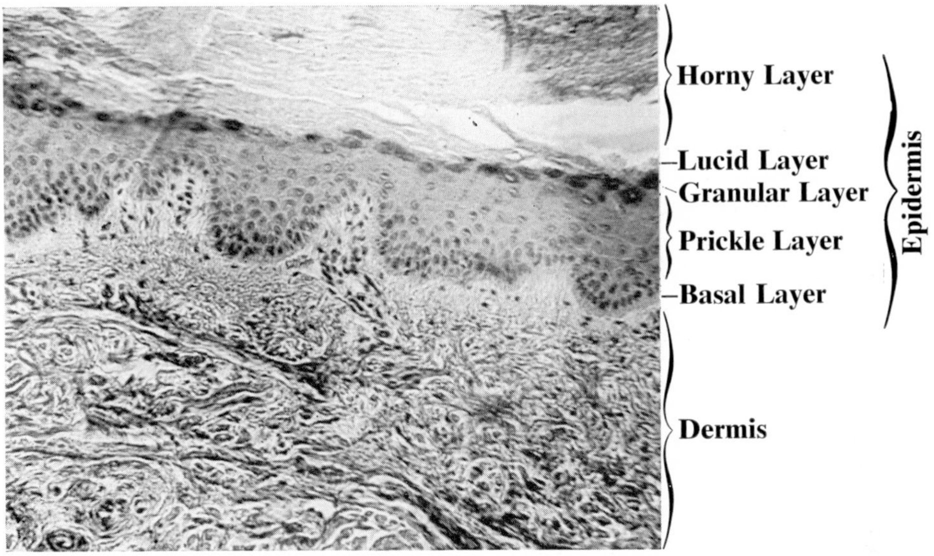

Fig. 2. Histology of the epidermis.
A microscopic section from the sole of the foot.
(*Dr. David Gibson*)

The *prickle layer* is made up of several layers of epidermal cells, chiefly of polyhedral shape. This layer gets its name from the existence of a network of cytoplasmic threads called prickles that extend between the cells. These prickles are most readily visible in this layer but, to a lesser extent, are present between all the cells of the epidermis.

The third layer is the *granular layer*. Here the cells are flatter and contain protein granules.

The *lucid layer* is next and appears as a translucent line of flat cells. This layer of the skin is present only on the palms and the soles. The granular and the lucid layers make up the transitional layer of the epidermis and act as a barrier to the inward transfer of noxious substances and outward loss of water.

The outermost layer of the epidermis is the *horny layer*. It is made up of stratified layers of dead keratinized cells that are constantly shedding. The chemical protein in these cells—keratin—is capable of absorbing vast amounts of water. This is readily seen during bathing when the skin of the palms and the soles becomes white and swollen.

VASCULAR SUPPLY

The vascular supply of the skin, while it is rich, is not unusual except for one special vascular body called the glomus. The glomus body is most commonly seen on the tips of the fingers, toes and under the nails. Each one of these organs contains a vessel segment which has been called the Sucquet-Hoyer canal. This canal represents a short circuit device connecting an arteriole with a venule without having to go through capillaries. The result is a marked increase in the blood flow through the skin. When this body grows abnormally the result is a very painful red glomus tumor, commonly occurring underneath a nail, that has to be removed by surgical means.

NERVE SUPPLY

The nerve supply of the skin consists of sensory nerves and motor nerves.

Sensory Nerves. The sensory nerves mediate the sensations of touch, temperature or pain. The millions of terminal, apparently nonspecific, free nerve endings have more to do with the specificity of skin sensation than the better-known highly specialized nerve endings, such as the Vater-Pacinian and the Wagner-Meissner tactile corpuscles.

Itching is certainly the most important presenting symptom of an unhappy patient. It may be defined simply as the desire to scratch. Itching apparently is a mild painful sensation that differs from pain in having a lower frequency of impulse stimuli. The release of proteinases (as follows itch powder application) may be responsible for the itch sensation. The pruritus may be of a pricking type or of a burning type and can vary greatly from one individual to another. Sulzberger called those abnormally sensitive individuals "itchish," analogous to the "ticklish" person. Itching can occur without any clinical signs of skin disease, or from circulating allergens or from local superficial contactants.

Motor Nerves. The involuntary sympathetic motor nerves control the sweat glands, the arterioles and the smooth muscles of the skin. Adrenergic fibers carry impulses to the arrectores pilorum muscles which produce goose flesh when they are stimulated. This is due to traction of the muscle on the hair follicle to which it is attached.

APPENDAGES

The appendages of the skin include both the cornified appendages (hairs and nails) and the glandular appendages.

Hairs are derived from the hair follicles of the epidermis. Since no new hair follicles are formed after birth, the different types of body hairs are manifestations of the effect of location and of external and internal stimuli. Hormones are the most important internal stimuli influencing the various types of hair growth. This growth is cyclic, with a growing phase and a resting phase. The average period of scalp hair growth ranges from 2 to 6 years. However, systemic stresses such as childbirth, may cause hairs to enter a resting stage prematurely. This postpartum effect is noticed most commonly in the scalp when these resting hairs are depilated during combing or washing; and the thought of approaching baldness causes sudden alarm on the part of the woman.

TYPES. The adult has two main types of hairs: the vellus hairs (lanugo hairs of the fetus) and the terminal hairs. The vellus hairs are the fine, short hairs of the body, whereas the terminal hairs are coarse, thick and pigmented. The latter hairs are developed most extensively on the scalp, the face and the extremities.

HAIR FOLLICLES. The hair follicle may be thought of as an invagination of the epidermis with its different layers of cells. These cells make up the matrix of the hair follicle and produce the keratin of the mature hair. The protein-synthesizing capacity of this tissue is enormous when one considers that at the rate of scalp hair growth of 0.35 mm. per day, over 100 linear feet of scalp hair is produced daily.

FACTS ABOUT HAIR AND ITS GROWTH. Certain facts should be stated concerning hair and its growth. (1) Shaving of excess hair on the extremities does not promote more rapid growth of coarse hair. The shaved stubs appear more coarse but, if allowed to grow normally, they would appear no different than before shaving. (2) The value of intermittent massage to stimulate scalp hair growth has not been proved. (3) Hair cannot turn gray overnight. The melanin pigmentation, which is distributed throughout the length of the nonvital hair shaft, takes weeks to be shed through the slow process of hair growth. (4) The common male type of baldness cannot safely be influenced by local and systemic measures, including hormones. Heredity is the greatest factor predisposing to baldness, and an excess of male hormone may contribute to hair loss in these people. Male castrates do not become bald.

Nails. The second cornified appendage, the nail, consists of a nail plate and the tissue that surrounds it. This plate lies in a nail groove which, similar to the hair follicle, is an invagination of the epidermis. Unlike hair growth, which is periodic, nail growth is continuous. Nail growth is about one third the rate of hair growth, or about 0.1 mm. per day. It takes approximately 3 months to restore a removed fingernail and about 3 times that long for the regrowth of a new toenail. Nail growth can be inhibited during serious illnesses or in old age, increased through nail-biting or occupational stress, and altered because of hand dermatitis or systemic disease. Topical treatment of nail disturbances is very unsatisfactory due to the inaccessibility of the growth-producing areas.

Glandular Appendages. TYPES. The glandular appendages of the skin are divided into two types: the sebaceous glands and the sweat glands (Fig. 3). The sebaceous glands form their secretion through distintegration of the whole glandular cell, whereas the sweat glands eliminate only a portion of the cell in the formation of secretion.

The *sebaceous glands* are present everywhere on the skin except the palms and the soles. The secretion from these glands is evacuated through the sebaceous duct to a follicle that may or may not contain a hair. This secretion is not under any neurologic control but is a continuous outflowing of the material of cell breakdown. These glands produce sebum, which covers the skin with a thin lipoidal film

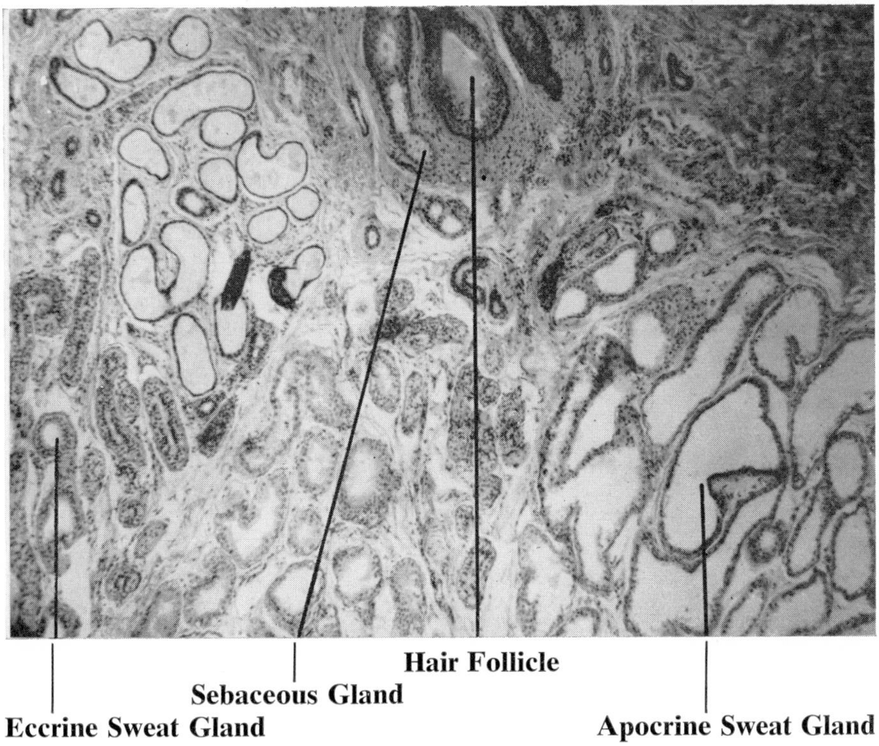

Fig. 3. Histology of the glands of the skin.
A microscopic section from the axilla.
(*Dr. David Gibson*)

that is mildly bacteriostatic and fungistatic and retards water evaporation. The scalp and the face may contain as many as 1,000 sebaceous glands per square centimeter. The activity of the gland increases markedly at the age of puberty and, in certain individuals, becomes plugged with sebum, debris and bacteria to form the blackheads and the pimples of acne.

The *sweat glands* are found everywhere in the human skin. They appear in greatest abundance on the palms and the soles and in the axillae. There are two main types of these glands. The eccrine or small sweat glands open directly onto the skin surface; the apocrine or large sweat glands, like the sebaceous gland, usually open into a hair follicle.

The *apocrine sweat glands* are found chiefly in the axillae and the genital region and do not develop until the time of puberty. These glands in man have very little importance except for the production of odor (the infamous "B.O."). Any emotional stresses which cause adrenergic sympathetic discharge produce apocrine sweating. This sweat is sterile when excreted but undergoes decomposition when contaminated by bacteria from the skin surface, resulting in a strong and characteristic odor. The purpose of the many cosmetic underarm preparations is to remove these bacteria or block the gland excretion. The main disease of the apocrine glands is hidradenitis suppurativa. This uncommon, chronic infection of these glands is caused by blockage of the duct which usually occurs in patients with the "acne-seborrhea complex."

The *eccrine sweat glands* and the cutaneous blood vessels are key factors in the maintenance of stable internal body temperatures despite marked environmental temperature changes. The eccrine glands flood the skin surface with water for cooling, and the blood vessels dilate or constrict to dissipate or to conserve body heat. The eccrine sweat glands are distributed everywhere on the skin surface, with the greatest concentration on the palms, the soles and the forehead. The prime stimulus for these small sweat glands is heat. Their activity is under the control of the nervous system, usually through the hypothalamic thermostat. Both adrenergic and cholinergic fibers innervate the glands. Blockage of the sweat ducts results in the disease entity known as prickly heat (miliaria).

Laboratory Procedures and Tests

CHAPTER **2**

IN ADDITION to the usual laboratory procedures used in the workup of medical patients, certain special tests are of importance in the field of dermatology. These include *skin tests, fungus examinations* and *biopsies*.

SKIN TESTS

There are 3 types of skin tests:

1. Intracutaneous
2. Scratch
3. Patch

The *intracutaneous tests* and the *scratch tests* can have two types of reactions: an immediate wheal reaction and a delayed reaction. The immediate wheal reaction develops to a maximum in 5 to 20 minutes. This type of reaction is elicited in testing for the cause of urticaria, atopic dermatitis and inhalent allergies. This immediate wheal reaction test is seldom used for determining the etiology of skin diseases.

The delayed reaction to intracutaneous skin testing is exemplified best by the tuberculin skin test. Tuberculin is available in two forms: Old Tuberculin Koch (OTK) or Purified Protein Derivative (PPD). Using OTK, the procedure is to start with 0.1 cc. of the 1:10,000 dilution (0.01 mg.) injected intracutaneously. This test is read in 48 hours and is positive if the redness at the site of the injection is 5 mm. greater than that at the control test site. If negative, the test can be repeated using a 1:1,000 dilution (0.1 mg.).

The PPD test is performed by using tablets that come in two strengths and injecting a solution of either one intracutaneously. If there is no reaction following the PPD No. 1 test, then the second strength may be employed.

Other intracutaneous skin tests with delayed reactions include the Ducrey vaccine test for the diagnosis of chancroid; the trichophytin test, which if positive shows an allergy to fungi of that type; and the Lygranum (Squibb) or Frei antigen (Lederle) skin tests which are used in the diagnosis of lymphogranuloma venereum.

Patch tests are used rather commonly in dermatology and offer a simple and accurate method of determining whether a patient is allergic to any of the testing agents (Figs. 4 and 5). There are two different reactions to this type of test: a primary irritant reaction and an allergic reaction. The primary irritant reaction occurs in the majority of the population when they are exposed to agents that have skin-destroying properties. Examples of these agents include soaps, cleaning fluids, bleaches, "corn" removers and counter-irritants. The allergic reaction indicates that the patient is more sensitive than normal to the agent being tested. It also shows that the patient has had a previous exposure to the agent being tested.

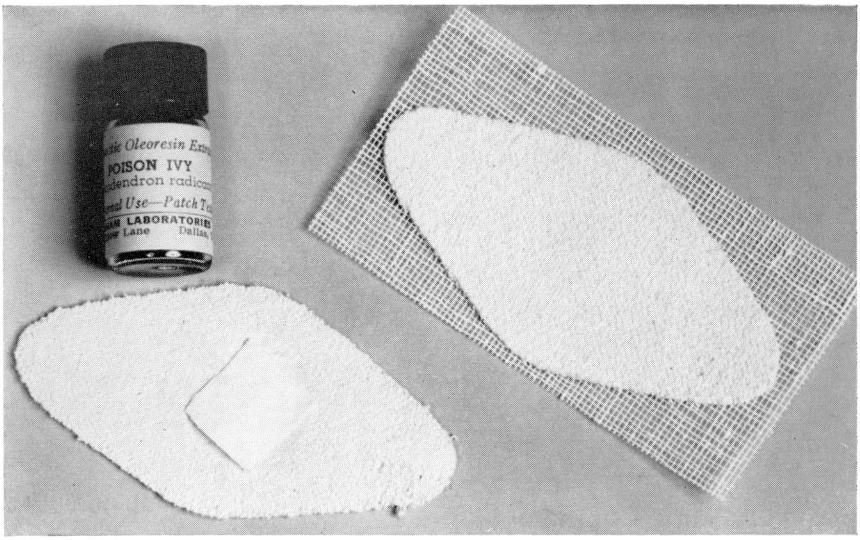

Fig. 4. Patch test material.

Diagnostic oleoresin extract of poison ivy (Graham) and Elastopatch (Duke). The Elastopatch is ready for application to the skin in the lower left-hand of the figure. The extract is placed on the square piece of sheeting.

(*K.U.M.C.*)

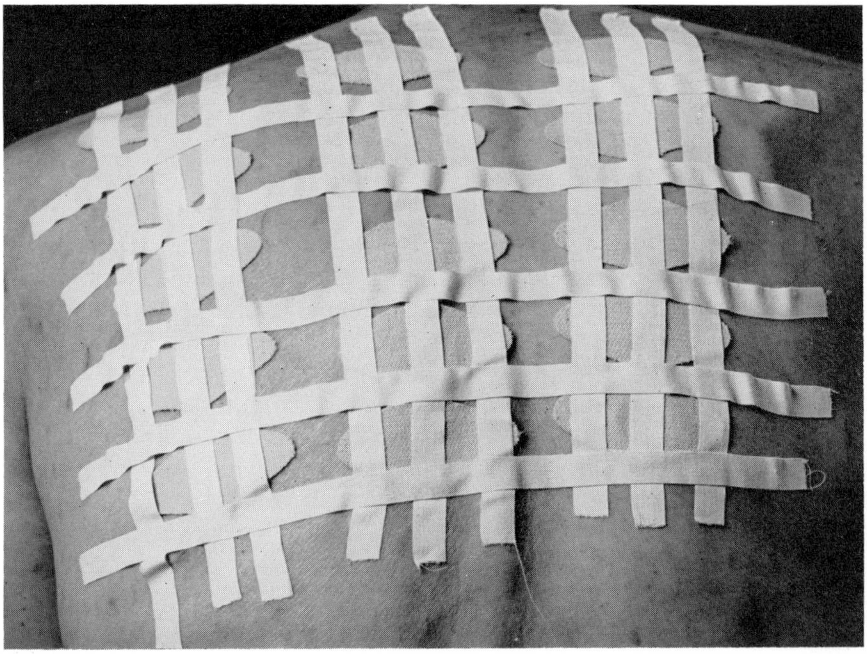

Fig. 5. Patch tests.

A series of patch tests on the back of a patient to establish the cause of chronic contact dermatitis in a farmer.

(*K.U.M.C.*)

The technic of the patch test is rather simple. For example, consider that a patient comes in with a dermatitis on the top of his feet and shoe leather or some chemical used in the manufacture of the leather is suspected as causing the reaction. The procedure for a patch test is to cut out a ½ inch square piece of the material from the inside of the shoe, moisten the material with distilled water, place it on the skin surface, and cover with an adhesive band or some patch-test dressing. The patch test is left on for 48 hours to 72 hours. When the test is removed the patient is considered to have a positive patch test if there is any redness or vesiculation under the site of the testing agent.

The patch test can be used to make or confirm a diagnosis of poison ivy dermatitis, ragweed dermatitis, or contact dermatitis due to medications, cosmetics, or industrial chemicals. Sulzberger and Baer[1] have compiled a list of chemicals, concentrations and vehicles to be used for eliciting the allergic type of patch test reaction. However, most tests can be performed very simply, as in the case of the shoe-leather dermatitis. One precaution is that the test must not be allowed to become wet in the 48-to-72-hour period.

A method of testing for allergy when food is suspected is to use the Rowe elimination diet.[2] The procedure is to limit the diet to the following basic foods which are known to be hypo-allergenic: lamb, lemon, grapefruit, pears, lettuce, spinach, carrots, sweet potato, tapioca, rice and rice bread, cane sugar, maple syrup, sesame oil, gelatin and salt. The patient is to remain on this basic diet for 5 to 7 days. At the end of that time one new food can be added every 2 days. The following foods may be added early: beef, white potatoes, green beans, milk along with butter and American cheese, and white bread with puffed wheat. If there is a flare-up of the dermatitis, which should occur within 2 to 8 hours after ingestion of an offending food, the new food should be discontinued for the present. More new foods are added until the normal diet, minus the allergenic foods, is regained.

FUNGUS EXAMINATIONS

Fungus examinations are a simple office laboratory procedure. They are accomplished by (1) scraping the diseased skin and examining the material directly under the microscope, (2) culturing the material and (3) examining the grown culture under the microscope. The skin scrapings are obtained by abrading a scaly diseased area with a knife blade, depositing the material on a slide, covering this residue with a 10 per cent aqueous potassium hydroxide solution and a cover slip. The preparation should be allowed to stand for 15 to 60 minutes to allow the keratin particles to dissolve. Then the slide is mounted on a microscope stage and examined for fungus elements with the low-power and the high-power lenses (Fig. 6).

For a culture preparation a part of the material from the scraping can be implanted in a test tube containing Sabouraud's media.[3] In 1 to 2 weeks a whitish or variously colored growth will be noted (Fig. 7). The species of fungus can be determined grossly by the color and the characteristics of the growth in the culture tube, and microscopically by study of a small amount of the culture material that has been removed and placed on a microscope slide. Most species of fungi have a characteristic microscopic appearance.

[1] Sulzberger, M. B., and Baer, R. L.: Office Immunology. Chicago, Yr. Bk. Pub., 1947, pp. 312-330. Baer, R. L., and Witten, V. H.: Year Book of Dermatology and Syphilology, 1957-1958 Series. Chicago, Yr. Bk. Pub., 1958, pp. 29-45.

[2] Sulzberger, M. B., and Baer, R. L.: Office Immunology. Chicago, Yr. Bk. Pub., 1947, p. 63.

[3] Tubes with this media can be obtained from most hospitals or from Derm Medical Co., P. O. Box 78595, W. Adams Station, Los Angeles 16, Calif.

BIOPSIES

The biopsy of a questionable skin lesion and microscopic examination of the biopsy section is another important laboratory procedure. The histopathology of many skin conditions is quite diagnostic, particularly when the biopsy specimen is studied by a pathologist who has some knowledge of dermatologic lesions.

The technics of performing surgical excision and punch biopsies of the skin are well known. Another simple way of removing skin tissue is to excise the piece with straight sharp-pointed scissors and stop the bleeding with light electrosurgery. This latter procedure is useful for certain types of elevated lesions and in areas where the cosmetic result is not important.

In addition to the above 3 special skin procedures, there are certain tests for specific skin conditions that will be discussed in connection with the respective diseases.

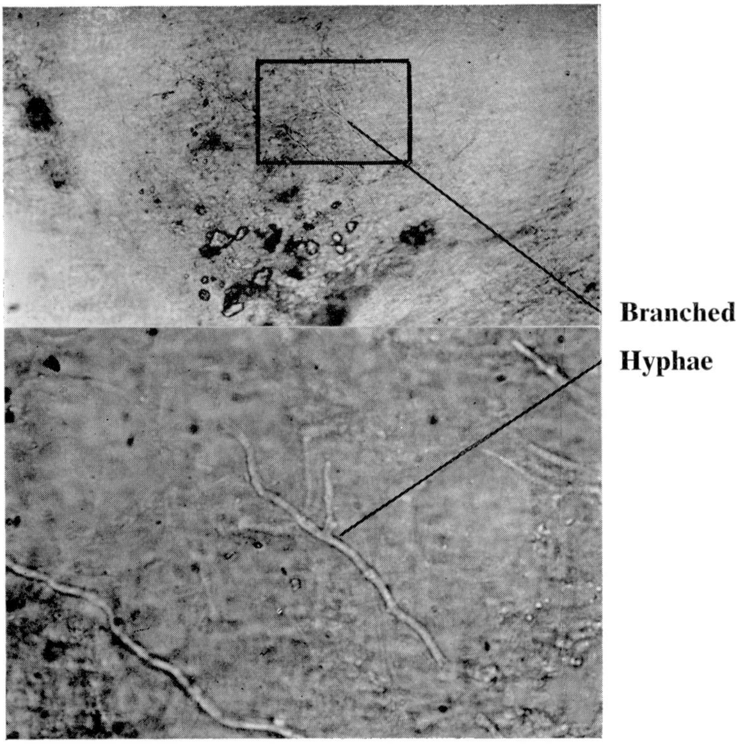

Fig. 6. Fungi from a skin scraping as seen with microscope in a KOH preparation.

(*Top*) Low power lens (× 100) view. (*Bottom*) High power lens (× 450) view of area outlined above.

(*Dr. David Gibson*)

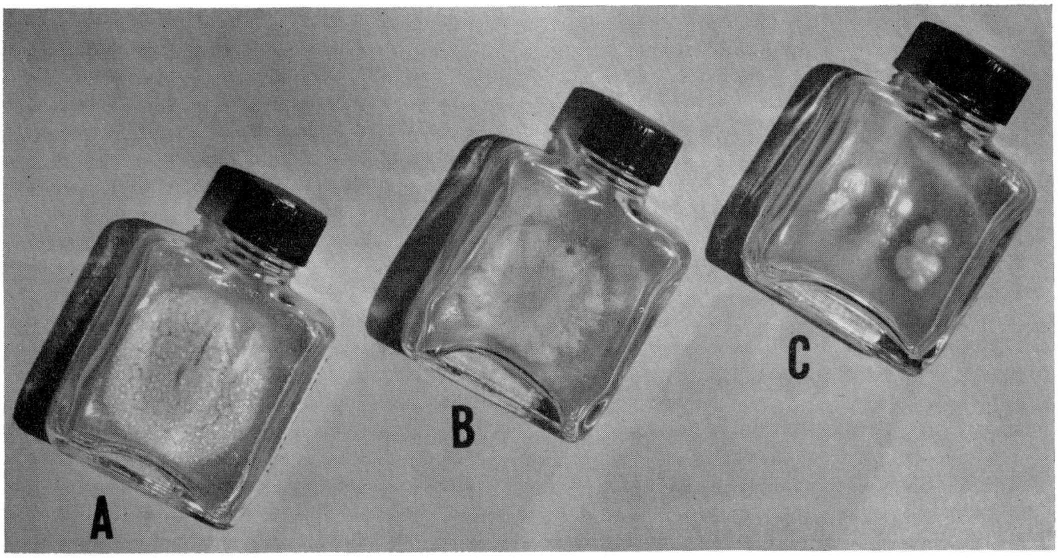

Fig. 7. Fungus cultures.
Cultures grown on disposable bottles of Sabouraud's media (Mycosel, Derm Medical). The three fungi are (A) *Trichophyton mentagrophytes,* (B) *Microsporum canis* (C) *Candida albicans.* (*K.U.M.C.*)

Dermatologic Diagnosis

CHAPTER 3

TO AID in determining the diagnosis of a presenting skin problem, this chapter will be concerned with discussions of primary and secondary lesions; also, diagnosis by location. It will contain lists of seasonal skin diseases, pediatric skin diseases, senile skin diseases, military dermatoses and dermatoses of Negroes.

PRIMARY AND SECONDARY LESIONS

No two skin diseases look alike, but most of them have some characteristic *primary* lesions and it is very important to examine the patient closely to find them. Commonly, however, the primary lesions have been obliterated by the *secondary* lesions of overtreatment, excessive scratching, or infection. Even in these cases it is usually possible by careful examination to find some primary lesions at the edge of the eruption or on other less irritated areas of the body. (Plates 1, 2, 3.)

A complete examination of the entire body is a necessity when confronted with a diffuse skin eruption or an unusual localized eruption.

Primary Lesions

A description of the basic primary lesions follows:

Macules are small, flat, circumscribed discolorations of the skin. Examples: freckles, measles rash, vitiligo, tattoos.

Papules are variously shaped, circumscribed, solid elevations; they are smaller than a pea. Examples: elevated moles, warts, lichen planus.

A *wheal* is a type of papule that is edematous and transitory. Examples: hives, insect bites.

Nodules are larger papules which may be above, level with, or beneath the skin surface. Examples: nodular secondary or tertiary syphilis, epitheliomas, xanthomas.

Large nodules are called *tumors.*

Vesicles are circumscribed, elevations of the skin containing serous fluid; they are smaller than a pea. Examples: early chickenpox, shingles, contact dematitis.

Bullae are larger vesicles. Examples: burns, pemphigus.

Pustules are circumscribed elevations of the skin containing purulent fluid. Examples: acne, impetigo.

Petechiae are discrete deposits of blood or blood pigments, smaller than a pea. Examples: drug eruptions, certain insect bites.

Purpura is a larger petechial lesion.

Secondary Lesions

Scales are shedding, dead epidermal cells which may be dry or greasy. Examples: dandruff, psoriasis.

Crusts are variously colored masses of

skin exudates. Examples: impetigo, infected dermatitis.

Excoriations are abrasions of the skin, usually superficial and traumatic. Examples: scratched insect bites, scabies.

Fissures are linear breaks in the skin, sharply defined with abrupt walls. Examples: congenital syphilis, athlete's feet.

Ulcers are irregularly sized and shaped excavations in the skin extending into the corium. Examples: stasis ulcers of legs, tertiary syphilis.

Scars are formations of connective tissue replacing tissue lost through injury or disease.

Keloids are hypertrophic scars.

Lichenification is a diffuse area of thickening and scaling with resultant increase in the skin lines and markings.

Several combinations of primary and secondary lesions commonly exist on the same patient. Examples: papulosquamous lesions of psoriasis, vesiculopustular lesions in contact dermatitis, and crusted excoriations in scabies.

DIAGNOSIS BY LOCATION

A physician is often confronted by a patient with skin trouble localized to one part of the body (Figs. 8 to 11). The following list of diseases with special localizations is meant to aid in the diagnosis of such conditions, but this list must not be considered as being all inclusive. Generalizations are the rule, and many of the rare diseases are omitted. For further information concerning the particular diseases consult the Dictionary-Index.

Scalp: Seborrheic dermatitis, contact dermatitis, psoriasis, folliculitis, pediculosis, and hair loss due to the following: male or female pattern, alopecia areata, tinea, chronic discoid lupus erythematosus, postpregnancy, or trichotillomania.

Ears: Seborrheic dermatitis, psoriasis, infectious eczematoid dermatitis, senile keratoses and, very rarely, fungus infection.

Face: Acne, rosacea, impetigo, contact dermatitis, seborrheic dermatitis, folliculitis, herpes simplex and, less commonly, lupus erythematosus and actinic dermatitis.

Eyelids: Contact dermatitis due to fingernail polish, seborrheic dermatitis, or atopic eczema.

Posterior Neck: Neurodermatitis, seborrheic dermatitis, or contact dermatitis.

Mouth: Aphthae, herpes simplex, geographic tongue, contact dermatitis and, less frequently, syphilis, lichen planus and pemphigus.

Axillae: Contact dermatitis, seborrheic dermatitis, hidradenitis suppurativa and, less commonly, granuloma due to deodorants, acanthosis nigricans and Fox-Fordyce disease.

Chest and Back (Fig. 12): Tinea versicolor, pityriasis rosea, acne, seborrheic dermatitis, psoriasis and secondary syphilis.

Groin and Crural Areas: Tinea infection, monilial infection, bacterial intertrigo, scabies, pediculosis and granuloma inguinale.

Penis (Fig. 13): Fusospirochetal balanitis, chancroid, herpes simplex, primary and secondary syphilis and, less frequently, scabies and balanitis xerotica obliterans.

Hands (Fig. 14): Contact dermatitis, dyshidrosis, id reaction to fungus infection of the feet, atopic eczema and, less commonly, pustular psoriasis, nummular eczema, erythema multiforme, secondary syphilis and fungus infection.

Cubital Fossae and Popliteal Fossae: Atopic eczema, contact dermatitis and prickly heat.

Elbows and Knees: Psoriasis and xanthomas.

Feet (Fig. 15): Fungus infection, primary or secondary bacterial infection, contact dermatitis from footwear or footcare and, less frequently, psoriasis, erythema multiforme and secondary syphilis.

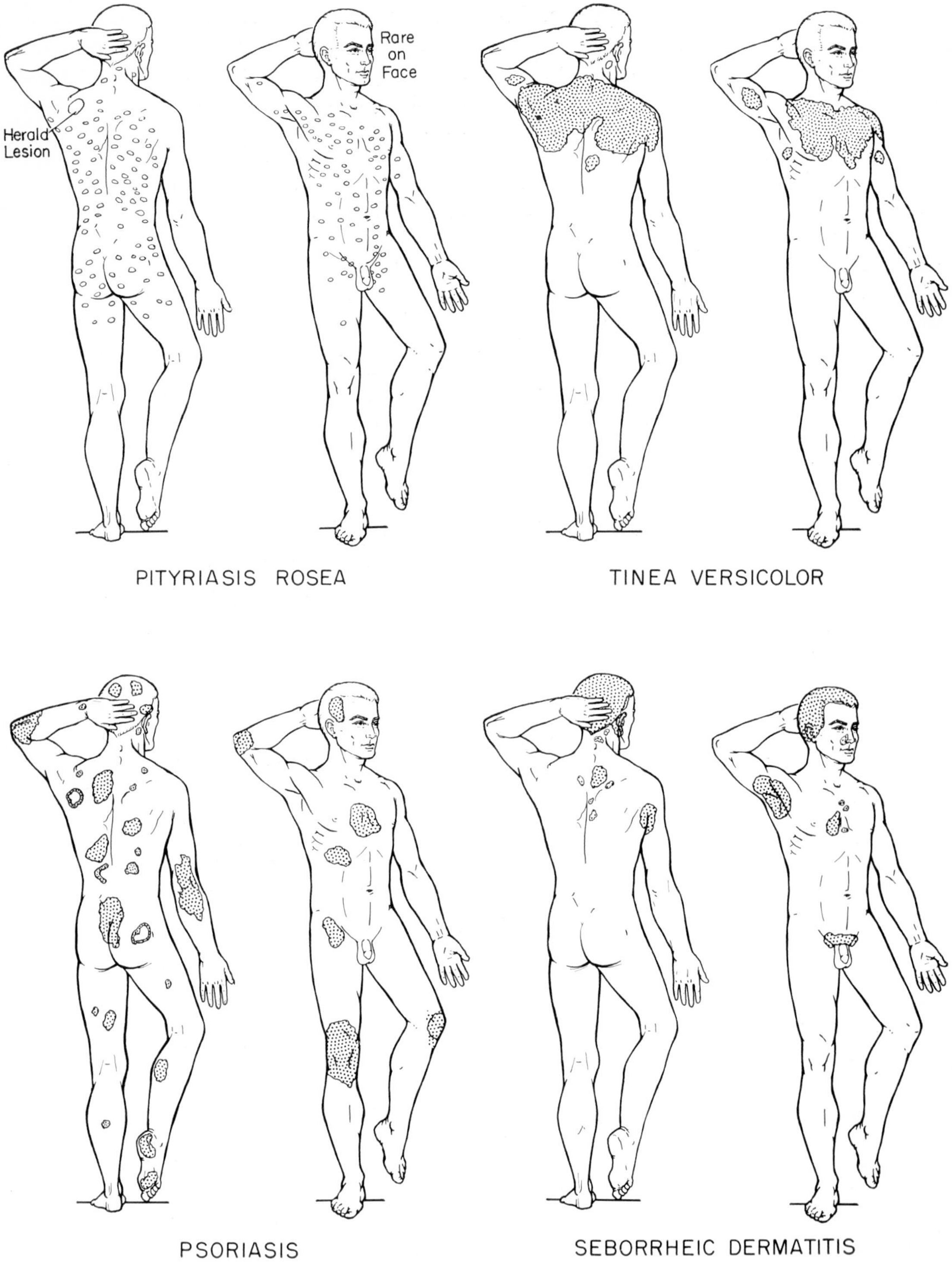

Fig. 8. Dermatologic silhouettes.

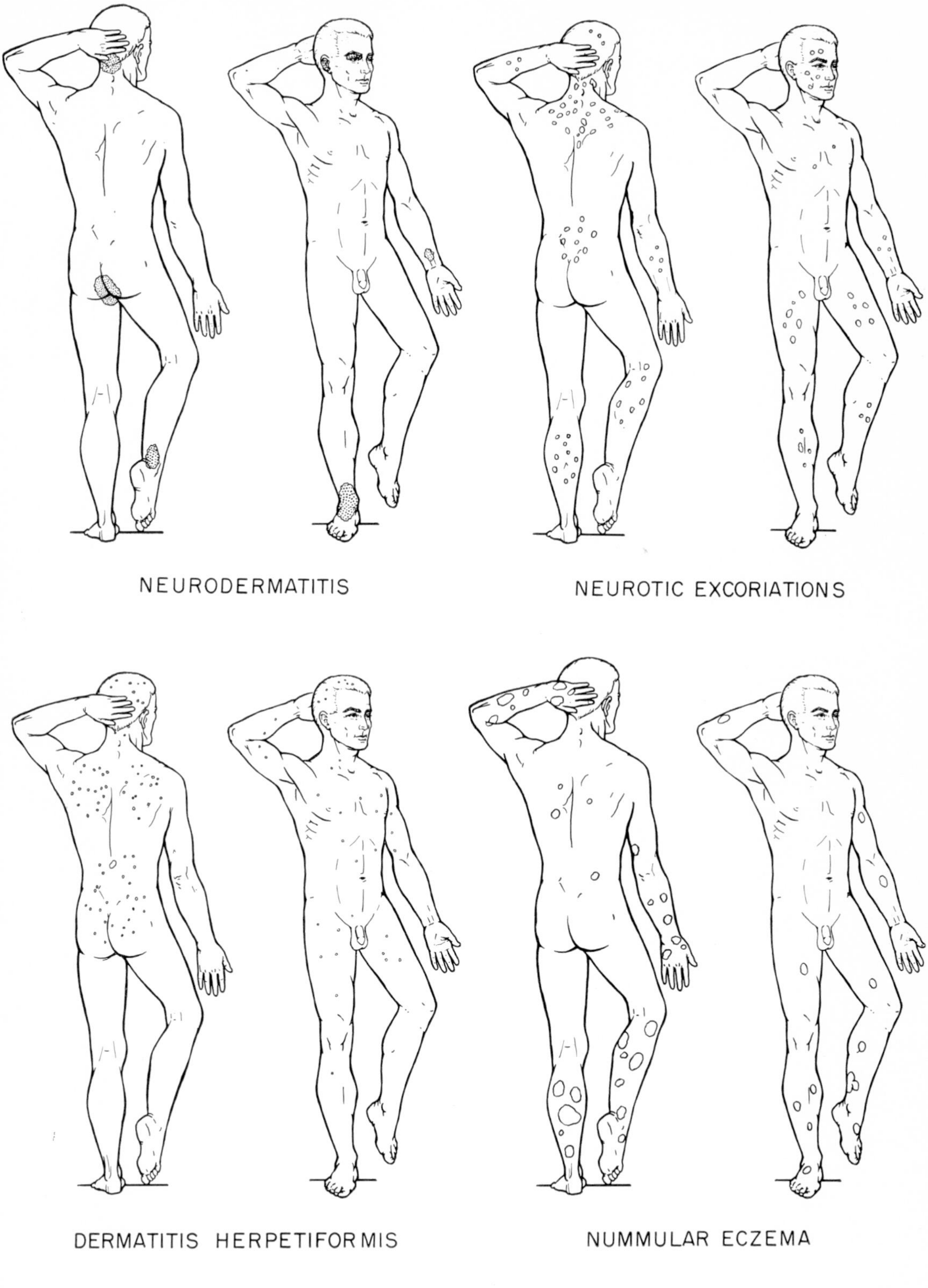

Fig. 9. Dermatologic silhouettes.

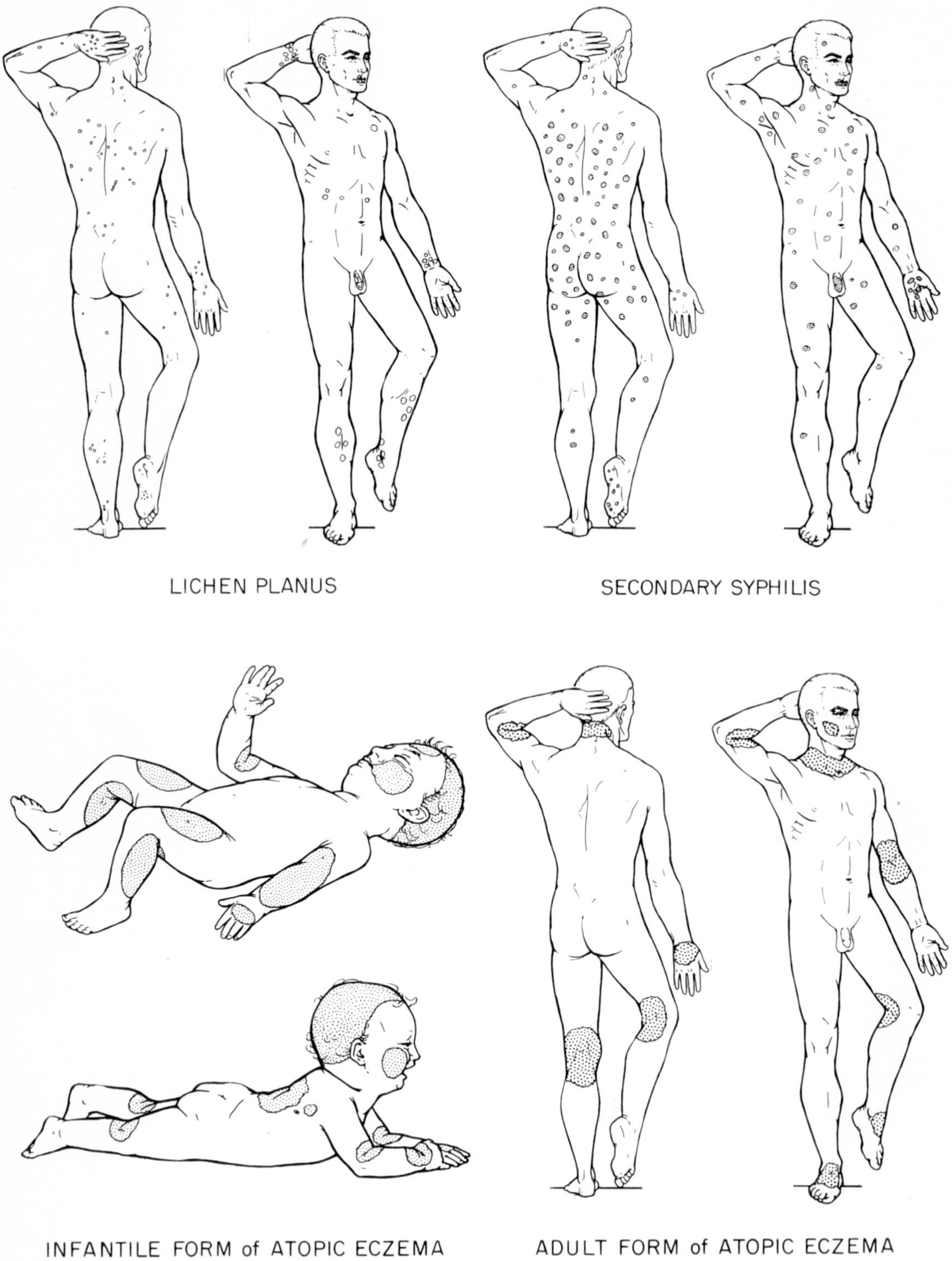

Fig. 10. Dermatologic silhouettes.

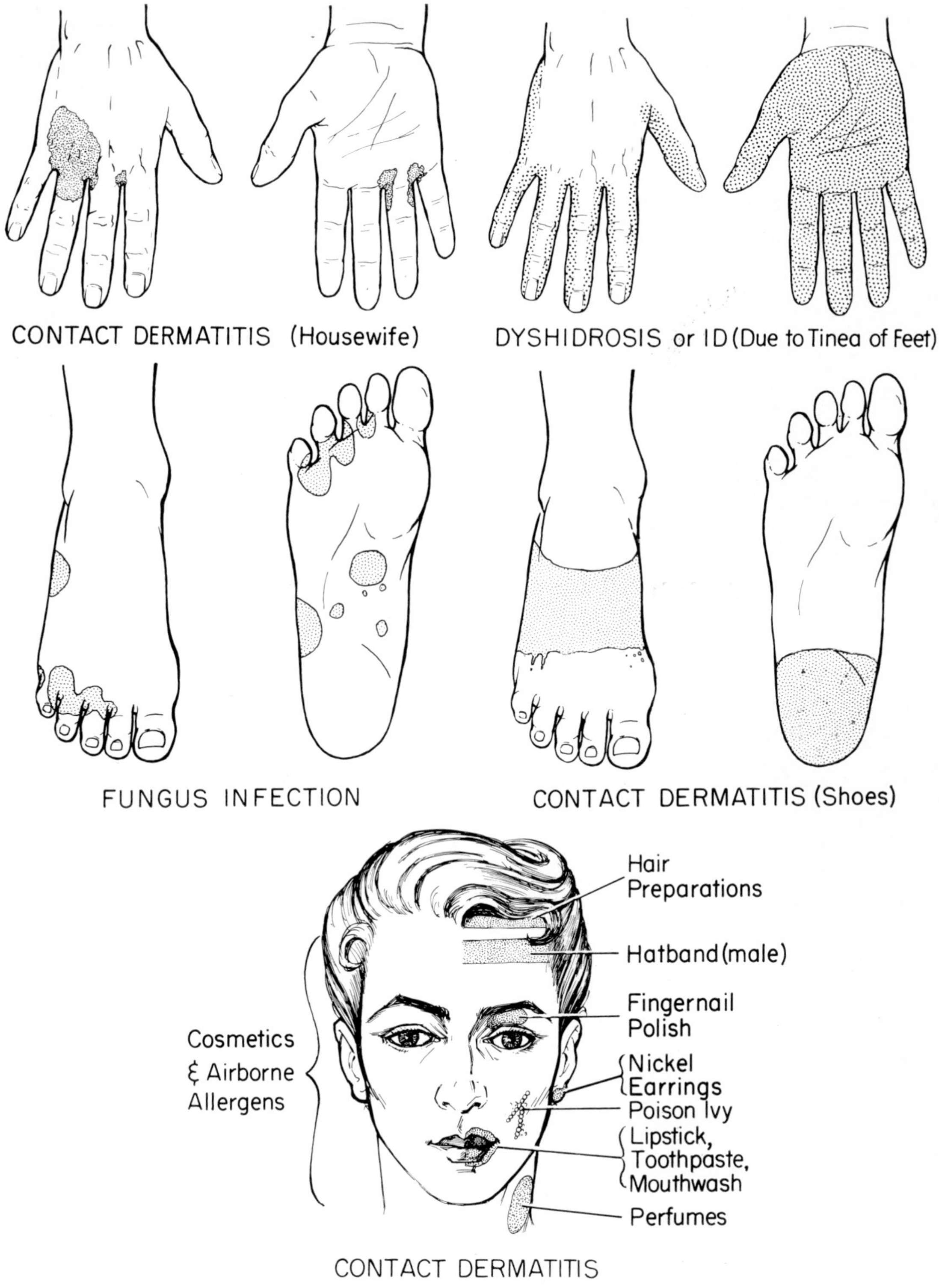

Fig. 11. Dermatologic silhouettes.

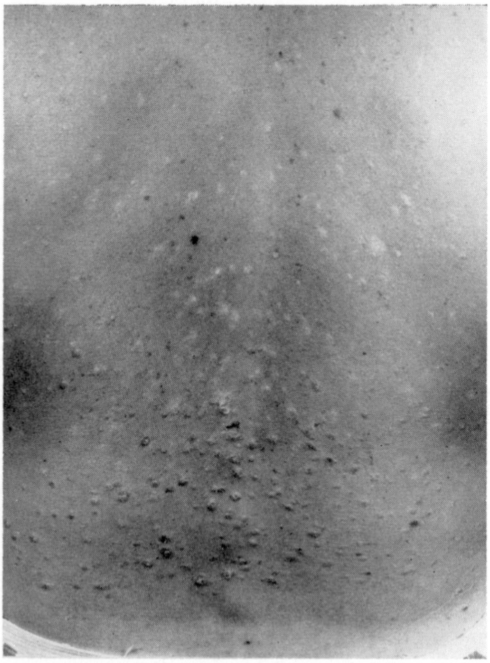

Psoriasis

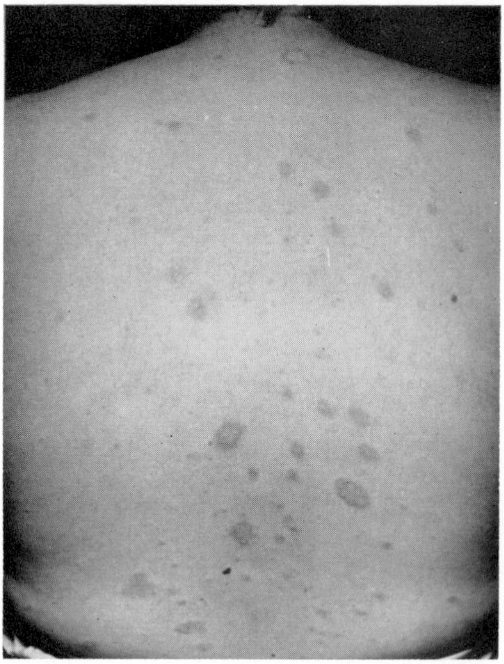

Pityriasis Rosea

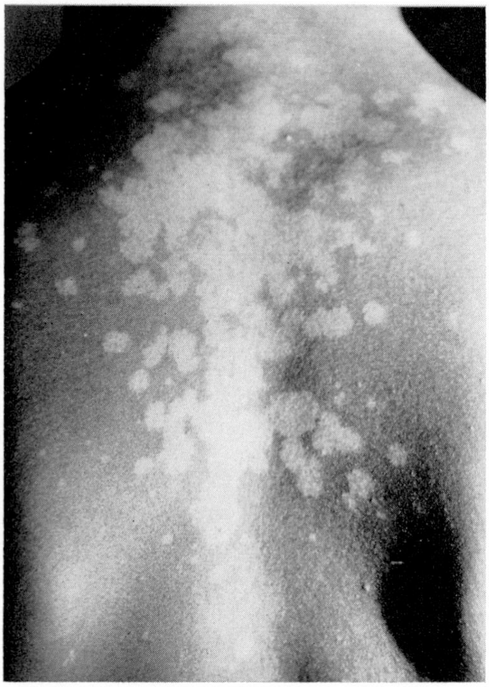

Tinea Versicolor (Negro)

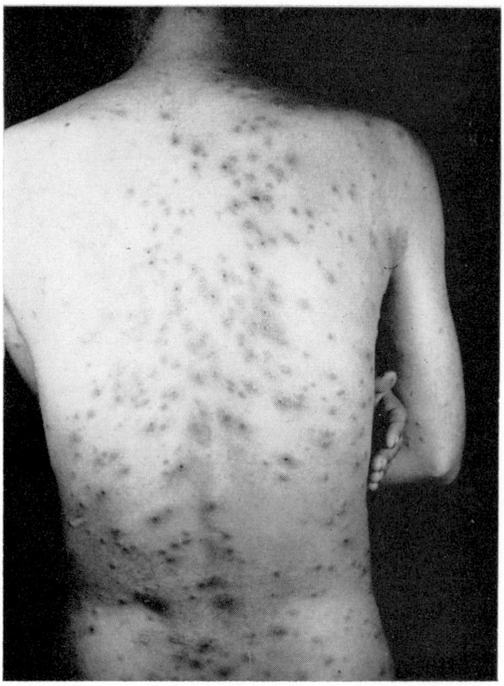

Secondary Syphilis

Fig. 12. Papulosquamous diseases on the back.

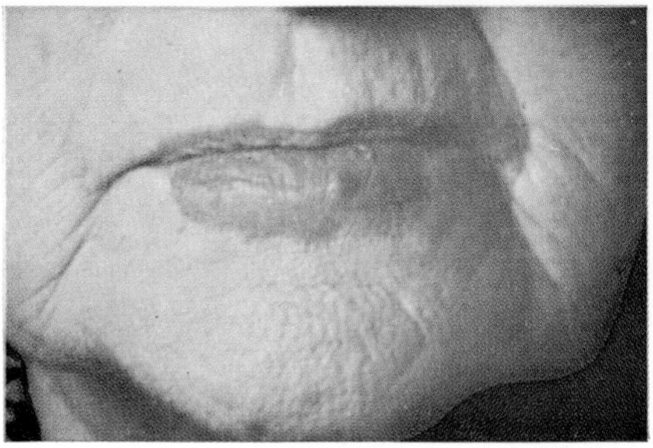

A. Macule

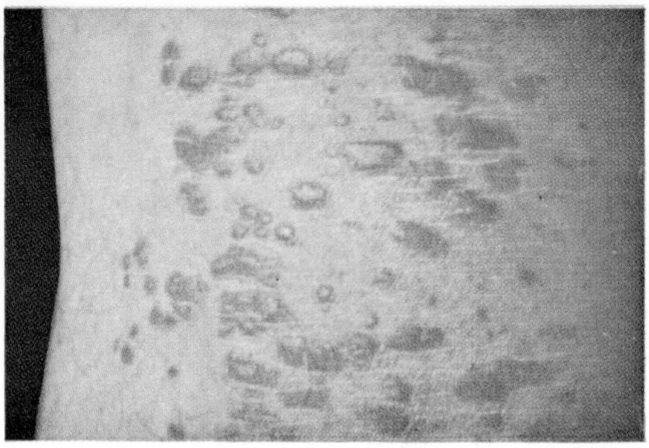

B. Papules

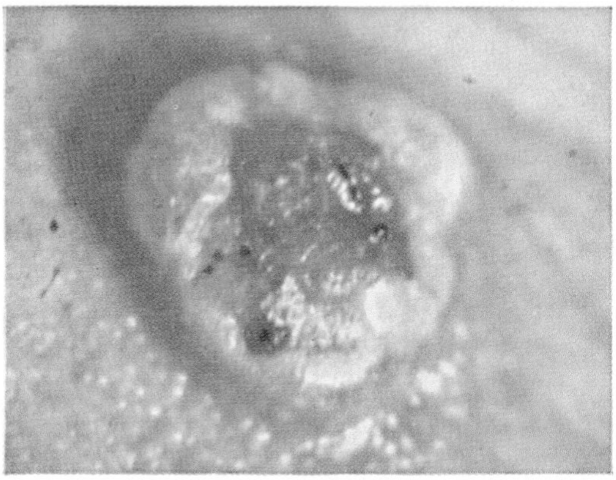

C. Nodule

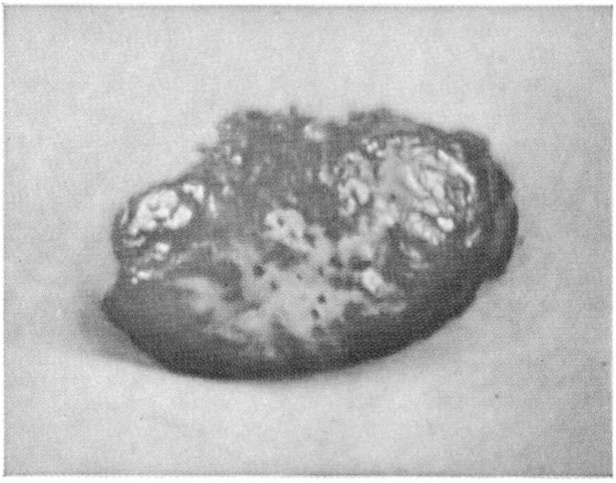

D. Tumor

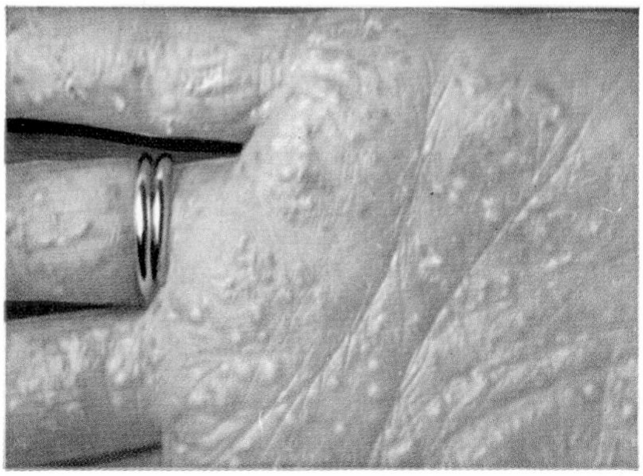

E. Pustules

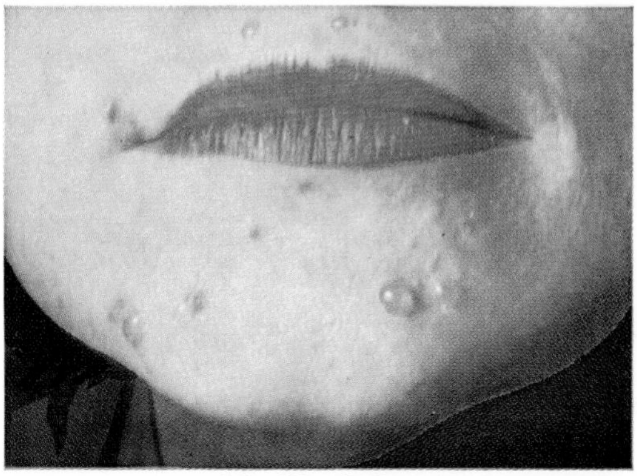

F. Vesicles

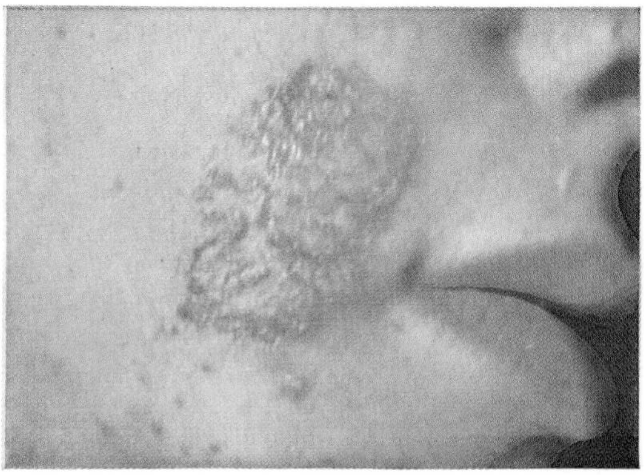

G. Crusts

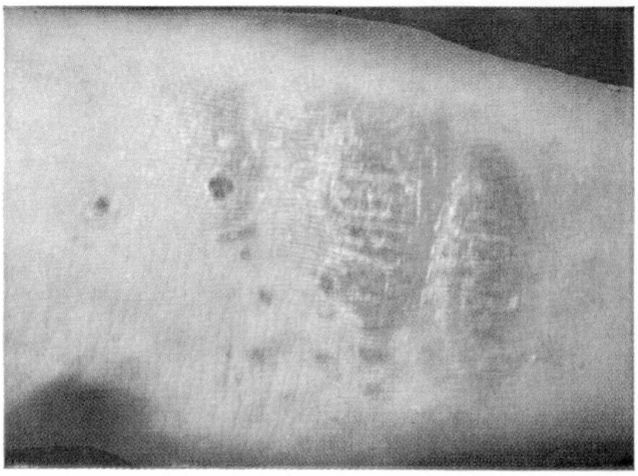

H. Lichenification

Plate 1. *(Caption on following page)*

Plate 1. Primary and secondary lesions.

A. Macular lesion on lip (port-wine hemangioma)
B. Papules on knee (lichen planus)
C. Nodule on lower eyelid (basal cell epithelioma)
D. Tumor of abdomen (mixed hemangioma)
E. Pustules on palm (pustular psoriasis)
F. Vesicles on face (pemphigus)
G. Crusted lesion on face (impetigo)
H. Lichenification on dorsum of ankle (neurodermatitis)

(*Geigy Pharmaceuticals*)

Plate 2. Nodular lesions.

A. Grouped nodular lesions with central scarring (tertiary syphiloderm)
B. Grouped warty, nodular lesions with central scarring (tuberculosis verrucosa cutis)

(*Marion B. Sulzberger: Folia Dermatologica, No. 1, Geigy Pharmaceuticals*)

Plate 3. Nodular lesions.

A. Polycyclic nodular lesion (superficial basal epithelioma)
B. Keloid

(*Marion B. Sulzberger: Folia Dermatologica, No. 1, Geigy Pharmaceuticals*)

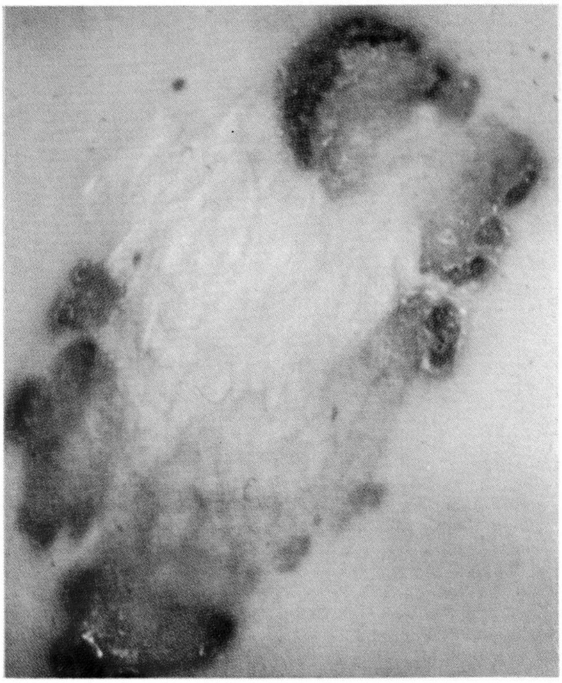

Plate 2A

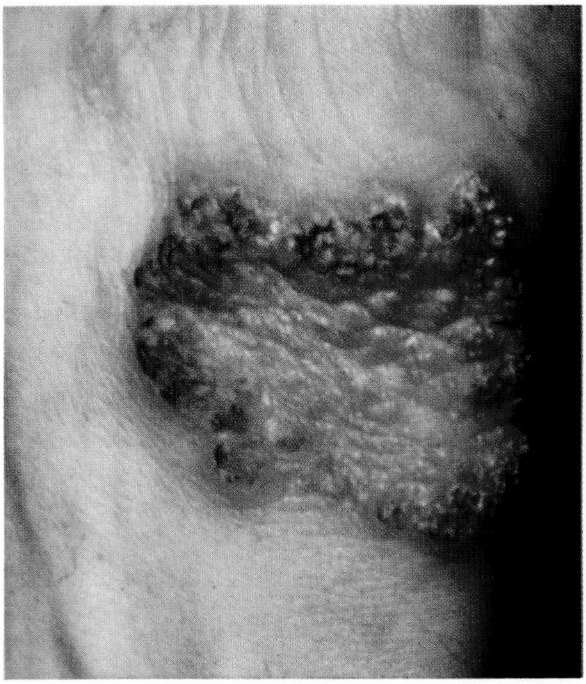

Plate 2B

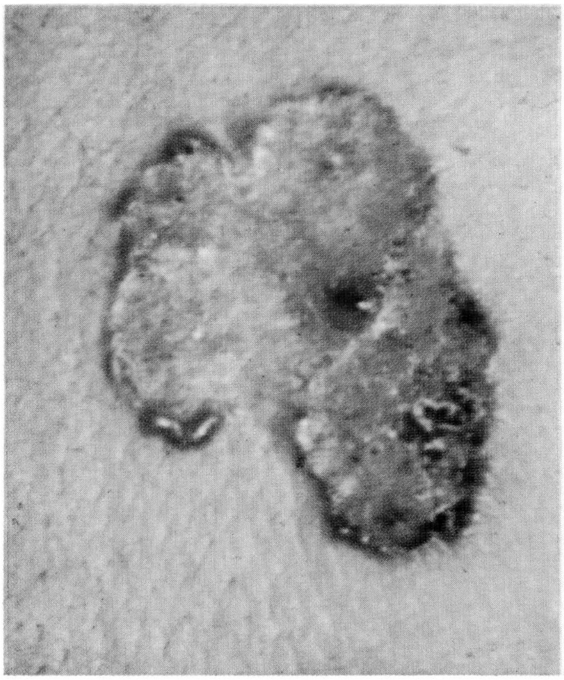

Plate 3A

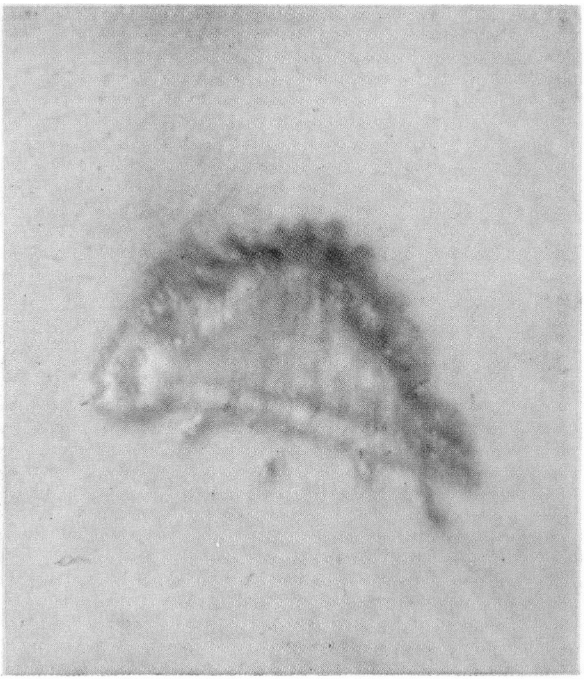

Plate 3B

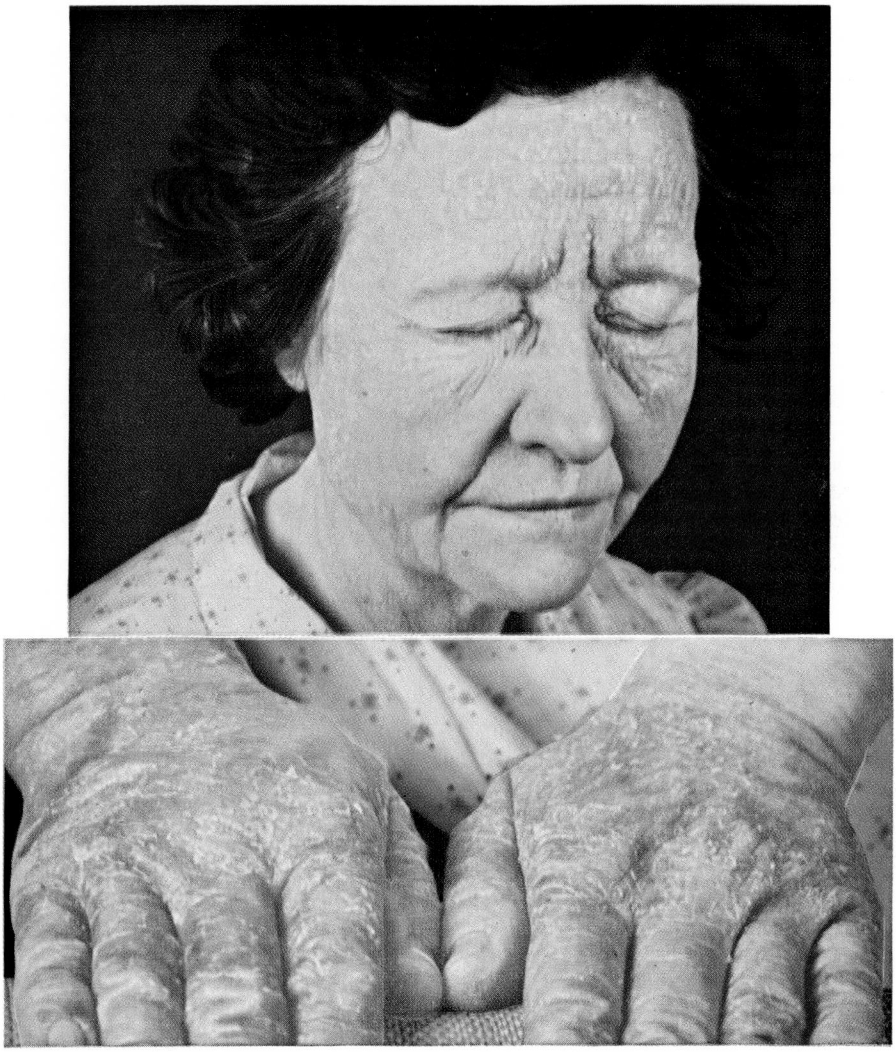

Plate 4. Contact dermatitis in a nurse due to chlorpromazine.

The hands and the face were involved most severely. This eruption was aggravated following exposure to sunlight. (K.U.M.C.)
(Burroughs Wellcome & Company, Inc.)

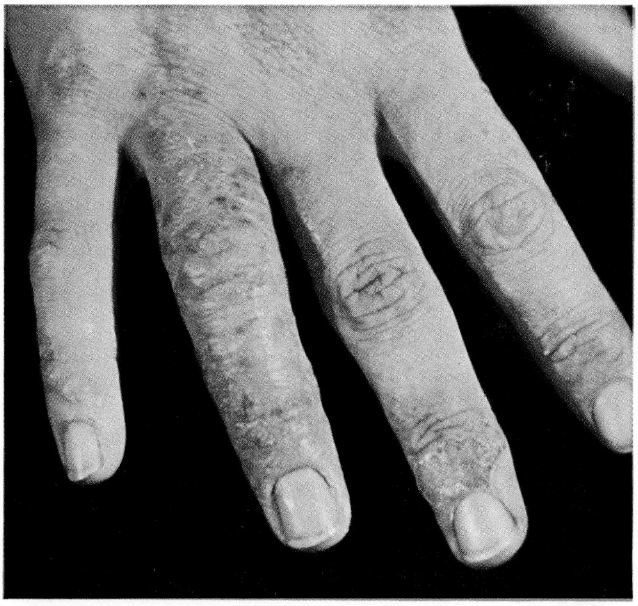

Plate 5. Contact dermatitis of the hand.

This common dermatitis is usually due to continued exposure to soap and water. (K.U.M.C.)
(Burroughs Wellcome & Company, Inc.)

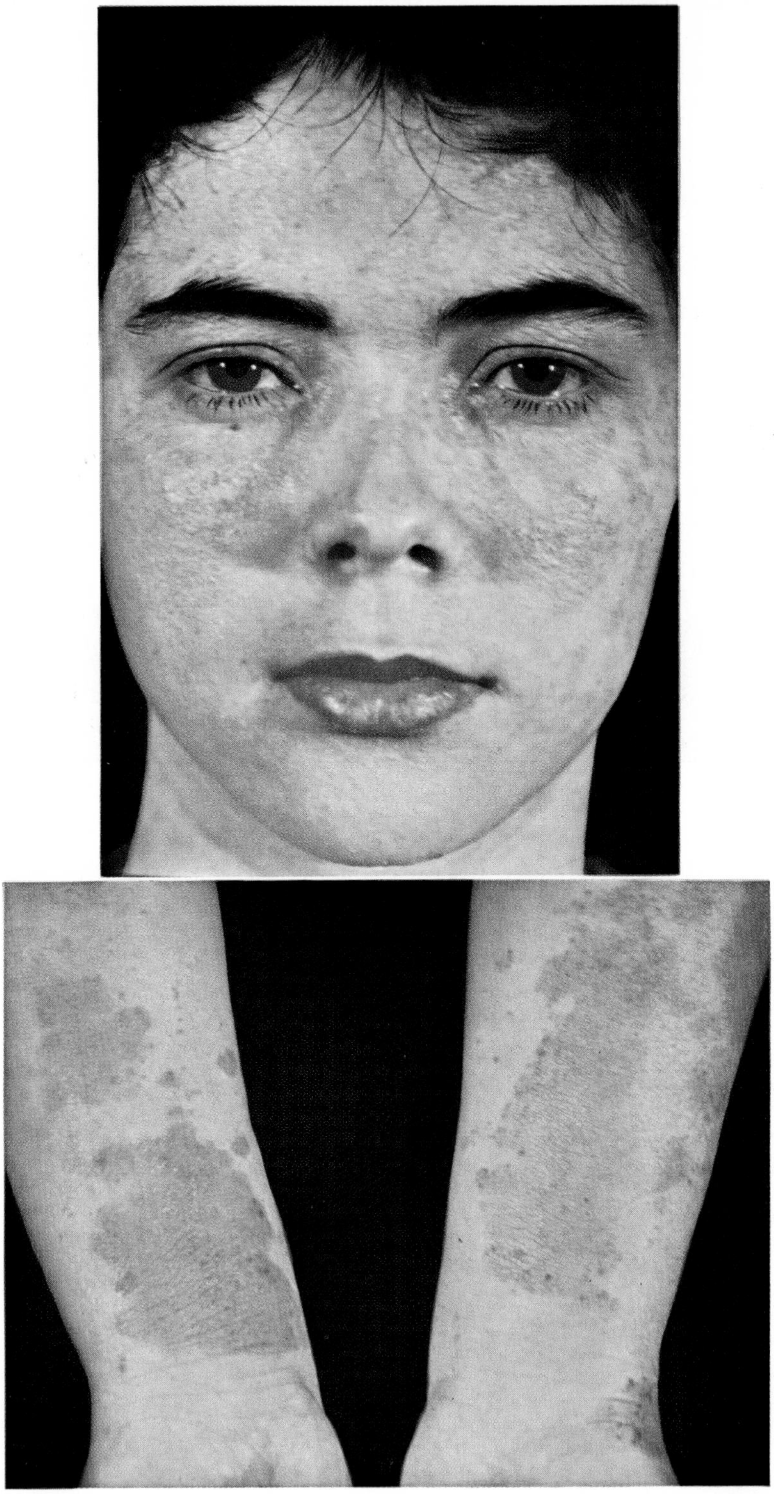

Plate 6. Atopic eczema.

This case of facial atopic eczema resembled acute lupus erythematosus. The arm eruption is on another patient and exemplifies the chronic lichenified form of atopic eczema. (K.U.M.C.)
(*Dome Chemicals*)

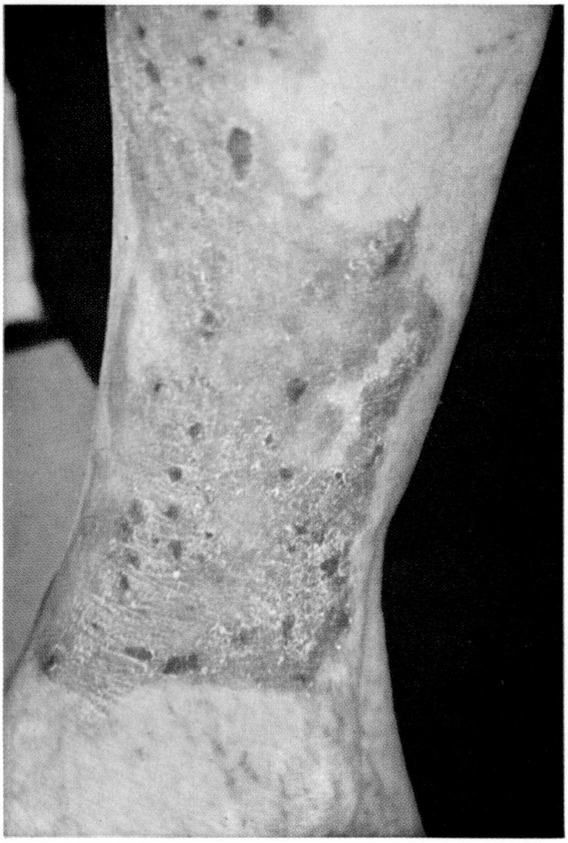

Plate 7. Neurodermatitis of the leg.

This is a common location for neurodermatitis. Note the lichenification and the excoriations due to the marked pruritus. (K.U.M.C.)
(Duke Laboratories)

In diagnosing a rather generalized skin eruption, the following 3 mimicking conditions must be considered first and ruled in or out by appropriate history or examination:
(1) Drug eruption (2) Contact dermatitis (3) Secondary syphilis

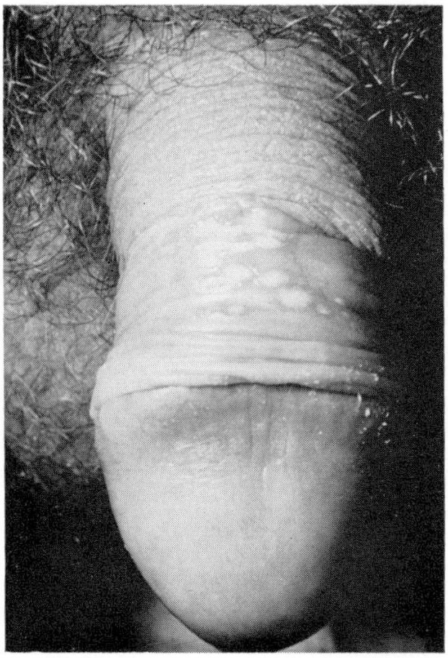

Herpes Simplex

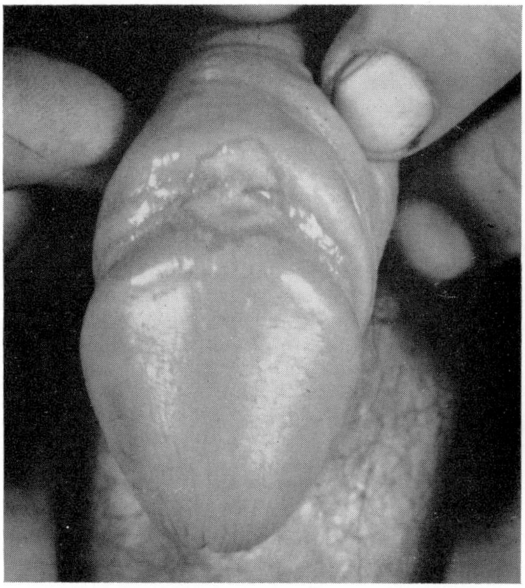

Primary Syphilis

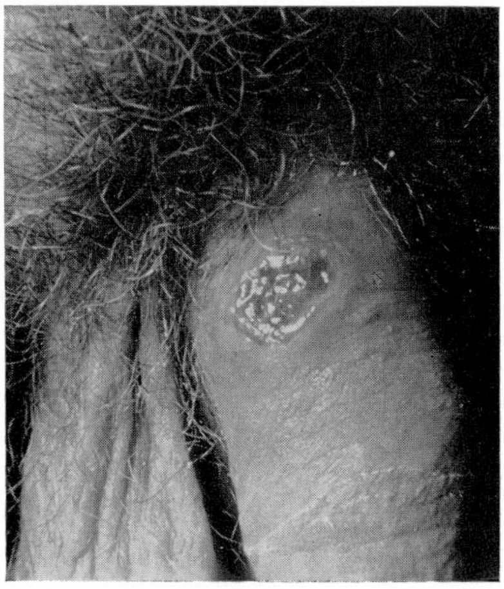

Furuncle

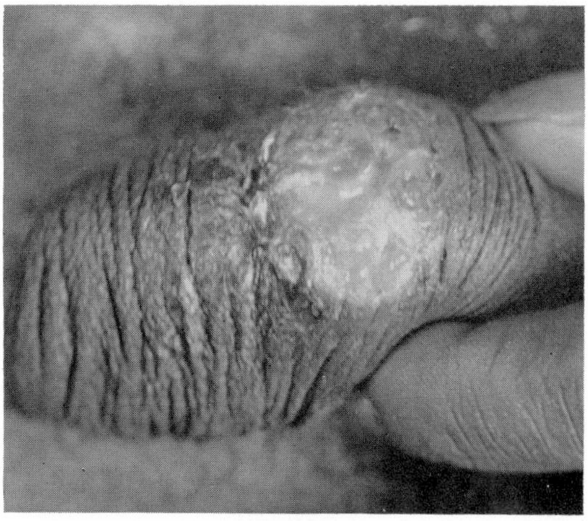

Chancroid

Fig. 13. Penile lesions.

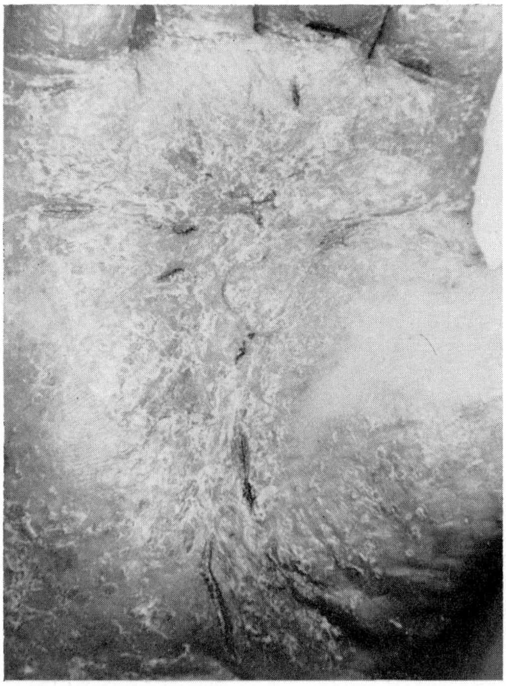

Contact Dermatitis

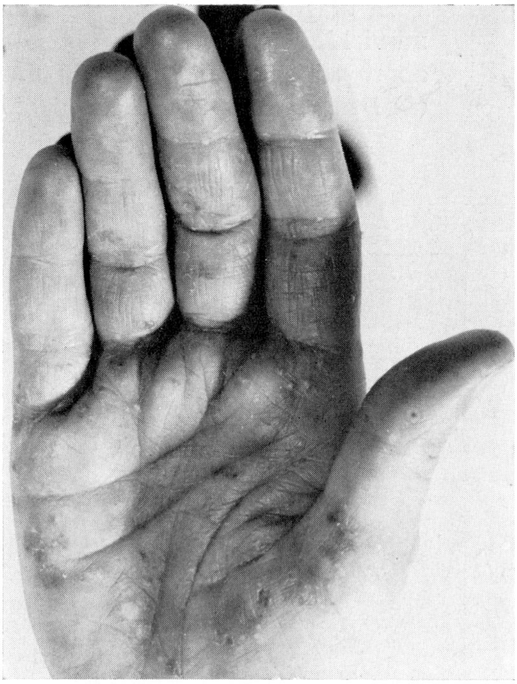

Tinea

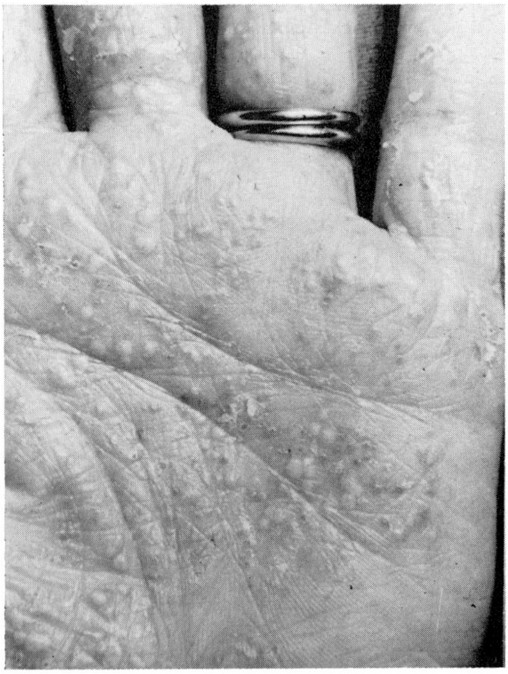

Pustular Psoriasis

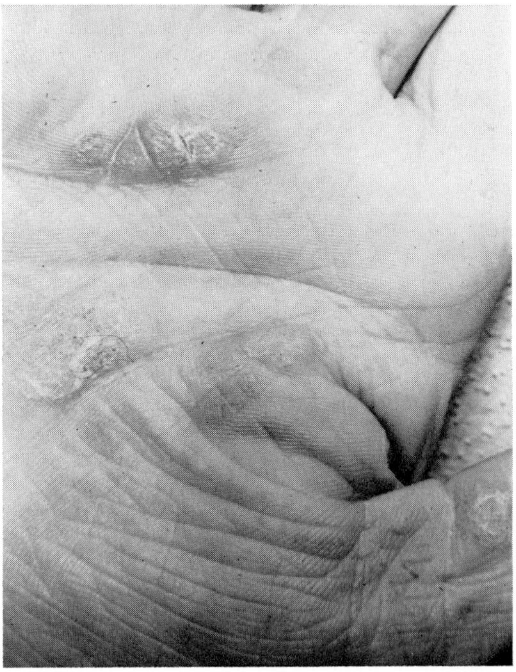

Psoriasis

Fig. 14. Palmar dermatoses

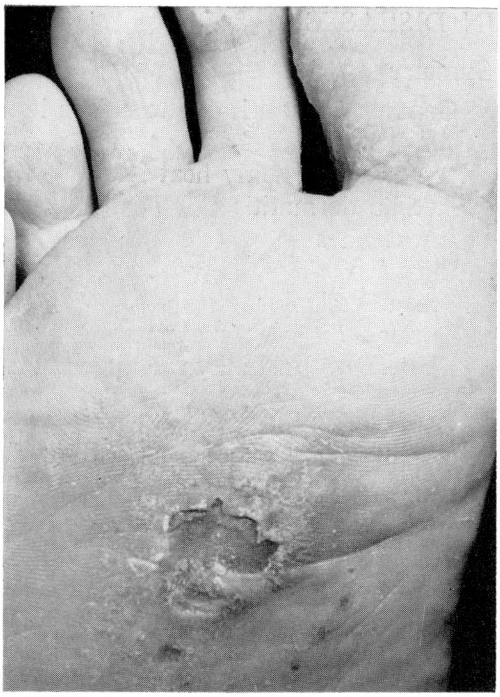

Acute Tinea

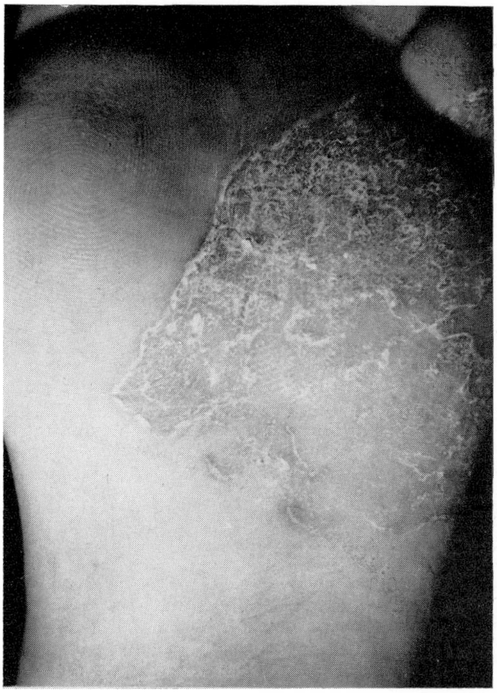

Chronic Tinea

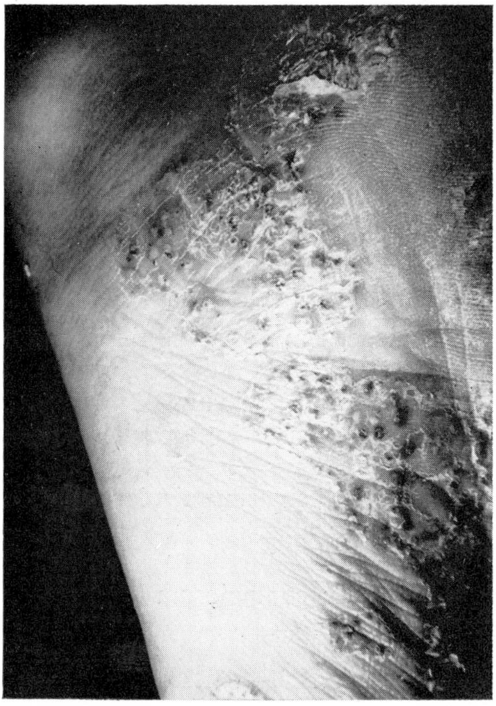

Pustular Psoriasis

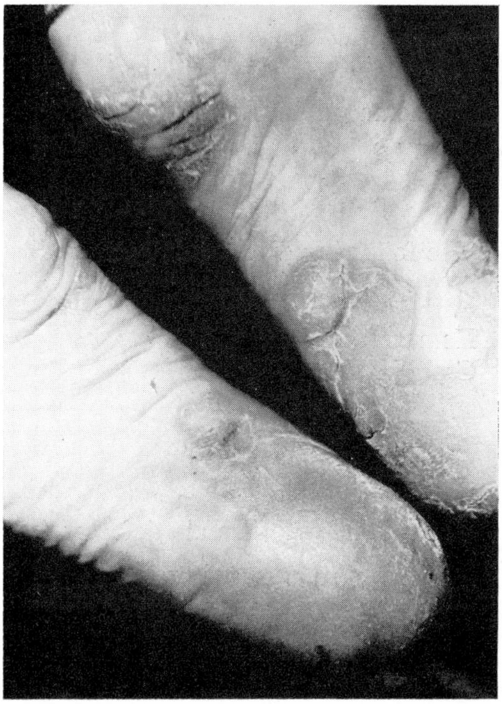

Psoriasis

Fig. 15. Plantar dermatoses.

SEASONAL SKIN DISEASES

Certain dermatoses have an increased incidence in various seasons of the year. In a busy dermatologist's office one sees literal "epidemics" of atopic eczema, pityriasis rosea, psoriasis and winter itch, to mention only a few. Knowledge of this seasonal incidence is helpful from a diagnostic standpoint. It will be sufficient to list only these seasonal diseases. Furthermore, specific information concerning them can be found elsewhere in the book. Remember that there are exceptions to every rule.

Winter

- Atopic eczema
- Psoriasis
- Nummular eczema
- Winter itch
- Seborrheic dermatitis
- Ichthyosis

Spring

- Pityriasis rosea
- Dyshidrosis
- Erythema multiforme (Hebra)

Summer

- Contact dermatitis due to poison ivy
- Tinea of the feet and groin
- Miliaria or prickly heat
- Actinic dermatitis
- Insect bites
- Impetigo
- Tinea versicolor
- Darier's disease (uncommon)
- Epidermolysis bullosa (uncommon)

Fall

- Winter itch
- Senile pruritus
- Atopic eczema
- Pityriasis rosea
- Contact dermatitis due to ragweed
- Tinea of the scalp (school children)

PEDIATRIC SKIN DISEASES

The following diseases have a predilection for the child (Fig. 16 & 17).

Infancy

- Hemangiomas
- Cradle cap
  - Seborrheic dermatitis
  - Atopic eczema
  - Moniliasis
- Intertrigo of diaper area
- Congenital ectodermal defects (uncommon)
- Epidermolysis bullosa (uncommon)

Childhood

- Atopic eczema and pityriasis simplex faciei
- Impetigo and ecthyma
- Contact dermatitis, especially due to poison ivy
- Tinea of all areas, particularly the body and scalp
- Warts
- Molluscum contagiosum
- Scabies
- Pediculosis
- Exanthems: Chickenpox, smallpox, scarlet fever, measles, etc.
- Urticaria pigmentosa (uncommon)
- Xanthogranuloma (uncommon)

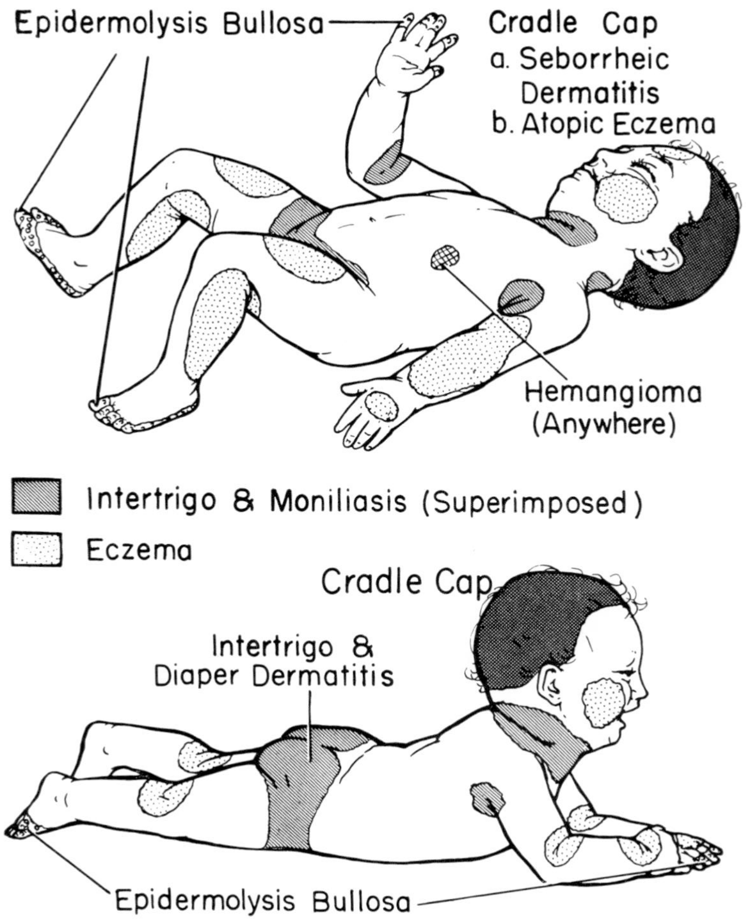

Fig. 16. Pediatric dermograms (infancy).

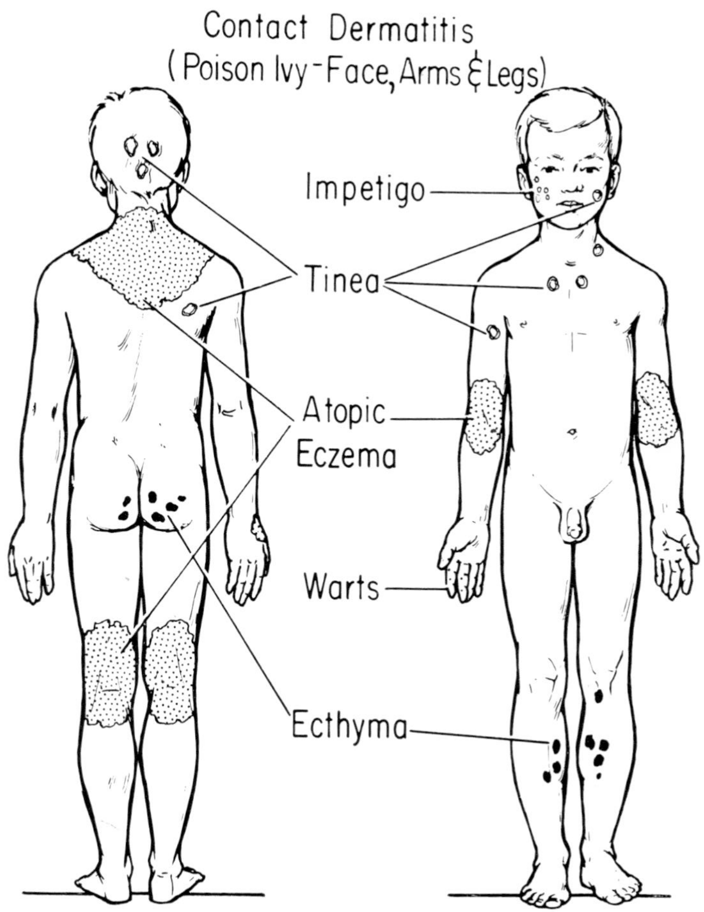

Fig. 17. Pediatric dermograms (childhood).

SENILE SKIN DISEASES

The care of the geriatric patient is becoming more dominant and certain skin diseases are seen with greater frequency in this group (Fig. 18).

Winter itch and dry skin
Stasis dermatitis and ulcers
Nummular eczema
Seborrheic keratoses
Senile keratoses and leukoplakia
Basal cell and prickle cell epitheliomas
Exfoliative dermatitis due to lymphoblastomas and other causes

MILITARY DERMATOSES

Under the ravages of war the lack of good personal hygiene, lack of adequate food, presence of overcrowding, injuries and pestilence, result in the aggravation of any existing skin disease and an increased incidence of the following skin diseases.

Scabies
Pediculosis
Syphilis and other venereal diseases
Bacterial dermatoses
Jungle rot in tropical climates:
  Tinea of the feet and the groin
  Pyoderma
  Dyshidroses
  Miliaria
  Atabrine drug eruption, lichen planuslike

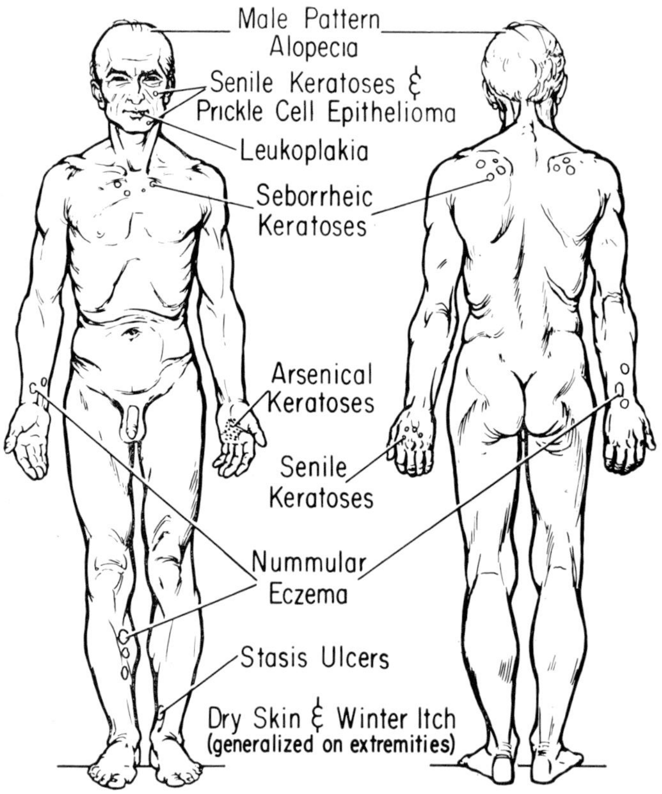

Fig. 18. Geriatric dermograms.

DERMATOSES OF NEGROES

The following skin diseases are seen with greater frequency in the Negro race as compared with the white race.

- Keloids
- Dermatosis papulosa nigra
- Pigmentary disturbances from many causes
- Traumatic marginal alopecia (from braids)
- Annular form of secondary syphilis
- Granuloma inguinale
- Mongolian spots

On the other hand, certain skin conditions are rarely seen in the Negro:

- Prickle cell or basal cell epitheliomas
- Senile keratoses

Your Introduction to the Patient

CHAPTER 4

FOLLOWING the usual conversation of introducing yourself to the new patient, the following might transpire.

DOCTOR: "What can I do for you, Mrs. Jones?"

MRS. JONES: "I have a bad breaking out on my hands."

DOCTOR (Writes on his chart under present complaint "hand dermatitis"): "How long have you had this breaking out?"

MRS. JONES: "Well, I've had this before, but what I have now has been here for only 3 weeks."

DOCTOR (Writes "duration, 3 weeks."): "When did you have this before, Mrs. Jones?"

MRS. JONES: "Let me see. I believe I had this twice before. The first time I had this breaking out was shortly after our wedding and I thought that it had to do with the fact that I had my hands in soap and water more than before. It took about a month to heal up. I treated it with salves that I had at home. It certainly wasn't bad then. The next time I broke out it was a little bit worse. This was after my first child was born. Johnnie is 3 years old now. I suppose I should have expected my hands to break out again now because I just had my second baby 3 months ago."

DOCTOR (Has just finished writing down the following, "The patient states that she has had this eruption on two previous occasions. Home treatment only. Both eruptions lasted approximately 1 month. Present eruption attributed to care of baby born 3 months ago."): "Mrs. Jones, what have you been putting on your hands for this breaking out?"

MRS. JONES: "Let me take off my bandages and I'll show you how my hands look."

DOCTOR: "Let me help you with these bandages. However, I want to ask you a few more questions before I look at your hands."

MRS. JONES: "Well, first I used a salve that I got over at the corner drugstore that said on the label it was good for athlete's foot. One of my neighbors told me that she used it for her hand trouble, and it had cured her hands. I don't think that her hands looked like mine though and I sort of feel that the salve made my hands worse. Then I decided I would burn out the infection, so I soaked my hands in some bleaching solution. This helped some with the itching, but it made the skin too dry. Then I remembered that you had given me some salve for Johnnie's 'infantigo,' so I put some of that on. That softened up my hands but didn't seem to help with the itching. So here I am, Doctor."

DOCTOR (Writing, "Treated with athlete's foot RX, bleach soaks, Johnnie's impetigo RX."): "How much itching are you having?"

MRS. JONES: "Well, my hands sting and burn when I get any soap and water on them, but I can sleep without them bothering me."

DOCTOR (Notes "mild itching."): "Are you taking any medicine by mouth now for anything? I even want to know about laxatives, vitamins, or aspirin. Have you had any shots recently?"

MRS. JONES: "No, I'm not taking any medicine."

DOCTOR: "Now, are you sure?"

MRS. JONES: "Well, I do take sleeping medicine at night occasionally, and, oh yes, I'm taking some reducing pills that Dr. Smith gave me about 2 months ago."

DOCTOR (Writes, "Drugs—takes sleeping medicine h.s. and reducing pills."): "Mrs. Jones, does anyone in your family have any allergies? Does anyone have any asthma, hayfever, or eczema? Your parents, brothers, sisters, children, etc."

MRS. JONES: "No, not that I can recall, Doctor."

DOCTOR: "Have you ever had any of those conditions? Any asthma, hayfever, or eczema?"

MRS. JONES: "No, I haven't had any of those. Sometimes I have a little sinus trouble though."

DOCTOR (Writes, "No atopy in patient or family."): "Now, let me have a good look at those hands. I also want you to remove your shoes and hose so that I can get a good look at your feet." (The doctor then examines the patient's hands and feet very carefully.) "Now are you sure that you don't have this anywhere else, Mrs. Jones?"

MRS. JONES: "No, I am positive I don't because I looked all over my skin this morning when I took a bath. However, I do have a mole on my back that I want you to look at, Doctor."

DOCTOR: "Has it been bothering you recently?"

MRS. JONES: "Well, no, but my bra strap rubs it occasionally."

DOCTOR (Examines the mole on Mrs. Jones's back.): "That certainly is a small mole, Mrs. Jones. It doesn't have any unusual color, and I see no reason for having it removed. It could be removed if you wish, but I don't think it is necessary."

MRS. JONES: "Well, I don't want it removed if you don't think it is necessary. Now, what do you think about my hands?"

DOCTOR: "Let me make a few notes about what I saw and then I'll tell you about your hands and the treatment."

The doctor writes, "Physical exam.: (1) A crusting, vesicular dermatitis is seen mainly in the webs of the fingers of both hands, worse on the right hand. There is no sharp border to the eruption. The nail of the right ring finger has several transverse furrows. The feet are clear. (2) In the mid-line of the upper back is a 3 x 3 mm. flat, faintly brownish lesion. Diagnosis: (1) Contact dermatitis, probably due to excess soap and water. (2) Pigmented compound nevus."

DOCTOR: "Mrs. Jones, you have a very common skin condition, commonly called housewives' eczema or housewives' dermatitis. I feel sure that it is aggravated by having your hands in soap and water so many times a day. Most housewives don't even have enough time to dry their hands carefully every time they are wet. Some people seem to be more sensitive to soaps than others. It isn't a real allergy but just a sensitivity due to the fact that the soap and the water have a tendency to remove the normal skin protective oils and fats. Some of those blisters are infected, and we will have to take care of that infection along with the other irritation. Here is what we will do to treat your hands." (The doctor then gives very careful instructions to Mrs. Jones, particularly with regard to the hand soaks, the way the salve is to be applied, advice concerning avoidance of excess soap and water, the use of rubber and cotton gloves, etc.)

In the above play-by-play description,

which is repeated many times a month in any busy practitioner's office, I have attempted to show some of the basic points in history-taking. The following factors should be stressed again:

1. *Local Treatment History*. Find out how much treatment and what kind of treatment has been given by the patient or by doctors.

2. *Drug History*. It is important to know if the patient is taking any medicine for any other disease for two reasons. First, you learn something about your patient from the drugs taken. For example, it is certainly important to know if a person is taking insulin for diabetes or digitalis for heart disease. This information can well influence your treatment of the patient. Secondly, drugs can cause many skin eruptions, and your index of suspicion of a drug eruption will be higher if you consistently request that information.

3. *Allergy History*. A family or a patient history of allergies can aid you in making a diagnosis of atopic dermatitis. Also if there is a positive allergy history, usually you can predict to the patient that her skin trouble will be slower in responding to treatment than a similar dermatitis in a nonallergenic patient. Atopic patients are more "itchish."

Topical Dermatologic Therapy

CHAPTER 5

MANY HUNDREDS of medications are available for use in treating skin diseases. However, most doctors have only a few favorite prescriptions that are prescribed day in and day out. These few prescriptions may then be altered slightly to suit an individual patient or disease.

The treatment of the majority of the common skin conditions can be made simpler if the doctor is aware of three basic principles.

1. The *type of skin lesion,* more than the cause, influences the kind of local medication used. The old adage "If it's wet, use a wet dressing, and if it's dry use a salve" is true for the majority of cases. For example, to treat a patient with an acute oozing, crusting dermatitis of the dorsum of the hand, whether due to poison ivy or soap, the doctor should prescribe wet soaks and a lotion. For a chronic-looking, dry, scaly patch of psoriasis on the elbow an ointment is indicated, since a lotion or a wet dressing would only be more drying. Bear in mind, however, that the type of skin lesion can change rapidly under treatment. The patient must be followed closely at the beginning of therapy. An acute oozing dermatitis treated with a lotion can change in 2 to 3 days to a dry scaly lesion that requires a paste or an ointment. Conversely, a chronic dry patch may become irritated with too strong therapy and begin to ooze.

2. The second basic principle in treatment is *never do any harm* and never overtreat. It is important for the physician to know which of the chemicals prescribed for local use on the skin are the greatest irritants and sensitizers. It is no exaggeration to say that the most commonly seen dermatitis is the overtreatment contact dermatitis. The overtreatment is often at the hands of the patient who has gone to his neighborhood drugstore or friend and used any and many of the medications available for the treatment of skin diseases. It is certainly not unusual to hear the patient tell of using a strong athlete's foot salve for the treatment of the lesions of pityriasis rosea.

3. The third principle is to *instruct the patient adequately regarding the application* of the medicine prescribed. The patient does not have to be told how to swallow a pill but does have to be told how to put on a wet dressing. Most skin patients are ambulatory, so there is no nurse to help them. They are their own nurse. The success or the failure of skin therapy rests upon adequate instruction of the patient or person responsible for the care. Even in hospitals, particularly when wet dressings or lotions are prescribed, it is wise for the doctor to instruct the nurse regarding the procedure.

With these principles in mind let us now turn to the medicine used. It is important to stress that I am endeavoring to present here only the most basic material necessary to treat the majority of skin diseases. For instance, there are many solutions for wet dressings, but boric acid solution is my preference. Other physicians have preferences different from the drugs listed, and their choices are respected; but to list all of them will not serve the purpose of this book. Two factors have guided me in the selection of medications presented in this formulary. First, the medication must be readily available in most drugstores; secondly, it must be a very effective medication for one or several skin conditions. The medications listed in this formulary will also be listed in a complete way in the treatment section concerning the particular disease. However, instructions for the use of the medications will be more nearly complete in this formulary.

One side of each page in this section has been left blank so that you can insert new or favorite prescriptions of your own.

THERAPY PEARLS

1. The type of skin lesion (oozing, infected, or dry), more than the cause, should decide the local medication that is prescribed.

2. Do no harm. Begin local therapy of a particular case with mild drugs. The concentration of ingredients can be increased as the acuteness subsides.

3. Carefully instruct the patient or the nurse regarding the local application of salves, lotions, wet dressings and baths.

4. Prescribe the correct amount of medication for the area and the dermatosis to be treated. This knowledge comes with experience.

5. Change the therapy as the response indicates. If a new prescription is indicated and the patient has some of the first RX left, use this up by instructing the patient to alternate using the old with the new prescription.

6. If a prescription is going to be relatively expensive, explain this fact to the patient.

7. Instruct the patient to telephone you if there are any questions, or if the medicine seems to irritate the dermatosis.

FORMULARY

A certain topical medication is prescribed to produce a specific beneficial effect.

Effects of Locally Applied Drugs

1. **Antipruritic agents** relieve itching in various ways. Commonly used chemicals and strengths include menthol 0.25%, phenol 0.5%, camphor 2%, and coal tar solution 2 to 10%. These chemicals are added to various bases for the desired effect. Numerous safe and unsafe proprietary preparations for relief of itching are also available. The unsafe preparations are those that contain antihistamines, benzocaine and related "caine" derivatives.

2. **Keratoplastic agents** tend to increase the thickness of the horny layer. Salicylic acid (1 to 2%) is an example of a keratoplastic agent, whereas stronger strengths of salicylic acid are keratolytic.

3. **Keratolytics** remove or soften the horny layer. Commonly used agents of this type include salicylic acid (4 to 10%), resorcinol (2 to 4%), and sulfur (4 to 10%). A *strong* destructive agent is trichloracetic acid, full strength.

4. **Antieczematous agents** remove oozing and vesicular excretions by various actions. The common antieczematous agents include 2% boric acid solution packs or soaks, coal tar solution (2 to 5%), and hydrocortisone and derivatives (0.5 to 1%) incorporated in lotions or salves.

5. **Antiparasitics** destroy or inhibit living infestations. Examples include Eurax lotion and cream for scabies, and Topicide lotion for scabies and pediculosis.

6. **Antiseptics** destroy or inhibit bacteria and fungi. Commonly used examples include Vioform (3%), Sterosan (3%), and antibiotics such as Neomycin (0.5%), Aureomycin (3%) and Terramycin (3%). Antifungal agents include Whitfield's ointment, Desenex ointment, Timofax ointment, Salundek ointment, and sulfur and ammoniated mercury in various bases.

7. **Emollients** soften the skin surface. Nivea oil, mineral oil and white petrolatum are good examples.

Types of Topical Dermatologic Medications

1. **BATHS:**
   A. Tar Bath
      Coal tar solution, U.S.P. (liquor carbonis detergens) 120.0
      Sig: 2 tablespoons to the tub of lukewarm water 6 to 8 inches deep
      Actions: Antipruritic, antieczematous
   B. Starch Bath
      Linit Starch, small box
      Sig: ½ box of starch to the tub of cool water 6 to 8 inches deep
      Actions: Soothing, antipruritic
      Indications: Generalized itching and dryness of skin, winter itch, urticaria

2. **SOAPS AND SHAMPOOS:**
   A. Oilatum Soap Unscented (Stiefel)
      Actions: Mild cleansing agent that leaves an oily film on the skin
      Indications: Dry skin, winter itch
   B. Dial Soap (Armour)
      Actions: Cleansing, antibacterial (contains hexachlorophene)
      Indications: Acne, pyodermas
   C. Selsun Suspension Shampoo (Abbott) 120.0
      Sig: Shampoo hair with 3 separate applications and rinses. Leave the last application on the scalp for 5 minutes before rinsing off. Do not use another shampoo as a final cleanser.
      Actions: Cleansing, antiseborrheic
      Indications: Dandruff, or itching scalp. Not toxic if used as directed.

3. **WET DRESSINGS OR SOAKS:**
Boric Acid Solution, 2%
Sig: 1 level tablespoon of boric acid crystals to 1 quart of tap water. Cover affected area with sheeting wet with solution and tie on with gauze bandage or string. Do not allow any wet dressing to dry out.
Actions: Acidifying, antieczematous, antiseptic
Indications: Oozing or vesicular skin conditions. Do not use over a large area of the body particularly in children.

4. **POWDERS:**
A. Purified Talc (U.S.P.) 60.0
Sig: Dust on locally b.i.d. (Supply in a powder can)
Actions: Absorbent, protective, cooling
Indications: Intertrigo, diaper dermatitis
B. Asterol Powder (Roche) 45.0
Sig: Dust on feet in A.M.
Actions: Absorbent, antifungal
Indications: Prevention or treatment of tinea pedis, tinea cruris

5. **SHAKE LOTIONS:**
A. Calamine Lotion (U.S.P.) 120.0
Sig: Apply locally to affected area t.i.d. with fingers or brush.
Actions: Antipruritic, antieczematous
Indications: Widespread, mildly oozing inflamed dermatoses
B. Nonalcoholic White Shake Lotion

Zinc oxide	24.0
Talc	24.0
Glycerin	12.0
Distilled water q.s.ad.	120.0

C. Alcoholic White Shake Lotion

Zinc oxide	24.0
Talc	24.0
Glycerin	12.0
Distilled water	
95% alcohol āā q.s.ad.	120.0

D. Colored Alcoholic Shake Lotion
To 5C above add: Almay Neutracolor (brunette shade) 2.4
To the above (5A, B, C, or D) you can add sulfur, resorcinol, menthol, phenol, etc. as indicated.

6. **OILS AND EMULSIONS:**
A. Zinc Oil

Zinc oxide	40%
Olive oil q.s.	120.0

Sig: Apply locally to affected area by hand or brush t.i.d.
Actions: Soothing, antipruritic and astringent
Indications: Acute and subacute eczematous eruptions
B. Nivea Skin Oil (Duke) 120.0
Sig: Apply to skin b.i.d. For nondrying bath put 2 tablespoonfuls in the tub of 6 to 8 inches of water.
Actions: Emollient, lubricating
Indications: Winter itch, dry skin

7. **TINCTURES AND AQUEOUS SOLUTIONS:**
A. Gentian Violet Solution

Gentian Violet	1%
Distilled Water q.s.	30.0

Sig: Apply with swab b.i.d.
Actions: Antifungal, antibacterial
Indications: Moniliasis, leg ulcers
B. Sodium Thiosulfate Solution

Sodium Thiosulfate	20%
Distilled Water q.s.	180.0

Sig: Apply nightly after bath.
Actions: Mildly antifungal
Indications: Tinea versicolor
C. Asterol Tincture (Roche) 30.0
Sig: Apply locally t.i.d.
Actions: Antifungal

Indications: Tinea cruris (stings!), tinea of nails

8. **PASTES:**

Zinc Oxide Paste (U.S.P.)
Sig: Apply locally b.i.d.
Actions: Protective, absorbent, astringent
Indications: Localized crusted or scaly dermatoses

9. **CREAMS AND OINTMENTS:**

A. The following are *water-washable cream bases* into which medications can be incorporated:
   a. Unibase (Parke-Davis)
   b. Neobase (Burroughs Wellcome)
   c. Acid Mantle Cream (Dome)
   d. Unscented cold cream (not water-washable)

B. The following are *ointment bases* to which medications can be added:
   a. White Petrolatum (U.S.P.)
   b. Zinc Oxide Ointment (U.S.P.)

C. Vioform Ointment or Cream, 3% (Ciba)
   Actions: Antiseptic, antiseborrheic

D. Pragmatar (Smith, Kline & French)
   Contains 3% sulfur, 3% salicylic acid and a tar, 4%
   Actions: Antifungal, keratolytic, antipruritic

E. Quotane Ointment (Smith, Kline & French)
   Actions: Antipruritic

F. Mixed antibiotic ointments:
   a. Neo-Polycin Ointment (Pitman Moore)
   b. Neosporin Ointment (Burroughs Wellcome)

G. Corticosteroid-antibiotic ointments. (The following are proprietary preparations, but hydrocortisone powder and antibiotics can be added to most ointments, creams or lotions in any strength. The following preparations can also be prescribed without the antibiotics.)
   a. Neo-Cortef Ointment (Upjohn) (1% hydrocortisone strength is usually adequate)
   b. Neo-Magnacort Ointment (Pfizer)
   c. Cortisporin Ointment (Burroughs Wellcome)
   d. Neo-Cort-Dome Creme and Lotion (Dome)
   e. Florinef-S Ointment and Lotion (Squibb)
   f. Neo-Hydeltrasol Ointment and Lotion (Merck, Sharpe and Dohme)
   Actions: Antibiotic, anti-inflammatory

H. Antifungal ointments
   a. Timofax Ointment (Burroughs Wellcome)
   b. Desenex Ointment (Wallace and Tiernan)
   c. Salundek Ointment (Wallace and Tiernan)
   d. Asterol Ointment (Roche)
   Actions: Antifungal
   e. Whitfield's Ointment (Benzoic and Salicylic Acid Ointment, U.S.P.)
   Actions: Antifungal, keratolytic. Use full or double strength. Be sure and specify "U.S.P." or you might get the older stronger 12% Benzoic and 6% Salicylic Acid Ointment.

I. Scabicide
   Eurax Cream and Lotion (Geigy)
   Actions: Scabicidal and antipruritic

J. Pediculocides and scabicides
   a. Benzyl Benzoate Lotion, U.S.P.
   b. Topocide (Lilly)
   c. Benzyl Benzoate Emulsion (Burroughs Wellcome)

K. Sun Screen Creams
   a. Skolex (Williams)
   b. A-fil (Texas Pharmacal)
      Sig: Apply to exposed areas before going outside.
      Actions: Screens out ultraviolet rays from 2,900 to 3,200 Ångströms.
      Indications: Actinic dermatitis, acute and chronic lupus erythematosus, possible prevention of skin cancers in light complexioned individuals. (These agents prevent skin tanning.)

10. **LOCAL AGENTS FOR OFFICE USE:**

A. Podophyllum in alcohol

Podophyllum Resin (U.S.P.)	25%
Alcohol q.s.ad.	30.0

Indications: For removal of venereal warts

Directions: Apply small amount to warts with cotton-tipped applicator every 4 to 5 days until warts are gone. Excess amount may be washed off in 6 hours after application to prevent irritation.

B. Chrysarobin Tincture

Chrysarobin	3%
Chloroform q.s.	30.0

Indications: Tinea of nails, tinea cruris.

Directions: Apply in office with cotton-tipped applicator every 5 to 7 days. It stings on crural area. Caution patient not to touch eyelids with treated fingers.

C. Trichloracetic Acid Solution (Saturated)

Indications: For removal by chemical cautery of warts on children, seborrheic keratoses and xanthelasma (with caution)

Directions: Apply with caution with cotton-tipped applicator. (Have water handy to neutralize.)

D. Modified Unna's Boot
   a. Dome Paste Bandage (Dome)
   b. Gelocast (Duke)
   Indications: For stasis ulcers, localized neurodermatitis

E. Ace Bandage, 3 inches in width (Becton, Dickinson)

Indications: For stasis dermatitis and leg edema

Physical Dermatologic Therapy

CHAPTER 6

THE FIELD of physical medicine embraces therapy with a variety of agents which include massage, therapeutic exercise, water, air, radiations (which include heat, light, ultraviolet, x-rays and radium), vibrations, refrigeration, and electricity of various forms. Many of these agents are used in the treatment of skin diseases.

HYDROTHERAPY

The physical agent most commonly used for dermatoses is hydrotherapy in the form of medicated or nonmedicated wet compresses and baths. Distilled water or tap water are the vehicles and may contain any of the following chemicals in varying strengths: sodium chloride, boric acid, aluminum acetate (Burow's solution), potassium permanganate, silver nitrate, tar, starch, oatmeal (Aveeno) and colloid (Soyaloid). The instructions and the dilutions for boric acid compresses, starch baths and tar baths are listed in the Formulary.

Wet Dressings

Wet dressings can be applied as open or closed dressings. The *open* compresses are used most frequently, since excessive maceration of tissue occurs when the dressings are "closed" with wax paper or rubber sheeting. The compresses can be *hot, cold* or at *room* temperature. Instructions to the patient or the nurse concerning correct application of the compresses should be explicit and detailed. For most conditions the area to be treated should be wrapped with 2 or 3 layers of clean sheeting or muslin. Then gauze 3 inches wide should be wrapped around the sheeting to hold it firmly in place. After that the dressing can be moistened with the solution by pouring it on or by squirting it on with a bulb syringe. In most instances the dressing is wet with the solution before it is wrapped on the affected area. The compresses should never be allowed to dry out and should be left on only for the time specified by the doctor. The solution used should be made fresh every day. For treating the face, the hands and the genitalia, special masks, gloves and slings can be improvised. The indications for wet compresses are any oozing, crusting, or pruritic dermatoses regardless of etiology.

Medicated Baths

Medicated baths should last from 15 to 30 minutes. Cool baths tend to lessen pruritus and are prescribed most frequently. Baths can be used for a multitude of skin diseases except those conditions where excessive dryness is to be avoided, such as for patients with atopic eczema, senile or winter pruritus and ichthyosis.

ELECTROSURGERY

Electrosurgery is employed very commonly in treating or removing a multitude of skin lesions. One of several different types of available current or instrument is employed to achieve a desired result. Five forms of electrosurgery are available.

Electrodesiccation or Fulguration

Electrodesiccation or fulguration is produced by an Oudin current of high voltage and low amperage, using a single or monoterminal electrode. The high frequency current wave is damped. Such a current is produced by the Hyfrecator and by the larger Bovie or Wappler units, using the spark-gap part of the machine. The effect on the skin is a charring of the tissues.

Electrocoagulation

Electrocoagulation is produced by a d'Arsonval current of relatively low voltage and high amperage, using biterminal electrodes. This current also is damped and can be obtained from the Bovie and the Wappler combination units, using the spark-gap part of the machine. Electrocoagulation is more destructive than electrodesiccation, due to the intense heat.

Electrosection

Electrosection or cutting is produced by a current which is undamped when delivered by a vacuum tube apparatus and moderately damped from a spark-gap apparatus. Biterminal electrodes are used. The large Bovie and Wappler combination units produce a moderately damped current from the spark-gap part of the machine and an undamped current from the vacuum tube part. When the vacuum tube cutting current is used the cut is clean with practically no coagulation, whereas the current from a spark-gap machine produces some coagulation of the cut skin edge. Any coagulation can be minimized by making a rapid stroke. Tissue skillfully removed in this manner can be studied histologically if necessary.

Electrocautery

Electrocautery is simply produced by applying heat to the skin. This can be supplied by many instruments, one of which is the Post Electric Cautery (Andover, N. J.). Many operators prefer this form of electrosurgery to electrodesiccation or electrocoagulation.

Electrolysis

Electrolysis utilizes a direct galvanic current to produce chemical cauterization of tissue due to the formation of sodium hydroxide in the tissues with liberation of free hydrogen at the negative electrode. Battery machines or rectified direct current instruments accomplish this. Electrolysis is used mainly to remove superfluous hair. A faster and less painful technic of hair epilation is to use the high frequency current set at a very low intensity where it will deliver a small electrodesiccation spark.

The dermatoses most commonly treated by electrosurgery are warts of all kinds, senile and seborrheic keratoses, leukoplakia, pigmented nevi, spider hemangiomas, hypertrichosis, and basal cell and prickle cell epitheliomas. The skill and the experience of the therapist will be the factor determining the scope of his use of the surgical diathermy machine.

Refrigeration

Therapeutic refrigeration can be accomplished by the use of liquid nitrogen, liquid oxygen, Freon 114, or solid carbon dioxide. The latter is used most commonly because of its availability from a tank of carbon dioxide, blocks from ice cream manufacturers, or from the Kidde Dry Ice Apparatus. The solid carbon dioxide is shaped into an appropriately sized "pencil" for treatment of superficial hemangiomas, warts or seborrheic keratoses. Freon 114 is used to freeze and immobilize the skin for dermabrasion removal of acne scars and senile keratotic skin.

RADIATION

Radiation agents are important in the field of skin diseases.

Ultraviolet Therapy

Ultraviolet therapy is most commonly utilized and available. The two sources of artificial ultraviolet radiation are the hot quartz mercury arc lamp, which operates at a high vapor pressure and relatively high temperature, and the cold quartz lamp which operates at a low vapor pressure and low temperature.

The *hot quartz lamp* is used mainly for the effect from its radiations at 2,900 to 3,200 Ångström units. These rays cause erythema and tanning of the skin. Modifications of these lamps are sold as sun lamps for use in the home. The dermatoses most commonly treated with the hot quartz lamp are psoriasis, acne, pityriasis rosea and seborrheic dermatitis, particularly when the last is of the generalized type on the body.

The *cold quartz lamp* has mainly disinfecting and desquamating effects on the skin, due to the predominance of rays at 2,537 Ångström units. Its use in dermatology and in general is limited.

X-Ray Therapy

Another of the physical therapeutic agents commonly used for skin diseases is x-ray therapy. A detailed discussion of x-ray therapy is not within the scope of this book, since it is a specialized subject of considerable magnitude. Radiation therapy should be administered only by an adequately trained dermatologist or radiologist. If correct shielding and dosage are observed, x-ray therapy is quite safe, as has been proved by many well-controlled studies.

X-ray or radium therapy finds its greatest use in the treatment of skin cancers, acne, various pruritic dermatoses, hemangiomas, cutaneous lymphoblastomas (particularly granuloma fungoides) and fungus infections of the scalp. X-ray therapy is contraindicated in the management of light sensitive eruptions (acute or chronic lupus erythematosus, actinic dermatitis), radiodermatitis, hypertrichosis and localized excessive perspiration. For the majority of dermatoses, excluding malignancies, the physical factors of superficial x-ray therapy are 70 to 100 kilovolt-peak, 2 to 5 milliamperes, 20 to 30 cm. focal skin distance and no filter. The half-value layer with these factors varies with the machine from 0.6 to 1.0 mm. of aluminum. The average superficial x-ray therapy dose for dermatoses is 75 r per week. This weekly dose can be given up to a maximum total of 600 to 1,000 r if absolutely indicated. The top maximum dose depends on many factors, such as seriousness of the lesion being treated, response of the dermatosis to therapy, complexion of the individual, and age of the individual. *Under no circumstances should such a maximum course of x-ray therapy ever be repeated.* Grenz ray therapy is an even more superficial form of radiation therapy and therefore it is potentially less harmful.

Dermatologic Allergy

CHAPTER 7

CONTACT dermatitis, industrial dermatoses, atopic eczema and drug eruptions are included in this chapter because of their obvious allergenic factors. Nummular eczema is also included because it resembles some forms of atopic eczema and may even be a variant of atopic eczema.

CONTACT DERMATITIS

(Plates 4 and 5)

Contact dermatitis, or dermatitis venenata, is a very common inflammation of the skin caused by the exposure of the skin to either primary irritant substances, such as soaps, or to allergenic substances, such as poison ivy resin. Industrial dermatoses will be considered at the end of this section.

Primary Lesions. See any of the stages from mild redness, edema or vesicles to large bullae with a marked amount of oozing.

Secondary Lesions. Crusting from secondary bacterial infection, excoriations and lichenification.

Distribution and Etiology. Any agent can affect any area of the body. However, certain agents commonly affect certain skin areas.

FACE AND NECK (Fig. 19): Cosmetics, soaps, insect sprays, ragweed, perfumes

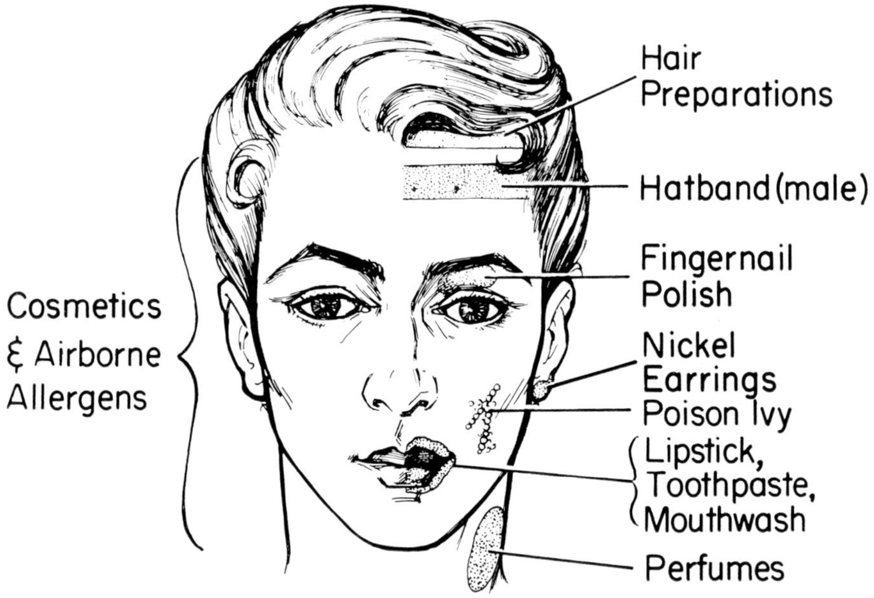

Fig. 19. Contact dermatitis of the face.

(sides of neck), fingernail polish (eyelids), hatband (forehead), mouthwashes, tooth paste or lipstick (perioral), nickel metal (earlobes), industrial oil (facial chloracne)

HANDS AND FOREARMS: Soaps, hand lotions, wrist bands, industrial chemicals, poison ivy and a multitude of other agents. Irritation from soap often begins under rings.

AXILLAE: Deodorants, dress shields, or dry cleaning solutions

TRUNK: Clothing (new, not previously cleaned), rubber or metal attached to or in clothing

ANOGENITAL REGION: Douches, dusting powder, contraceptives, colored toilet paper, poison ivy, or too strong salves for treatment of pruritus ani and fungal infections

FEET: Shoes, foot powders, too strong salves for "athlete's feet" infection

GENERALIZED ERUPTION: Volatile airborne chemicals (paint spray, ragweed), medicaments locally applied to large areas, bath powder, or clothing

Determine the site of the INITIAL eruption and think of the agents that touch that area.

Course. Duration very short to very chronic. As a general rule, successive recurrences become more chronic (i.e., seasonal ragweed dermatitis can become a year-round dermatitis). An established hypersensitivity reaction is never lost. Also, certain individuals have greater susceptibility for allergic and irritant contact dermatitis.

Season. A very careful seasonal history of the onset in chronic cases may lead to discovery of an unsuspected causative agent, such as ragweed.

Family Incidence. Not evident.

Contagiousness. The eczematous reaction, for instance the blister fluid of poison ivy, contains no allergen that can cause the dermatitis in another individual. However, if the poison ivy oil or other

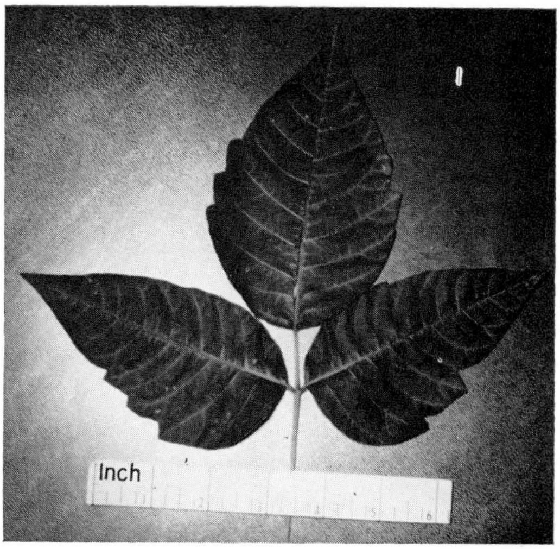

Fig. 20. Large leaves of the poison ivy plant.

allergen remains on the skin of the affected person, contact of the allergen with a susceptible individual could cause a dermatitis.

Laboratory Findings. Patch tests (p. 7) are of value in eliciting the cause in a problem case. Careful interpretation is a necessity.

Differential Diagnosis. A contactant reaction must be thought of and ruled in or out in any case of eczematous dermatitis on any body area.

Treatment. Two of the commonest contact dermatoses seen in the doctor's office are *poison ivy dermatitis* and *hand dermatitis.* The treatment of these two conditions will be discussed.

TREATMENT OF CONTACT DERMATITIS DUE TO POISON IVY

A patient comes into your office with a linear, vesicular dermatitis of the feet, the hands and the face. He states that he spent the week-end fishing and that the rash broke out the next day. The itching is rather severe but not enough to keep him awake at night. He had "poison ivy" 5 years ago. (Fig. 20.)

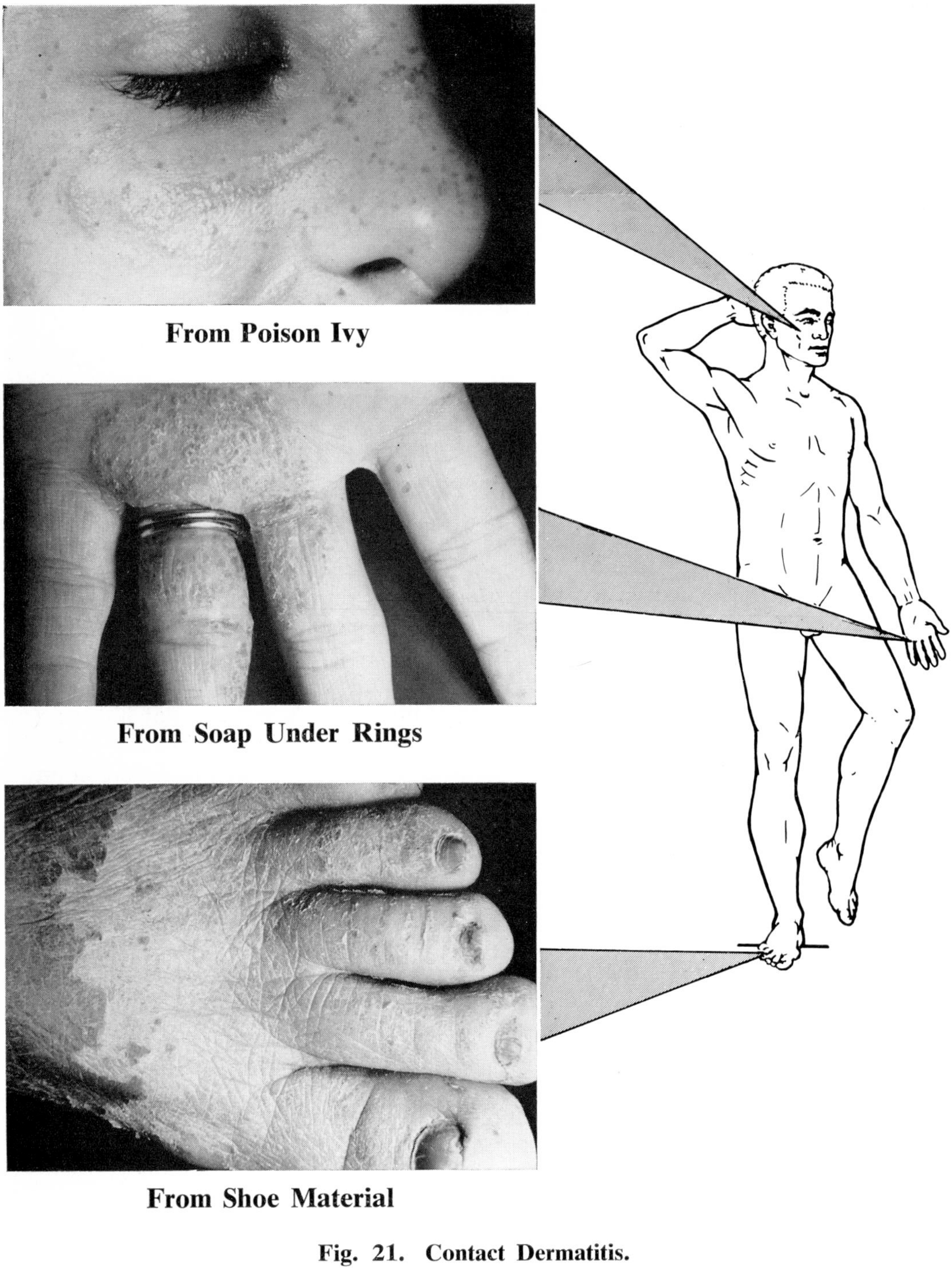

From Poison Ivy

From Soap Under Rings

From Shoe Material

Fig. 21. Contact Dermatitis.

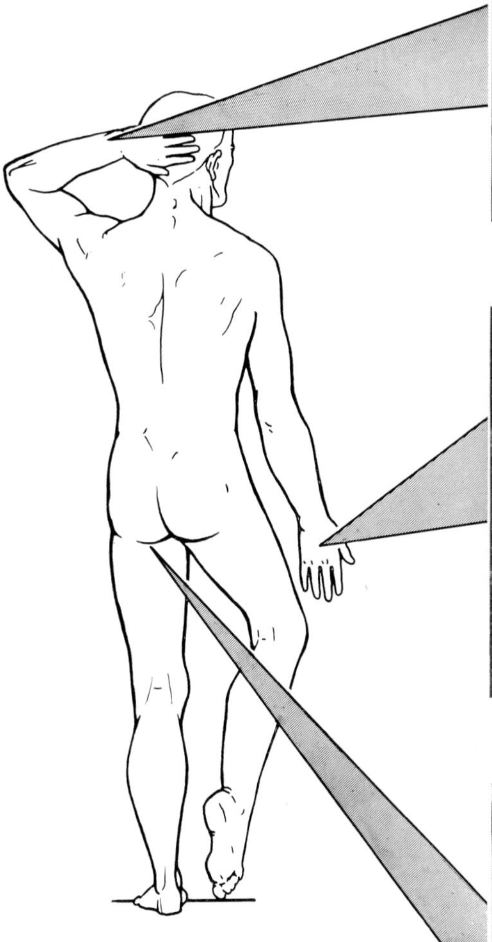

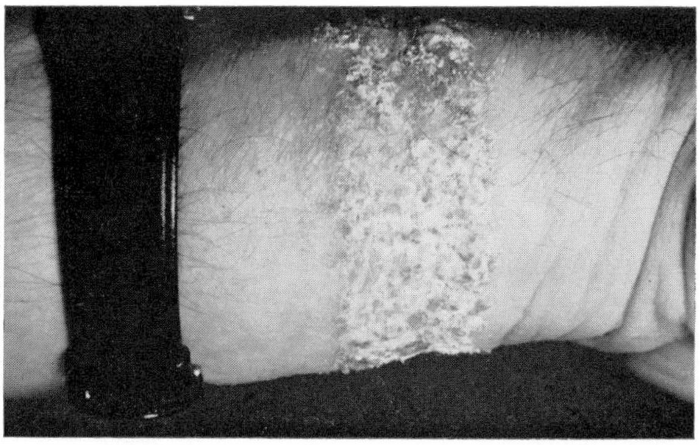

From Leather Watch Band

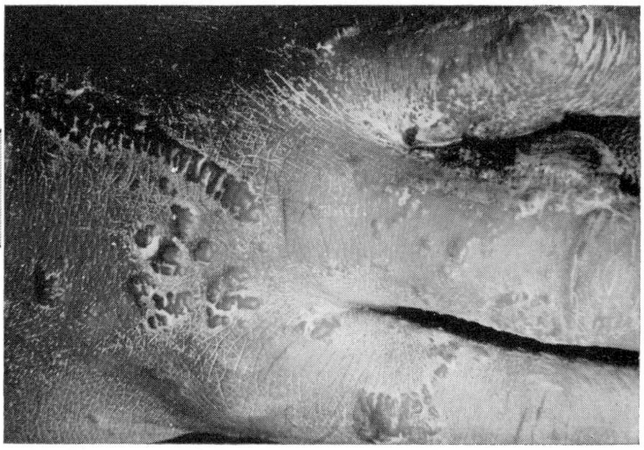

From Poison Ivy. Note linear vesicles.

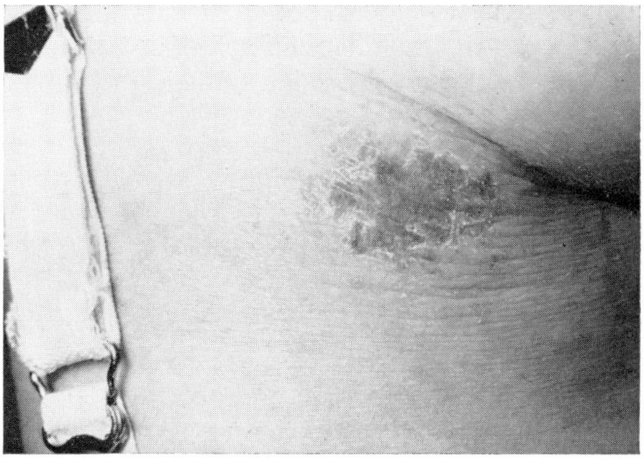

From Nickel Metal in Garter Strap

Fig. 22. Contact dermatitis.

Treatment on First Visit

1. Assure the patient that he cannot give the dermatitis to his family or spread it on himself from the blister fluid.

2. Suggest that the clothes worn while fishing be washed or cleaned to remove the allergenic resin.

3. Débridement. The blisters should be opened with manicure scissors and not by sticking with a needle. Cutting the top open with the scissors will prevent that blister from reforming.

4. Boric acid solution (2%) wet packs

Sig: 1 tablespoon of boric acid crystals to 1 quart of cool water. Apply sheeting or toweling, wet with the solution, to the blistered areas for 20 minutes twice a day. The wet packs need not be removed during the 20-minute period.

(For a more widespread case of poison ivy dermatitis, cool starch baths, ½ box of Linit Starch to the tub, give considerable relief from the itching.)

5. Nonalcoholic white shake lotion q.s. 120.0

Sig: Apply 3 times a day to the affected areas.

(The patient probably has been to the corner drugstore and obtained calamine lotion, so the nonalcoholic white shake lotion has the added value of being of a different color.)

6. Pyribenzamine tablets, 50 mg., or Temaril, 2.5 mg. #30

Sig: 1 tablet t.i.d. a.c. (For relief of itching.)

Subsequent Visits

1. Continue the wet packs only as long as there are blisters and oozing. Extended use is too drying for the skin.

2. After 3 to 4 days of use the lotion may be too drying. Substitute:

Hydrocortisone	0.5%
Menthol	0.25%
White petrolatum q.s.	30.0

Sig: Apply small amount locally t.i.d., or more often if itching is present.

Severe Cases of Poison Ivy Dermatitis

1. Triamcinoline (Kenacort or Aristocort), 4 mg. #20

Sig: 1 tablet q.i.d. for 3 days then 1 tablet b.i.d. for 4 days.

2. Hospitalization of a severe case might be indicated for more intensive wet packs, ACTH injections, etc.

The use of poison ivy vaccine orally or intramuscularly is contraindicated during an acute episode. Desensitization may occur following a long course of oral ingestion of graduated doses of the allergin. Desensitization does not occur following a short course of intramuscular injections of the vaccine.

Treatment of Contact Dermatitis of the Hand Due to Soap

A young housewife states that she has had a breaking-out on her hands for 5 weeks. The dermatitis developed about 4 weeks after the birth of her last baby. She states that she had a similar eruption after her previous two pregnancies. She has used a lot of local medication of her own, and the rash is growing worse instead of better. The patient and her immediate family never have had any asthma, hay fever or eczema.

Examination of her hands reveals small vesicles on the sides of all of her fingers with a 5-cm.-sized area of oozing and crusting around her left ring finger.

Treatment on the First Visit

1. General instructions must always be given to these patients.

A. Assure the patient that the hand eczema is not contagious to her family.

B. Inform the patient that soap irritates the dermatitis and that it must be avoided as much as possible. A housewife will find this avoidance very difficult. One of the best remedies is to wear protective gloves when extended soap-and-water contact is unavoidable. Rubber gloves alone produce a considerable amount of irritating perspiration, but this is absorbed when thin white cotton gloves are worn under the rubber gloves. Lined rubber gloves are not as satisfactory, because the lining eventually becomes dirty and soggy and cannot be cleaned easily.

C. For body cleanliness any mild soap can be used, or the following:

Oilatum Soap (Stiefel)
Basis Soap (Duke)

D. Tell the patient that the above prophylactic measures will have to be adhered to for several weeks after the eruption has apparently cleared or there will be a recurrence. Injured skin is sensitive and needs to be babied for an extended time.

2. Boric Acid Soaks

Sig: 1 tablespoon of boric acid crystals to 1 quart of cool water. Soak hands for 15 minutes twice a day.

3. Corticosteroid Ointments

A. Neo-Magnacort ointment 15.0
B. 1% Neo-Cortef ointment 15.0

In place of the above or other available proprietary steroid ointments, hydrocortisone powder can be mixed with white petrolatum or water-washable bases. This cuts down the cost of the prescription. Example:

Hydrocortisone powder 0.5%
White petrolatum q.s. 15.0
Sig: Apply sparingly locally q.i.d.

Housewive's eczema cannot usually be cured with a steroid salve alone without observing the other protective measures.

Treatment of Resistant, Chronic Cases

1. To the corticosteroid ointment add as indicated sulfur 3 to 5%, coal tar solution 3 to 10%, or an antipruritic agent such as menthol, 0.25%, or camphor 2%.

2. Oral Corticosteroid Therapy. A short course of such therapy will often improve or cure a chronic dermatitis.

3. Superficial x-ray therapy administered by a competent dermatologist or radiologist is valuable for chronic persistent cases. Usually 3 or 4 treatments given at weekly or semiweekly intervals are effective. There is no danger from superficial x-ray radiation if it is given correctly and the total dosage is not excessive (see p. 41).

INDUSTRIAL DERMATOSES

Sixty-five percent of all the industrial diseases are dermatoses. The average case of occupational dermatitis is compensated for 10 weeks, resulting in a total cost of over $100,000,000 a year in the United States. The commonest cause of these skin problems is contact irritants, of which cutting oils are the worst offenders. Lack of adequate cleansing is a big contributing factor.

It is not possible to list the thousands of different chemicals used in the hundreds of varied industrial operations which have the potential of causing a primary irritant reaction or an allergic reaction on the skin surface. The most complete text on this entire subject of occupational dermatoses is that by Schwartz, Tulipan, and Birmingham, entitled *Occupational Diseases of the Skin* (ed. 3, Philadelphia, Lea and Febiger, 1956).

Management of Industrial Dermatitis

A cutting-tool laborer presents himself with a pruritic red, vesicular dermatitis on his hands, forearms and face of 2 months duration.

1. Obtain a careful detailed history of his type of work, and any recent change such as use of new chemicals, new cleansing agents, exposure at home with hobbies, painting, etc. Question him concerning remission of the dermatitis on week ends, or while on vacation.

2. Question concerning the first-aid care given at the plant. Too often this care

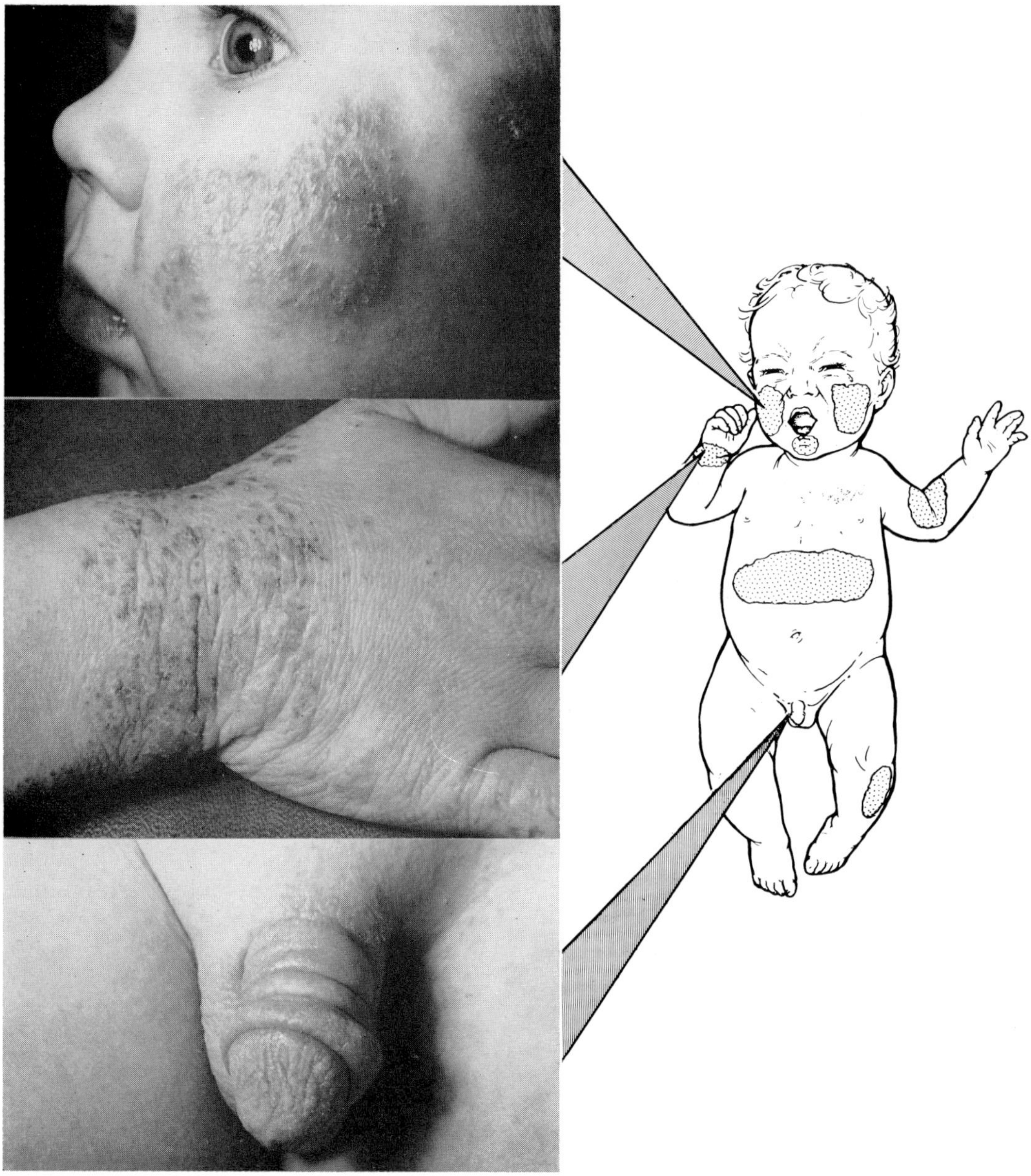

Fig. 23. Atopic eczema (infant).

aggravates the dermatitis. Bland protective remedies should be substituted for potential sensitizers, such as sulfonamide and penicillin salves, antihistamine creams, benzocaine ointments, nitrofuran preparations, and strong antipruritic lotions and salves.

3. Treatment of the dermatitis with wet compresses, bland lotions, or salves is the same as for any contact dermatitis (see previous discussion). Unfortunately, many of the occupational dermatoses respond slowly to therapy. This is due in part to the fact that most patients continue to work and are re-exposed repeatedly to small amounts of the irri-

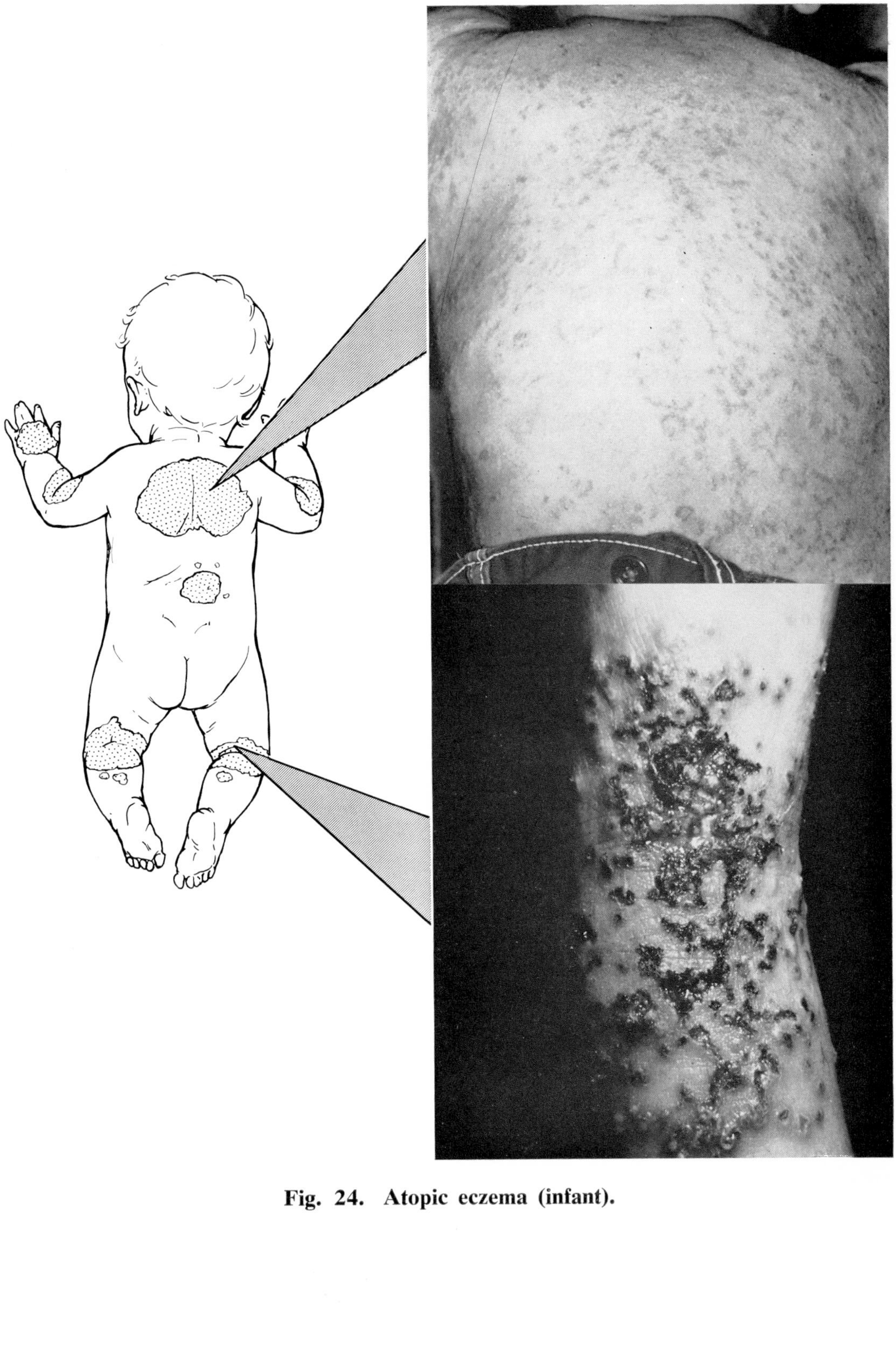

Fig. 24. Atopic eczema (infant).

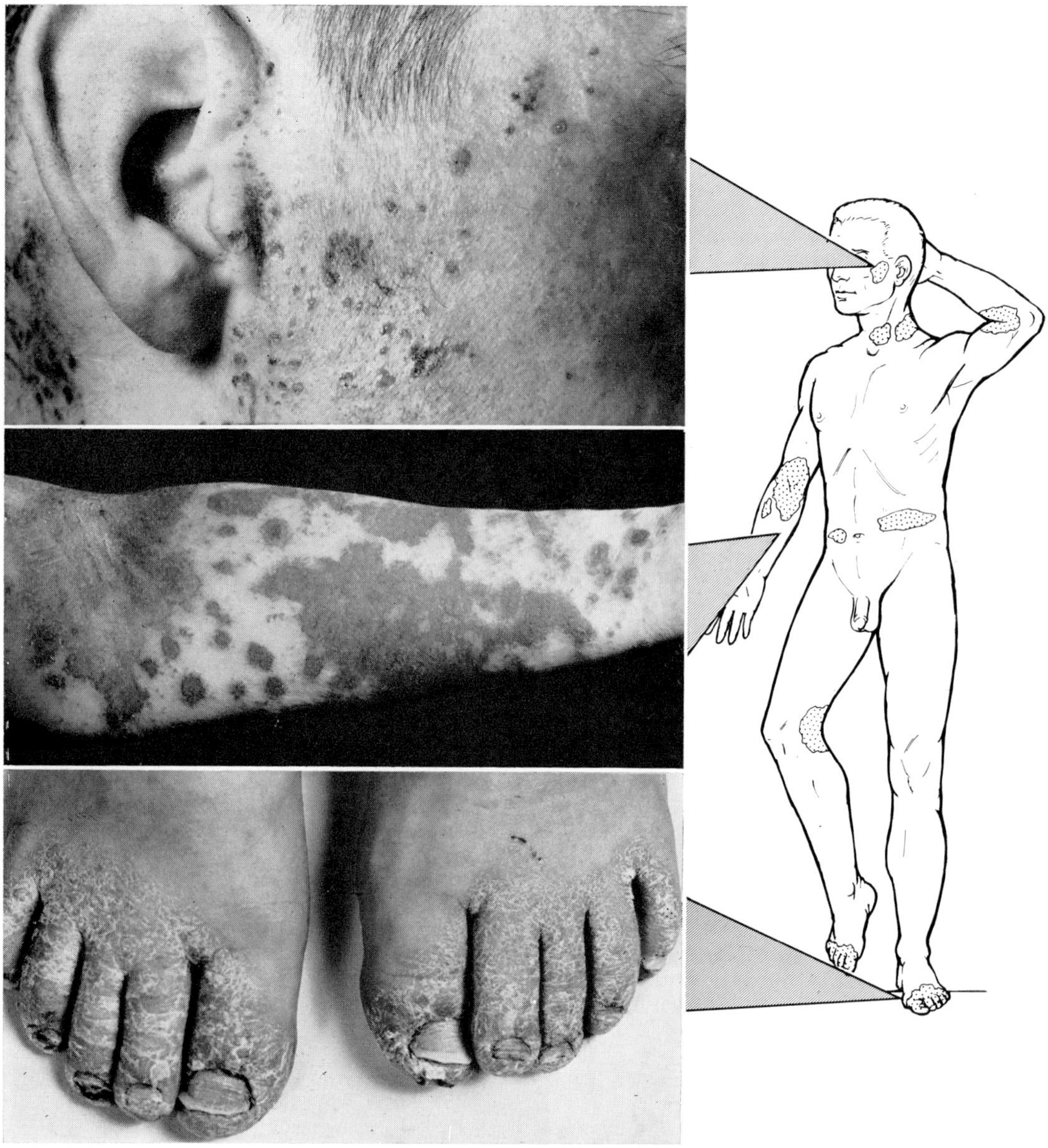

Fig. 25. Atopic eczema.

tating chemicals, even though precautions are taken. Also, certain industrial chemicals, such as chromates, beryllium salts and cutting oils, injure the skin in such a way as to prevent healing for months and years.

4. The legal complications with compensation boards, insurance companies, the industry and the injured patient can be discouraging, frustrating and time-consuming. However, most patients are not malingerers but they do expect and deserve proper care and compensation for their injury.

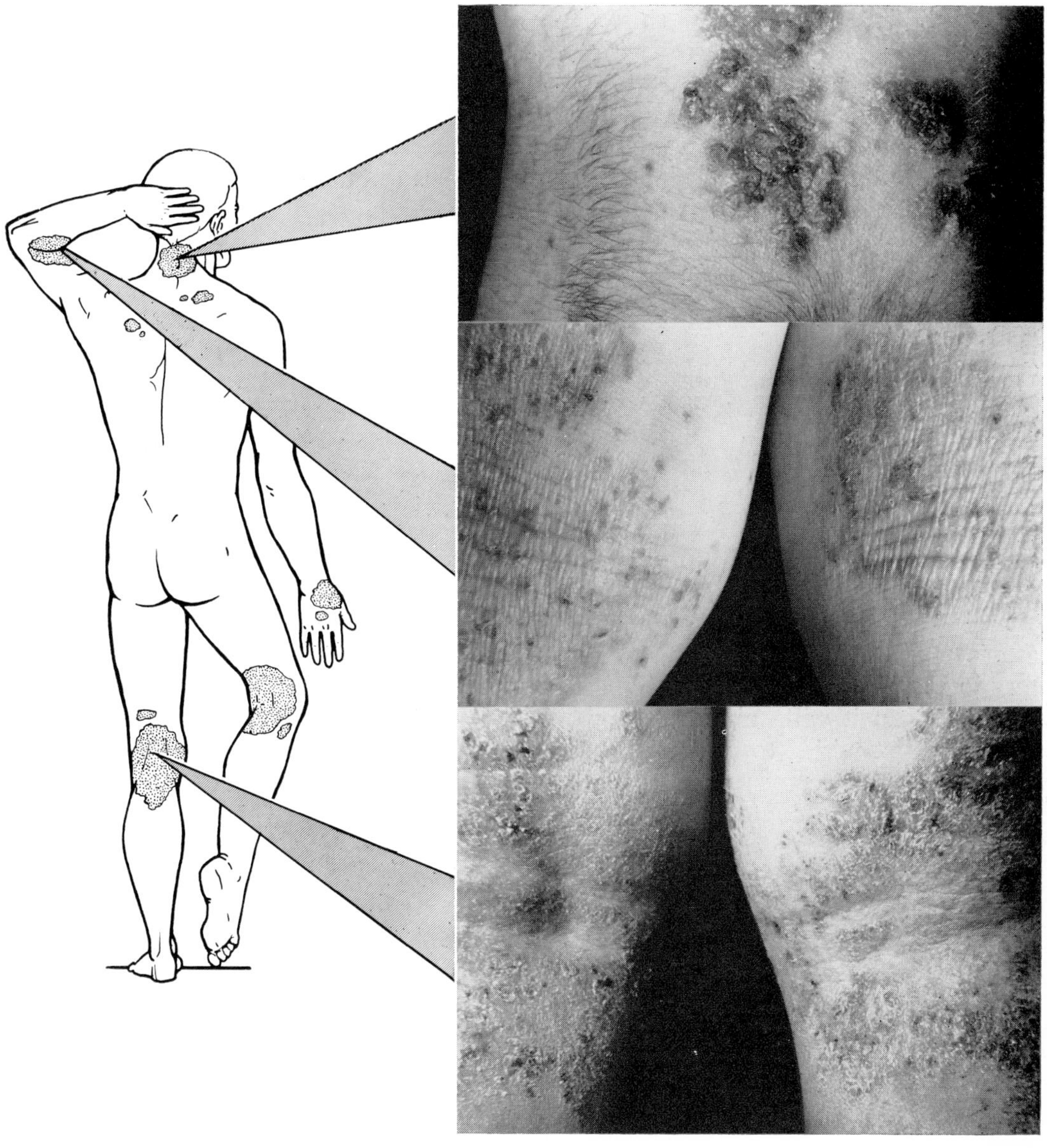

Fig. 26. Atopic eczema.

ATOPIC ECZEMA
(Plate 6)

Atopic eczema is a rather common, markedly pruritic, chronic skin condition that occurs in two clinical forms: *infantile* and *adult* (Figs. 23-26).

Clinical Lesions. Infantile form—blisters, oozing and crusting with excoriation. Adolescent and adult forms—marked dryness, thickening (lichenification), excoriation and even scarring.

Distribution. Infantile form—on face, scalp, arms and legs, or generalized. Adolescent and adult form—on cubital and popliteal fossae and less commonly on dorsum of hands and feet, ears, or generalized.

Course. Varies from mild single episode to severe chronic, recurrent episodes resulting in the "psychoitchical" individual. The infantile form usually becomes milder or even disappears after the age of 3 or 4. At the age of puberty and the late teens flare-ups or new outbreaks can occur. Young housewives may have their first recurrence of atopic eczema since childhood due to their new job of dishwashing and baby care. Thirty per cent of patients with atopic dermatitis eventually develop allergic asthma or hay fever.

Etiology. The following factors are important.

1. *Heredity* is the most important single factor. The family history is usually positive for one or more of the triad of allergic diseases, asthma, hay fever, or atopic eczema. Determination of this history in hand dermatitis cases is important because often it will enable you, on the patient's first visit, to prognosticate a more drawn-out recovery than if the patient had a simple contact dermatitis.

2. *Dryness of the skin* is important. Most often atopic eczema is worse in the wintertime. The factor here is the decrease in home or office humidity that causes a drying of the skin. For this reason bathing and the use of soap and water should be reduced.

3. *Wool and lanolin* (wool fat) commonly irritate the skin of these patients. The wearing of wool clothes may be another reason for an increased incidence in the winter.

4. *Allergy to foods* is a factor often overstressed, particularly with the infantile form. The mother's history of certain foods causing trouble should be your guide for eliminating foods. The correctness of her belief can be tested by adding these incriminated foods to the diet, one new food every 48 hours, when the dermatitis is stable. Scratch tests and intracutaneous tests uncover very few dermatologic allergens.

5. *Emotional stress and nervousness* aggravate any existing condition such as itching, duodenal ulcers, or migraine headaches. Therefore, this "nervous" factor is important but not causative enough to label this disease *disseminated neurodermatitis.*

Differential Diagnosis

Dermatitis venenata (positive history usually of contactants, no family allergic history, distribution rather characteristic, p. 42).

Psoriasis (patches localized to extensor surfaces, mainly knees and elbows, p. 83).

Seborrheic dermatitis in infants (absence of family allergy history, lesions scaling and greasy, p. 73).

Localized neurodermatitis (single patches mainly, no family allergy history, p. 63).

Treatment of Infantile Form: FIRST VISIT. Child aged 6 months with mild oozing, red, excoriated dermatitis on face, arms and legs.

1. Follow regular diet except for the avoidance of any foods which the mother believes aggravate the eruption.

2. Avoid exposure of baby to excessive bathing with soaps and to contact with wool and products containing lanolin.

3. Coal tar solution 120.0
Sig: ½ tablespoon to the lukewarm bath water. Bathe only once or twice a week.

4. Hydrocortisone powder 1%
White petrolatum q.s. 15.0
Sig: Apply sparingly locally b.i.d. to affected areas.

(Proprietary corticosteroid-antibiotic preparations are listed in the Formulary, p. 31.)

5. Benadryl elixir 90.0
Sig: 1 teaspoonful b.i.d.

SUBSEQUENT VISITS

1. Add coal tar solution, 3% to 10%, to the above ointment.

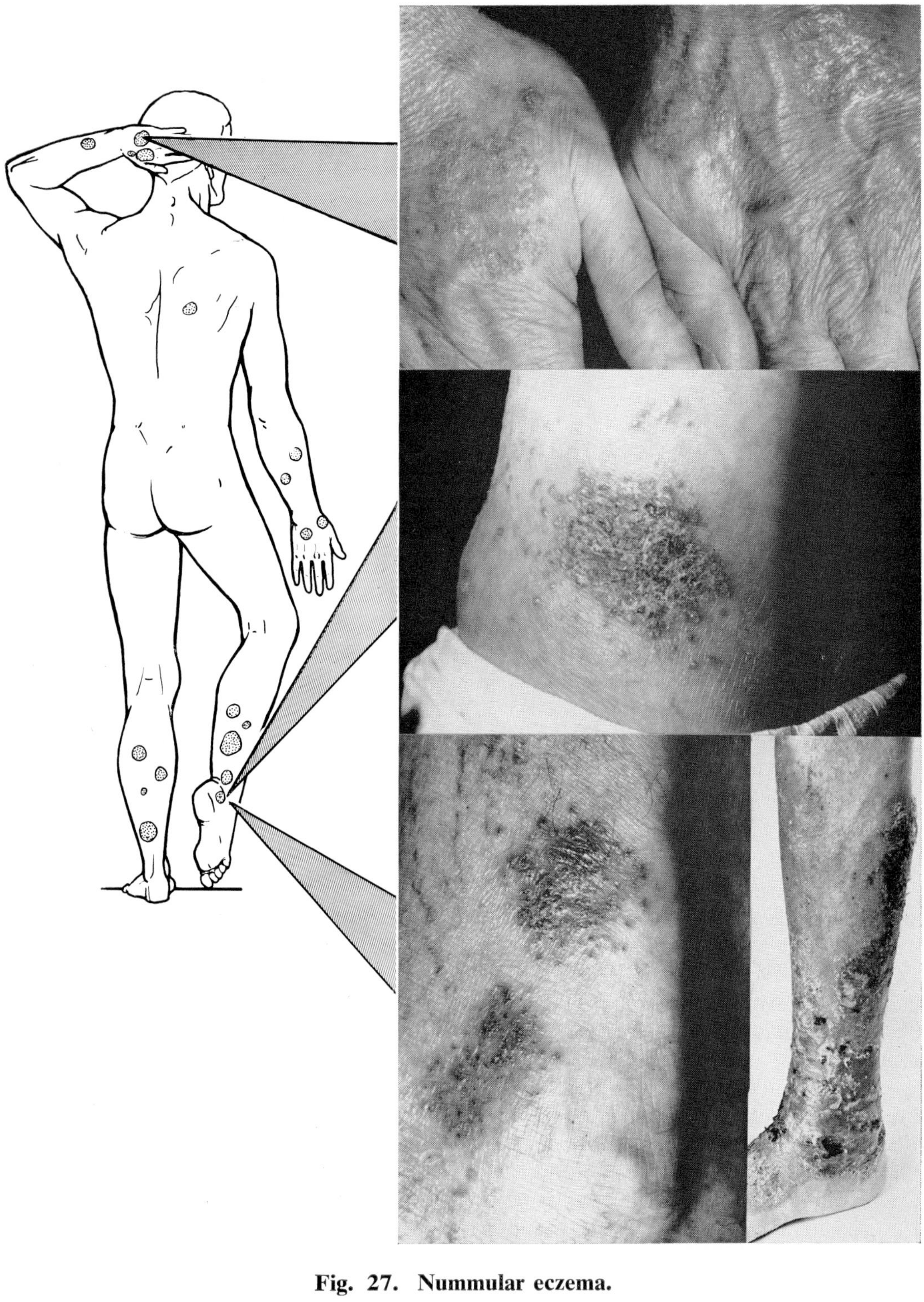

Fig. 27. Nummular eczema.

SEVERE OR RESISTANT CASES

1. Restrict diet to milk only, and after 3 days add one different food every 24 hours. An offending food will cause a flare-up of the eczema in several hours.

2. Hydrocortisone liquid (Fluid Cortef) 90.0

Sig: 1 teaspoonful (10 mg.) q.i.d. for 3 days, then 1 teaspoonful t.i.d. for 1 week. (Decrease the dose or discontinue as improvement warrants. Vary the dosage according to age of the child.)

3. Hospitalization with change of environment may be necessary for severe case.

Treatment of Adult Form: FIRST VISIT. Young adult with dry, scaly lichenified patches in cubital and popliteal fossae:

1. Stress avoidance of excess soap and water for bathing, avoidance of lanolin preparations locally, and contact with wool.

2. Menthol ¼%
Coal tar solution 5%
Quotane oint. q.s. 30.0
Sig: Apply b.i.d. locally or p.r.n.

3. Phenergan tab., 12.5 mg. #15
Sig: 1 tab. h.s.

SUBSEQUENT VISITS

1. To the above salve:

A. Increase concentration of the coal tar solution up to 10%.

B. Add hydrocortisone, 0.25% to 1%.

C. If the salve is too drying, change the base (Quotane oint.) to white petrolatum.

2. Nonspecific protein injections are of some value, such as: Piromen, beginning with 0.1 cc. of the 10 gamma per cc. dilution.

3. Unfiltered superficial x-ray therapy is often beneficial for chronic cases, given once a week for 4 to 6 treatments of 75 r each by a dermatologist or a radiologist.

4. Systemic ACTH or corticosteroid therapy may be indicated for severe and resistant cases.

NUMMULAR ECZEMA

This is a moderately common distinctive eczematous eruption characterized by coin-shaped (nummular), papulovesicular patches mainly on the arms and the legs of young adults and elderly patients. (Fig. 27.)

Primary Lesions. Coin-shaped patches of vesicles and papules usually on the extremities.

Secondary Lesions. Lichenification and bacterial infection.

Course. Very chronic, particularly in the older age group. Recurrences are common.

Subjective Complaints. Itching is usually quite severe.

Etiology. Nothing definite, but these factors are important:

1. History is usually positive for asthma, hay fever or atopic eczema, particularly in the young adult group.

2. Ingestion of iodides and bromides aggravates the disease.

3. Bacterial infection of the lesions is common.

4. In the older age group a history of a low-protein diet is common.

5. The low indoor humidity of wintertime causes dry skin which intensifies the itching, particularly in the elderly patients.

Differential Diagnosis

Atopic eczema (mainly in cubital and popliteal fossae, not coin-sized lesions, p. 51).

Psoriasis (not vesicular, see scalp and fingernail lesions, p. 83).

Contact dermatitis (will not see coin-sized lesions on both arms and legs, p. 42).

"Id" reaction, from stasis dermatitis of legs or a localized contact dermatitis (clinically impossible to differentiate this from nummular eczema but have history of previous primary dermatitis that suddenly became aggravated.

Treatment. First visit in the winter of an elderly male with 5 to 8 distinct, coin-shaped, excoriated, vesicular, crusted lesions on the arms and the legs.

1. Instruct the patient to avoid excess bathing with soap and water.

2. Tell the patient to avoid these foods, which are rich in iodides and bromides: salted nuts, cheeses (except cottage cheese), sea foods, iodized salt (can use plain salt), tomatoes, melons and spinach.

3. Increase the intake of protein-rich foods such as beef products, liver and gelatin.

4. Hydrocortisone powder 1%
White petrolatum, q.s. 30.0
Sig: Apply t.i.d. locally.

5. Benadryl, 50 mg. #15
Sig: 1 capsule h.s. for antipruritic and sedative effect.

Treatment of Resistant Cases

1. Add coal tar solution, 3% to 10%, to the above salve.

2. A short course of oral corticosteroid therapy is effective, but relapses are common.

3. Depo-Testosterone (Upjohn), 50 mg. per cc.
Sig: Give 1 cc. intramuscularly weekly for 3 to 4 weeks. Quite effective for resistant cases.

DRUG ERUPTIONS

It can be stated almost without exception that any drug systemically administered is capable of causing a skin eruption. *Any patient with a rather generalized skin eruption should be questioned concerning the use of oral or parenteral drugs.* To jog the memory of patients I often ask, "Do you take any medicine for any condition? What about medicated tooth paste, laxatives, vitamins, aspirin and tonics? Have you received any shots in the past month?" As stated in Chapter 4, this questioning also gives the doctor some general information regarding other ills of the patient which might influence the skin problem. An eruption due to allergy or primary irritation from *locally* applied drugs is a contact dermatitis.

Any of the larger dermatologic texts have extensive lists of common and uncommon drugs with their common and uncommon skin reactions. These books must be consulted for the rare reactions, but the following paragraphs will cover 95% of these idiosyncrasies.*

Drugs and Their Dermatoses

Drug eruptions are usually not characteristic for any certain drug or group of drugs. However, the following drugs most commonly cause the associated skin lesions. Systemic drug reactions will not be stressed in this chapter. (Fig. 28.)

Acetophenetidin (Phenacetin). In Empirin Compound, Phenaphen, A.S.A. Compound, A.P.C., Anacin, Nembudeine, Bromo Quinine, Coricidin, Super-Anahist and many other remedies. See urticaria and erythematous eruptions.

ACTH. See Cushing's syndrome, hyperpigmentation, acneiform eruptions, seborrheic dermatitislike eruptions and hirsutism.

Amphetamine (Benzedrine). Coldness of extremities and redness of neck and shoulders; it increases itching in neurodermatitis.

Antabuse. Redness of face and possible acne.

Antibiotics. Various agents have different reactions, but in general see monilial overgrowth in oral, genital and anal orifices resulting in pruritus ani, pruritus vulvae and generalized pruritus. Monilial skin lesions may spread out from these foci. Also commonly see urticaria, and erythema-multiformelike eruptions, particularly from penicillin.

Antihistamines. In Coricidin, Super-Anahist and many other preparations. See urticaria, eczematous dermatitis and pityriasis-rosealike rash.

* A very extensive list of drugs and their reactions is found in Sutton, R. L., Jr.: Diseases of the Skin, St. Louis, Mosby, 1956.

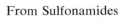

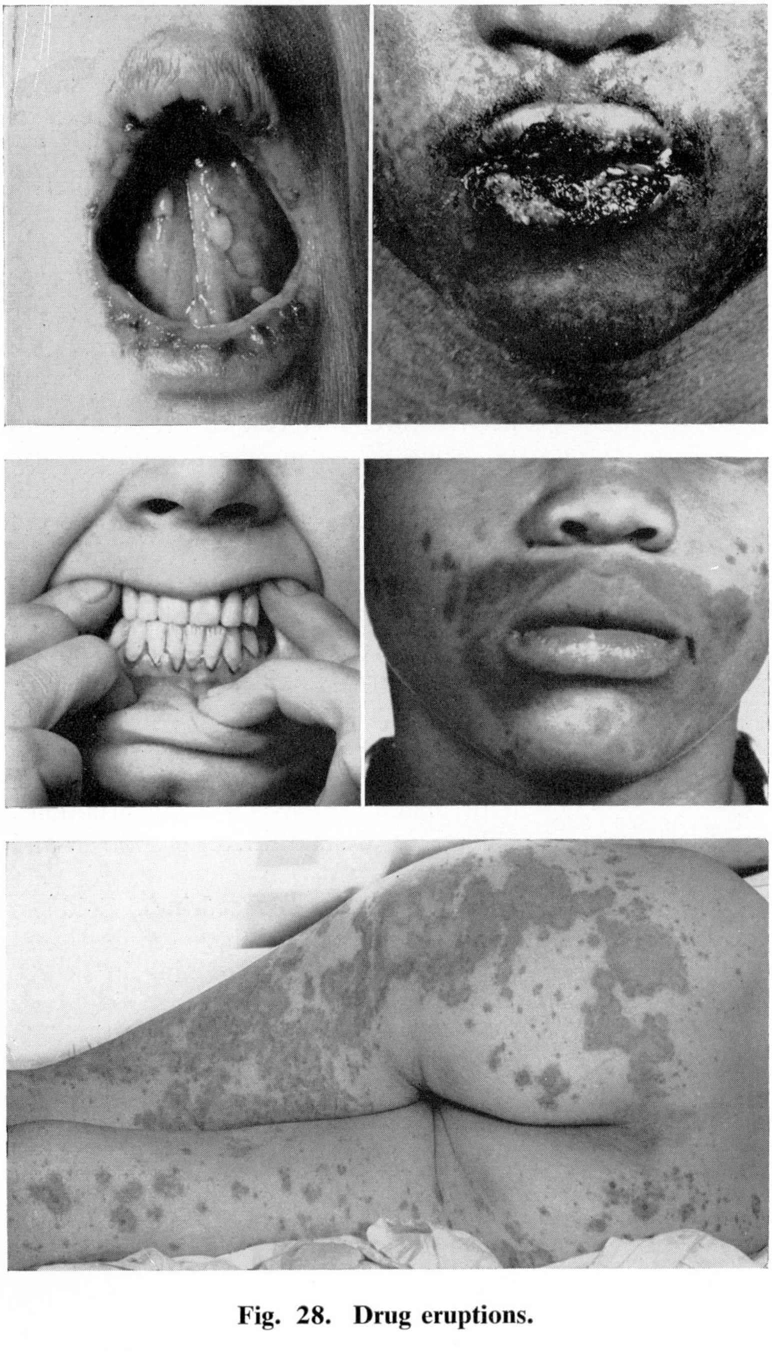

From Sulfonamides

(*Left*) Bismuth Line of Gums

(*Right*) Phenolphthalein Fixed Eruption

Penicillin Urticarial-like Eruption

Fig. 28. Drug eruptions.

Antitoxin. Get immediate reaction with skin manifestations of pruritus, urticaria and sweating; and delayed serum sickness reaction with urticaria, redness and purpura.

Apresoline. Causes systemic lupus erythematosuslike reaction.

Arsenic. Inorganic arsenic (Fowler's solution, Asiatic pills) causes erythematous, scarlatiniform, vesicular, or urtica-

From Iodide
(Same patient)

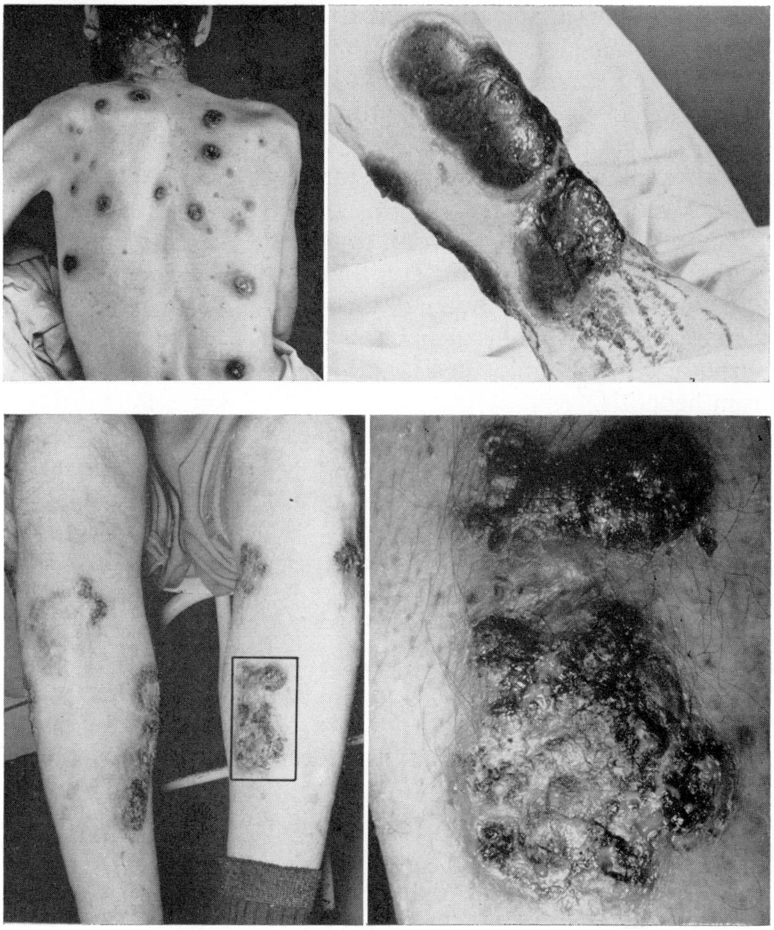

From Bromide

Fig. 29. Drug eruptions.

rial rashes. Delayed reactions include palmar and plantar keratoses and eventual carcinomatous changes. Organic arsenic (Mapharsen, Neo-arsphenamine, Tryparsamide) causes similar skin changes plus a severe form of exfoliative dermatitis. A mild erythema on the 9th day of therapy is not unusual. British Anti-lewisite (BAL) is effective therapy if given early for the skin reactions due to organic arsenicals.

Aspirin and Salicylates. Aspirin is found as an ingredient in a multitude of cold and antipain remedies. Pepto-Bismol contains salicylates. See urticaria, purpura and bullous lesions.

Atabrine. See universal yellow pigmentation, blue macules on face and mucosa, and lichen planuslike eruption.

Atropine. Scarlet feverlike rash.

Barbiturates. See urticarial, erythematous, bullous, or purpuric eruptions and fixed drug eruptions.

Bismuth. See bluish pigmentation of gums, and erythematous, papulosquamous and urticarial skin eruptions.

Boric Acid. Accidental oral ingestion can cause exfoliative dermatitis and severe systemic reaction.

Bromides. (See Iodides.) In Neurosine, Bromo Quinine, Bromo-Seltzer, Shut-eye and other drugs. Mainly see acnelike pustular lesions that can spread to form deep granulomatous pyodermas that heal with marked scarring. These must be differentiated from other granulomas (Fig. 29).

Butazolidin. Widespread erythematous, bullous eruptions.

Choral Hydrate. Urticarial, papular, erythematous and purpuric eruptions.

Chlorpromazine (Thorazine). See maculopapular rash, increased sun sensitivity, purpura with agranulocytosis, and icterus from hepatitis.

Chloroquine (Aralen). Erythematous or lichenoid eruptions with pruritus.

Codeine and Morphine. Erythematous, urticarial, or vesicular eruption.

Cortisone and Derivatives. Rarely see any cutaneous allergy.

Diasone. Red, maculopapular, vesicular eruption with agranulocytosis, occasionally like erythema nodosum.

Dicumarol. Hair loss and purpura.

Digitalis. Rarely, an erythematous, papular eruption is seen.

Digitoxin. Thrombocytopenic purpura.

Dilantin. Hypertrophy of gums, and erythema multiformelike eruption.

Estrogenic Substances and Stilbestrol. Edema of legs with cutaneous redness progressing to exfoliative dermatitis.

Gold. Eczematous dermatitis of hands, arms, legs, etc., or pityriasis rosealike eruption. Seborrheiclike eruption, urticaria, or purpura.

Insulin. See urticaria with serum sickness symptoms; also fat atrophy at injection site.

Iodides. (See Bromides.) Papular, pustular, ulcerative, or granulomatous lesions mainly on acne areas or legs (Fig. 29). Administration of chloride hastens recovery.

Isoniazid. Pruritus of legs and head with scaliness.

Liver Extract. See urticaria, diffuse redness and itching.

Meprobamate. Small purpuric lesions and erythema multiformelike eruption.

Mercury. Erythema, pruritus, scarlatiniform eruption; also stomatitis.

Mesantoin. See macular rash and severe bullous eruption.

Morphine. (See Codeine.)

Para-aminosalicylic Acid. Scarlatiniform or morbilliform rash and also fixed drug eruption.

Phenacetin. (See Acetophenetidin.)

Phenolphthalein. Found in 4 Way Cold Tablets, Exlax, Bromo Quinine, Phenolax, Petrogalar with Phenolphthalein, Agarol, Caroid and Bile Salts, Alophen, and pink icing on cakes. See fixed drug eruption which consists of hyperpigmented or purplish, flat or slightly elevated, discrete, single or multiple patches.

Quinidine. See edema, purpura, scarlitiniform eruption that may go on to exfoliative dermatitis.

Quinine. See any kind of diffuse eruption.

Salicylates. (See Aspirin.)

Silver. See diffuse bluish or grayish pigmentation of skin and gum margins due to a deposit of silver salts.

Stilbestrol. (See Estrogenic Substances.)

Sulfonamides. Urticaria, scarlatiniform eruption, erythema nodosum, eczematous flare of exudative dermatitis, erythema multiformelike bullous eruption or fixed eruption.

Tridione. Acneiform eruption of face.

Triethylene Melamine (TEM). Pruritic maculopapular eruption.

Thorazine. (See Chlorpromazine.)

Vitamins

Vitamin A. Due to long-term therapy with large doses, see scaly, rough, itchy skin with course, dry, scant hair growth and systemic changes.

Vitamin D. Rare skin lesions, but see headache, nausea, diarrhea, increased urination, sore gums and joints.

Vitamin B Group. See urticaria, pruritic redness and even anaphylactic reactions following I.M. or I.V. administration. Nicotinic acid quite regularly causes a red flush, pruritus and less often hives within 15 to 30 minutes after oral ingestion of 50 to 100 mg. The patient should be warned concerning this flush to eliminate unnecessary alarm.

Dermatoses and Their Drugs

As stated above, drug eruptions are usually not characteristic for any particular chemical, but experience has shown that certain *clinical pictures* commonly follow absorption of certain drugs. (For description of these eruptions see the disease mentioned.)

Measleslike Eruption. Barbiturates, arsenic, sulfonamides, quinine and many others.

Scarlet Feverlike Eruption or "Toxic Erythema." Arsenic, barbiturates, codeine, morphine, mercury, quinidine, salicylates, sulfonamides and others.

Pityriasis Rosealike Eruption. Bismuth, gold, barbiturates and antihistamines.

Eczematous Eruption. Quinine, procaine, antihistamines, gold, mercury, sulfonamides, penicillin and organic arsenic.

Urticaria. Penicillin, salicylates, serums, sulfonamides, barbiturates and opium group.

Fixed Drug Eruption. (See the drug "phenolphthalein," p. 58, for description.) Phenolphthalein, acetophenetidin, barbiturates, organic arsenic, gold, salicylates, sulfonamides and many others.

Erythema Multiformelike Eruption. Penicillin and other antibiotics, sulfonamides, phenolphthalein, barbiturates, Dilantin and meprobamate.

Erythema Nodosumlike Eruption. Sulfonamides, iodides, bromides, salicylates and Diasone.

Acnelike or Pustular Lesions. Bromides, iodides, Tridione and ACTH.

Vesicular or Bullous Eruptions. Sulfonamides, penicillin, Butazolidin and Mesantoin.

Purpuric Eruptions. Barbiturates, salicylates, meprobamate, organic arsenic, sulfonamides and Dicumarol.

Exfoliative Dermatitis. See in course of any severe generalized drug eruption particularly due to arsenic, penicillin, sulfonamides and barbiturates.

Lichen Planuslike Eruption. Atabrine, arsenic and gold.

Seborrheic Dermatitislike Eruption. Gold and ACTH.

Photosensitivity Reaction. Sulfonamides, chlorpromazine, quinidine, and Oxsoralen and Meloxine.

Pigmentary Changes. Silver salts and Atabrine.

Keratoses and Epitheliomas. Arsenic and mercury.

Course of Drug Eruptions. This depends on many factors, including the type of drug, severity of the cutaneous reaction, systemic involvement, general health of the individual, and efficacy of corrective therapy. Most cases with bullae, purpura, or exfoliative dermatitis have a serious prognosis and a protracted course.

Treatment

1. Eliminate the drug. This simple procedure is often delayed, with resulting serious consequences, because a careful history is not taken. *When confronted with any diffuse or puzzling eruption, routinely question the patient regarding ANY medication taken by ANY route.*

2. Further therapy depends on the seriousness of the eruption. Most barbiturate measleslike eruptions subside with no therapy. An itching drug eruption should be treated to relieve the itch (starch baths and a nonalcoholic calamine lotion or white shake lotion). Cases of exfoliative dermatitis or severe erythema multiformelike lesions require corticosteroid and other supportive therapy (see pp. 69 and 165).

Pruritic Dermatoses

CHAPTER 8

PRURITUS or itching brings more patients to the doctor's office than any other skin disease symptom. Itchy skin is not easily cured or even alleviated. Many hundreds of proprietary over-the-counter and prescription drugs are touted as effective anti-itch remedies, but not one is 100% effective. However, many are partially effective, but it is unfortunate that the most effective locally applied chemicals frequently irritate or sensitize the skin.

Pruritus is a symptom of many of the common skin diseases such as contact dermatitis, atopic eczema, seborrheic dermatitis, hives, some drug eruptions and many other dermatoses. Relief of itching is of prime importance in treating these diseases.

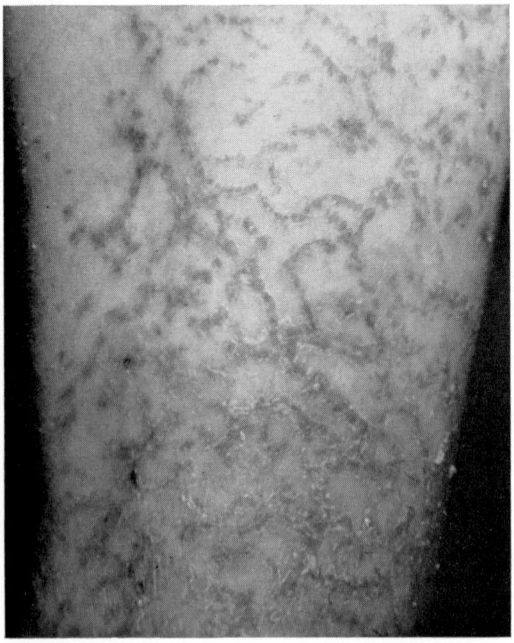

Fig. 30. Senile dry skin of the leg.

In addition to the pruritus occurring as a symptom of many skin diseases, there are other clinical forms of pruritus that deserve special consideration. These special types include *generalized pruritus* of the winter, senile and essential varieties, and *localized pruritus* of the neurodermatitis type, of the ears, the anal area and the genitalia.

GENERALIZED PRURITUS

Diffuse itching of the body without perceptible skin disease usually is due to wintertime dry skin, senile skin or to unknown causes.

Winter pruritus or **pruritus hiemalis** is a common form of generalized pruritus, although most patients complain of itching confined mainly to their legs. Every autumn of the year a certain number of elderly patients, and occasionally young ones, will walk into the doctor's office complaining bitterly of the rather sudden onset of itching of their legs. These patients have dry skin due to the low humidity in their furnace-heated homes. Clinically, the skin shows excoriations and dry curled scaling plaques resembling a sun-baked muddy beach at low tide. The dry skin associated with winter itch is to be differentiated from *ichthyosis,* a congenital dermatosis of varying severity

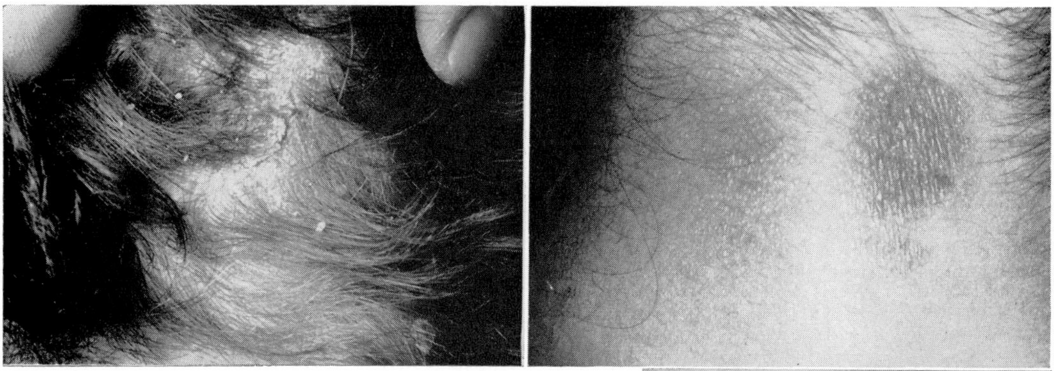

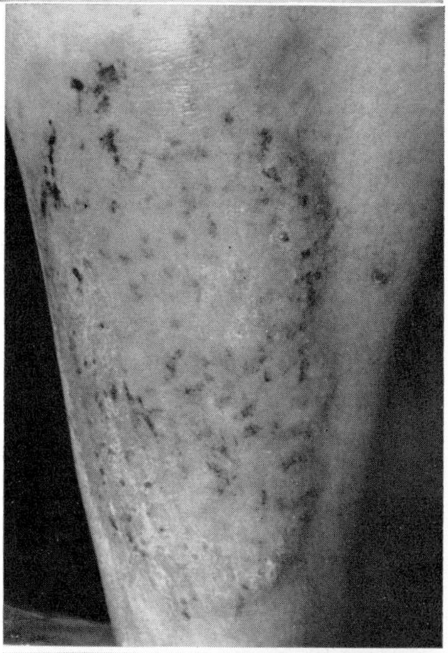

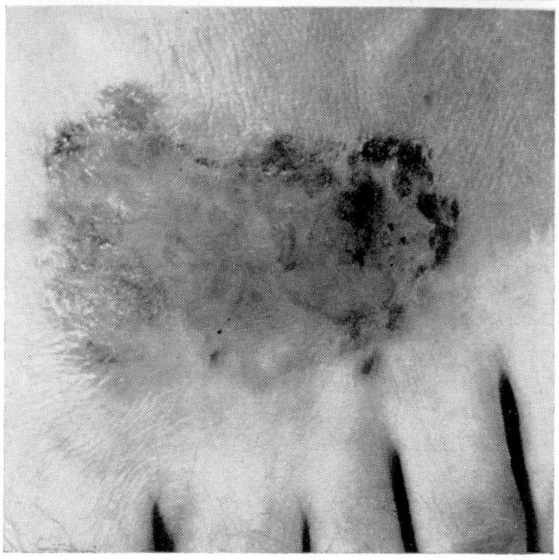

Fig. 31. Neurodermatitis.

(*Top, left*) In occipital area of scalp.
(*Top, right*) On posterior neck region. Note lichenification. (Dr. David Morgan.)
(*Center*) On anterior tibial area. Note excoriation. (K.C.G.H.)
(*Bottom*) On dorsum of foot with secondary infection.

which is also worse in the wintertime. Treatment of winter pruritus consists of (1) limiting general bathing to once a week; (2) use of a bland soap such as Ivory, Oilatum or Basis; (3) local application twice daily of white petrolatum, Nivea Skin Oil or Cream, or Lowilla Emollient; and (4) oral antihistamines which are sometimes effective such as Chlor-trimeton 4 mg. q.i.d., Temaril 2.5 mg. q.i.d., or Dimetane 4 mg. q.i.d.

Senile pruritus is a resistant form of generalized pruritus in the elderly patient (Fig. 30). It can occur at anytime of the year and may or may not be associated with dry skin. This form of itch occurs most commonly on the scalp, the shoulder, the sacral areas and the legs. Clinically, some patients have no cutaneous signs of the itch, but others may have linear excoriations. *Scabies* should be ruled out, as well as the diseases mentioned under the next form of pruritus to be considered, essential pruritus. Treatment is usually not very satisfactory. In addition to the agents mentioned previously in connection with winter pruritus, the injection of testosterone (Depo-Testosterone, 50 mg. intramuscularly) once a week for 2 to 4 weeks is often beneficial.

Essential pruritus is the rarest form of the generalized itching diseases. No age is exempt, but it occurs most frequently in the elderly patient. The itching is usually quite diffuse, with occasional "bites" in certain localized areas. All diffuse itching is worse at night, and no exception is made for this form of pruritus. Before a diagnosis of essential pruritus is made the following diseases must be ruled out by appropriate studies: *drug reaction, diabetes mellitus, uremia, lymphoblastoma* (granuloma fungoides, leukemia, or Hodgkin's disease), *liver disease,* or *intestinal parasites.* Treatment is the same as for senile and winter pruritus.

LOCALIZED PRURITIC DERMATOSES

Neurodermatitis
(Plate 7)

A few words must be said concerning the nomenclature of this disease. Other common terms for this condition include *lichen chronicus simplex* and *lichenified dermatitis.* There are pros and cons for all of the terms, but the term "neurodermatitis" has been selected because it is already being used rather universally, it stresses (perhaps too strongly) the emotional nervous habit of scratching, and it is simpler to use than the next best term, lichen chronicus simplex.

Neurodermatitis is a common skin condition characterized by the occurrence of single, or less frequently multiple, patches of chronic, itching, thickened, scaly, dry skin in one or more of several classic localizations (Fig. 31). It is unrelated to atopic eczema, which unfortunately has the synonym "disseminated neurodermatitis," a term that should be abandoned.

Primary Lesions. This disease begins as a small, localized, pruritic patch of dermatitis that might have been an insect bite, a chigger bite, contact dermatitis, or other minor irritation which may or may not be remembered by the patient. Because of various etiologic factors mentioned below, a cycle of itching, scratching, more itching and more scratching supervenes, and the chronic dermatosis develops.

Secondary Lesions. These include excoriations, lichenification and, in severe cases, marked verrucous thickening of the skin with pigmentary changes. In these severe cases healing is bound to be followed by some scarring.

Distribution. This condition is seen most commonly at the hairline of the nape of the neck, on the wrists, the ankles, the ears (see external otitis), anal area (see pruritus ani), etc.

Course. Quite chronic and recurrent. The majority of cases respond quickly to correct treatment, but some can last for years and defy all forms of therapy.

Subjective Complaints. Intense itching, usually worse at night, even during sleep.

Etiology. The initial cause (a bite, stasis dermatitis, contact dermatitis, seborrheic dermatitis, tinea cruris, psoriasis) may be very evanescent, but it is generally agreed that the chronicity of the lesion is due to the nervous habit of scratching. It is a rare patient who will not volunteer the information or admit it if questioned that the itching is worse when he or she is upset, nervous, or tired. Why some people with a minor skin injury respond with the development of a lichenified patch of skin and others do not is due to the personality make-up of that individual.

Age Group. It is very common to see neurodermatitis of the posterior neck in menopausal women. Other clinical types of neurodermatitis are seen at any age.

Family Incidence. Unrelated to allergies in patient or family, thus differing from atopic eczema.

Related to Employment. Recurrent exposure and contact to irritating agents at work can lead to neurodermatitis.

Differential Diagnosis

Psoriasis (several patches on the body in classic areas of distribution, family history of disease, see classic whitish scales, sharply circumscribed patch, p. 83).

Atopic eczema (allergic history in patient or family, multiple lesions, classically seen in cubital and popliteal areas and face, p. 51).

Contact dermatitis (acute onset, contact history positive, usually red, vesicular and oozing; may see acute contact dermatitis overlying neurodermatitis due to overzealous therapy, p. 42).

Lichen planus, hypertrophic form on anterior tibial area (also see lichen planus in mouth and on other body areas, biopsy usually characteristic, p. 92).

Seborrheic dermatitis of scalp (does not itch as much, is better in summer; a diffuse, scaly, greasy eruption, p. 73).

Treatment. A 45-year-old female patient with severely itching, scaly, red lichenified patch on back of the neck at the hairline.

1. Explain the condition to the patient and tell her that your medicine will be directed toward stopping the itching. If this can be done, and if she will cooperate by keeping her hands off the area, the disease will disappear. Emphasize this effect of scratching by stating that if both arms were broken, the eruption would be gone when the casts were removed. However, this is not a recommended form of therapy.

2. For severe bouts of intractable itching:

Ice cold boric acid packs

Sig: 1 tbsp. of boric acid crystals to 1 quart of ice cold water. Apply cloth wet with this solution for 15 minutes p.r.n.

3. A corticosteroid ointment 15.0

Sig: Apply q.i.d. or more often as itching requires.

TREATMENT ON RETURN VISIT

1. Add menthol 0.25% or coal tar solution 3% to 10% to above ointment for greater antipruritic effect.

2. Phenobarbital, 15 mg. #50

Sig: 1 tablet a.c. and 2 h.s.

TREATMENT OF RESISTANT CASES

1. Meprobamate, 400 mg. #30

Sig: 1 tablet q.i.d., a.c. and h.s.

2. Triamcinolone or methylprednisolone, 4 mg. #24

Sig: 1 tablet q.i.d. for 3 days, then 1 b.i.d. for 4 days.

3. X-ray therapy as given by a competent dermatologist or radiologist.

4. Dome Paste Boot. Apply in office for cases of neurodermatitis localized to arms and legs. This is a physical deterrent to scratching. Leave on for a week at a time.

5. Psychotherapy is of questionable value.

EXTERNAL OTITIS

External otitis is a descriptive term for a common and persistent dermatitis of the ears due to several causes. The agent most frequently blamed for this condition is "fungus," but pathogenic fungi are rarely found in the external ear. The true causes of external otitis, in order of frequency, are as follows: seborrheic dermatitis, neurodermatitis, contact dermatitis, atopic eczema, psoriasis, pseudomonas bacterial infection (which is usually secondary to other causes) and, lastly, fungus infection which also can be primary or secondary to other factors. For further information on the specific processes refer to each of the diseases mentioned.

Treatment. Primarily, this should be directed toward the specific cause, such as care of the scalp for seborrheic cases, or avoidance of jewelry for contact cases. However, when this is done, certain special technics and medicines must be used in addition to clear up this troublesome area.

An elderly woman comes in with an oozing, red, crusted, swollen left external ear with a wet canal but an intact drum. A considerable amount of seborrheic dermatitis of the scalp is confluent with the acutely inflamed ear area. The patient has had itching ear trouble off and on for 10 years, but in the past month it has become most severe.

1. Always inspect the canal and the drum with an otoscope. If excessive wax and debris are present in the canal, or if the drum is involved in the process, the patient should be treated for these problems or referred to an ear specialist. Salves should not be placed in the ear canal. An effective liquid to dry up the oozing canal is as follows:

   Hydrocortisone powder 0.5%
   Boric acid 2%
   Burow's Solution, 1:10 strength, q.s. 15.0
   Sig: 2 drops in ear t.i.d.

2. Boric acid solution wet packs

   Sig: 1 tablespoon of boric acid to 1 quart of cool water. Apply wet cloths to external ear for 15 minutes 3 times a day.

3. A corticosteroid-antibiotic ointment 5.0

   Sig: Apply locally to external ear t.i.d., not in canal.

SUBSEQUENT THERAPY. Several days later following decreased swelling, cessation of oozing and lessening of itching, institute the following changes in therapy:

1. Decrease the boric acid soaks to once a day.
2. Sulfur, ppt. 5%

   A cortiscosteroid-antibiotic oint. q.s. 15.0
   Sig: Apply locally t.i.d. to ear.

For persistent cases, a short course of oral corticosteroid or antibiotic therapy often removes the fire so that local remedies will be effective. X-ray therapy, correctly administered, is also useful for chronic cases.

PRURITUS ANI

Itching of the anal area is a common malady that can vary in severity from mild to marked. The patient with this very annoying symptom is apt to resort to self-treatment and therefore delay the visit to the physician. Usually, he has overtreated the sensitive area, and the immediate problem of the physician is to quiet down the acute contact dermatitis. The original cause of the pruritus ani is often difficult to ascertain.

Primary Lesions. These can range from slight redness confined to a very small area, to an extensive contact dermatitis with redness, vesicles and oozing of the entire buttock.

Secondary Lesions. Excoriations from the intense itching are very common and after a prolonged time they progress toward lichenification. A generalized papulovesicular id eruption can develop from an acute flare-up of this entity.

Course. The majority of cases of pruritus ani respond rapidly and completely to proper management, especially if the cause can be ascertained and eliminated. However, every physician will have his problem case that will continue to scratch and defy all therapy.

Etiology. The proper management of this socially unacceptable form of pruritus consists in searching for and eliminating the several factors that contribute to the persistence of this symptom-complex. These factors can be divided into general and specific etiologic factors.

1. GENERAL FACTORS

A. *Diet.* The following irritating

foods should be removed from the diet: chocolate, nuts, cheeses and spicy foods. Coffee, because of its stimulating effect on any form of itching, should be limited to 1 cup a day. Rarely, certain other foods will be noted by the patient to aggravate the pruritus.

B. *Bathing*. Many patients have the misconception that the itching is due to uncleanliness. Therefore, they resort to excessive bathing and scrubbing of the anal area. This is harmful and irritating and must be stopped.

C. *Toilet Care*. Harsh toilet papers contribute greatly to the continuance of this condition. Cotton or a proprietary cleansing cloth called "Tucks" must be used for wiping. Mineral oil can be added to the cotton if necessary. Rarely, an allergy to the pastel tint in colored toilet tissues is a factor causing the pruritus.

D. *Scratching*. As with all of the diseases of this group, chronic scratching is a vicious cycle. The main purpose of the physician is to give relief from this itching, but a gentle admonishment to the patient to keep his hands off is indicated. With the physician's help, the itch-and-scratch habit can be broken. The emotional and mental personality of the patient regulates the effectiveness of this suggestion.

2. SPECIFIC ETIOLOGIC FACTORS

A. *Oral Antibiotics*. Pruritus ani from this cause is being seen with increasing frequency. It may or may not be due to an overgrowth of monilial organisms. The physician who automatically questions his patients about recent drug ingestion will not miss this diagnosis.

B. *Neurodermatitis*. It is always a problem to know which comes first, the itching or the "nervousness." In most instances the itching comes first, but there is no denying that once pruritus ani has developed it is aggravated by emotional tensions and "nerves." However, it is a rare case that has a "deep-seated" psychotic problem.

C. *Psoriasis* in this area is common. Usually, other skin surfaces are also involved.

D. *Atopic eczema* of this site in adults is rather unusual. A history of atopy in the patient or family is helpful in establishing this etiology.

E. *Fungus Infection*. Contrary to old beliefs, this cause is quite rare. Clinically, a raised, sharp, papulovesicular border is seen that commonly is confluent with tinea of the crural area. If a scraping or a culture reveals fungi, then stronger local therapy than usual is indicated for cure.

F. *Worm Infestation*. In children pinworms can usually be implicated. A diagnosis is made by finding eggs on morning anal smears or by seeing the small white worms when the child is sleeping. Worms are a rare cause of adult pruritus ani.

G. *Hemorrhoids*. In the lay person's mind this is undoubtedly the commonest cause. Actually, it is an unimportant primary factor but may be a contributing factor. Hemorrhoidectomy alone is rarely successful as a cure for pruritus ani.

H. *Cancer*. This is a very rare cause of anal itching, but a rectal or proctoscopic examination may be indicated.

Treatment. FIRST VISIT. A patient states that he has had anal itching for 4 months. It followed a 5-day course of an antibiotic for the Asian flu. Many local remedies have been used; the latest, a supposed remedy for athlete's foot, aggravated the condition. Examination reveals an oozing, macerated, red area around the anus.

1. Initial therapy should include removal of the general factors listed under "Etiology" and giving instructions as to diet, bathing, toilet care and scratching.
2. Boric acid wet packs.

Sig: 1 tablespoon of boric acid crystals to 1 quart of cool water. Apply wet cloths to the area b.i.d. while lying in bed for 20 minutes, or more often if necessary for severe itching. Ice cubes may be added to the solution for more anti-itching effect.

3. Nonalcoholic white shake lotion

℞ 60.0

Sig: Apply to area b.i.d. (May burn slightly on first few applications.)

4. Benadryl, 50 mg. #15

Sig: 1 capsule h.s. (For itching and sedation.)

SECOND VISIT. After the acute contact dermatitis has subsided:

A corticosteroid ointment q.s. 15.0
Sig: Apply locally t.i.d.

SUBSEQUENT VISITS

1. As tolerated, add increasing strengths of sulfur, coal tar solution, or menthol 0.25%, or phenol 0.5% to the above ointment or to any of the following:

Quotane ointment 15.0

Vioform ointment, with or without hydrocortisone 15.0

Sterosan ointment, with or without hydrocortisone 15.0

2. A short course of oral corticosteroid therapy may be indicated for resistant cases.

3. X-ray therapy is sometimes beneficial. It should be administered by a competent dermatologist or radiologist in a dose of 75 to 100 r weekly, of unfiltered, superficial radiation for a total dose of only 400 to 600 r.

GENITAL PRURITUS

Itching of the female vulva or the male scrotum can be treated in much the same way as pruritus ani, if these special considerations are borne in mind.

Vulvar Pruritus. Etiologically, it is due to monilia or trichomonas infection; contact dermatitis from douche chemicals, contraceptive jellies and diaphragms; chronic cervicitis; neurodermatitis; menopausal or senile atrophic changes; or leukoplakia. Pruritus vulvae is frequently seen in patients with diabetes mellitus and during pregnancy. Treatment can be adapted from that for pruritus ani (p. 64) with the addition of a daily douche such as vinegar, 2 tablespoons to 1 quart of warm water.

Scrotal Pruritus. Etiologically, it is due to tinea infection; contact dermatitis from soaps, powders, clothing; or neurodermatitis. Treatment is similar to that given for pruritus ani (p. 64).

Vascular Dermatoses

CHAPTER 9

URTICARIA, erythema multiforme and its variants, and erythema nodosum are included under this heading because of their vascular reaction patterns. Stasis dermatitis is included because it is a dermatosis due to venous insufficiency in the legs.

URTICARIA

The commonly seen entity of urticaria or hives can be acute or chronic and due to known or unknown causes. The urticarial wheal results from liberation of histamine from damaged mast cells located around the smaller cutaneous blood vessels. There are many physical and chemical agents which can damage these mast cells and cause a sudden liberation of histamine.

Lesions can vary from pea-sized red papules to large circinate patterns with red borders and white centers that can cover an entire side of the trunk or the thigh. Vesicles and bullae are seen in severe cases along with hemorrhagic effusions. Edema of the glottis is a serious complication which can occur in the severe form of urticaria labeled *angioneurotic edema*.

Course. Acute cases may be mild or explosive but usually disappear with or without treatment in a few hours or days. The chronic form has remissions and exacerbations for months and years.

Etiology. Many cases of hives, particularly of the chronic type, after careful questioning and investigation are concluded to result from no apparent causative agent. Other cases, mainly the acute ones, have been found to result from the following factors or agents:

DRUGS. Penicillin is probably the commonest cause of acute hives, but any other drug, whether ingested, injected, inhaled or, rarely, applied on the skin, can cause the reaction. (See Drug Eruption, p. 55.)

FOODS are a common cause of acute hives. The main offenders are sea foods, strawberries, chocolate, nuts, cheeses, pork, eggs, wheat and milk. Chronic hives can be caused by traces of penicillin in milk products.

INSECT BITES AND STINGS. From mosquitoes, fleas, spiders and contact with certain moths, leeches and jellyfish.

PHYSICAL AGENTS. Due to heat, cold, radiant energy and physical injury. *Dermographism* is a term applied to a localized urticarial wheal produced by scratching the skin of certain individuals (Fig. 32).

INHALANTS. Nasal sprays, insect sprays, dust, feathers, pollens and animal danders comprise a partial list of offenders.

INFECTIONS. A focus of infection is always considered sooner or later in chronic cases of hives, and in unusual instances it is causative. The sinuses, the teeth, the tonsils, the gallbladder and the genitourinary tract should be checked.

INTERNAL DISEASE. Urticaria has been seen with liver disease, intestinal parasites, cancer and rheumatic fever.

"NERVES." After all other causes of

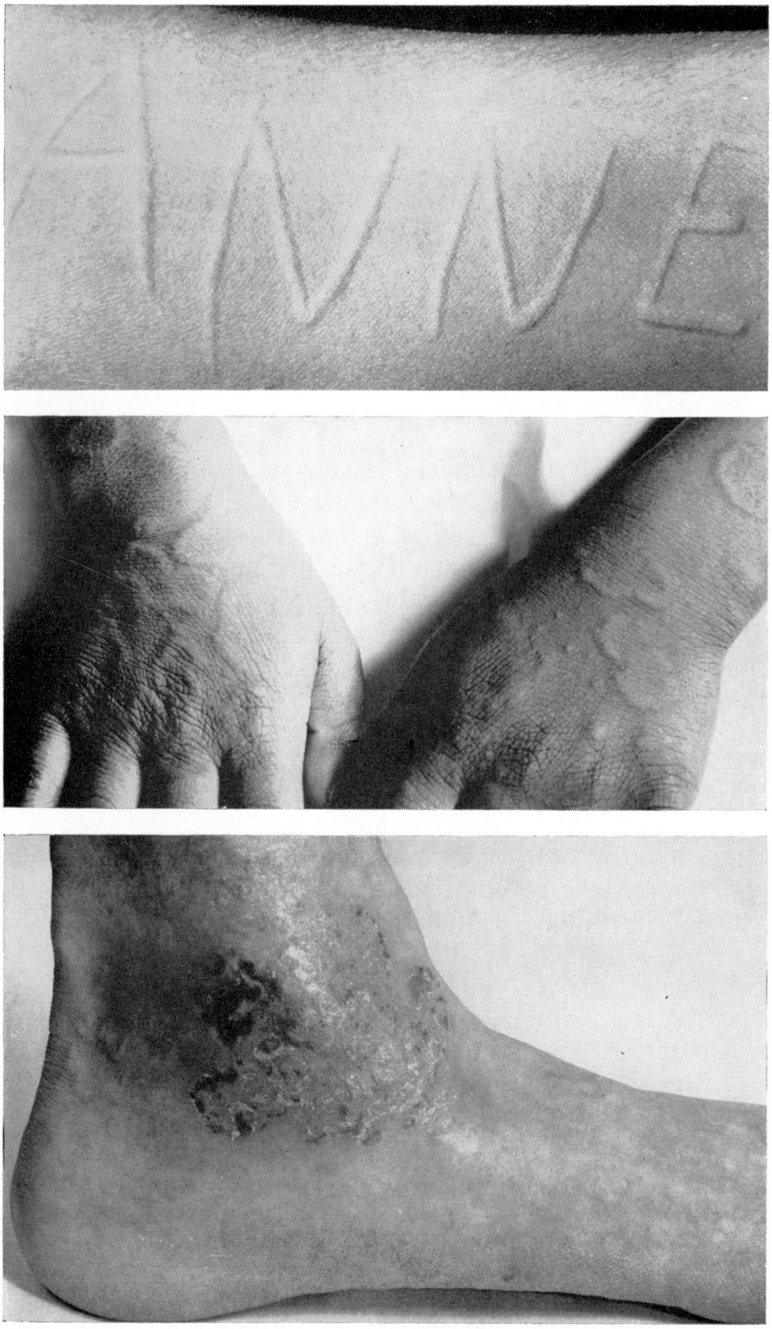

Dermographism (arm).

Erythema multiforme in Negro boy.

Stasis dermatitis and ulcer of ankle.

Fig. 32. Vascular dermatoses.

chronic urticaria have been ruled out there remain a substantial number of cases that appear to be related to nervous stress, worry, or fatigue. These cases benefit most from the establishment of good rapport between the patient and the doctor.

Differential Diagnosis. *Hebra's ery-*

thema multiforme (see systemic fever, malaise, and mouth lesions in children and young adults, p. 69).

Treatment

1. A case of *acute* hives due to penicillin injection one week previously for a "cold."

A. Linit starch bath

Sig: ½ box of Linit starch (small sized) to 6 to 8 inches of lukewarm water in the tub. Bathe for 15 minutes once or twice a day.

B. Camphor 1%

Alcoholic white shake lotion, q.s. 120.0

Sig: Apply b.i.d. locally for itching.

C. Chlor-trimeton, 4 mg. #30

Sig: 1 tablet t.i.d., a.c.

D. Benadryl, 50 mg. #15

Sig: 1 capsule h.s.

2. *For a more severe case of acute hives:*

A. Benadryl injection. Give 2 cc. (20 mg.) subcutaneously, or

B. Epinephrine hydrochloride. Give 0.3 to 0.5 cc. of 1:1,000 solution subcutaneously, or

C. Acthargel. Give 40 U. or 80 U. intramuscularly, or

D. Hydrocortisone tablets, 20 mg. (or newer related corticosteroid) #20

Sig: 1 tablet q.i.d. for 3 days then 1 tablet t.i.d.

E. Penicillinase (Neutrapen). Give 800,000 U. intramuscularly if hives are known to be due to penicillin. This therapy occasionally causes severe constitutional reactions.

3. Treatment for patient with *chronic* hives of 6 months duration. Cause undetermined after careful history and examination.

A. Phenergan, 12.5 mg. #20

Sig: 1 tablet h.s.

B. Diet. Suggest avoidance of chocolate, nuts, cheese and other milk products, sea foods, strawberries, pork, excess spicy foods, and excess of coffee or tea.

C. Staphylococcus Toxoid (Merck Sharp & Dohme), Dilution No. 1. Give 0.1 cc. subcutaneously and increase by 0.1 cc. twice or once a week up to 1.0 cc. (This is a mild form of nonspecific protein therapy that apparently is curative in some cases. Other agents that could be used are: Piromen, autohemotherapy, and crude liver injections.)

D. A mild sedative or tranquilizer such as meprobamate 200 mg. t.i.d. or phenobarbital 15 mg. t.i.d.

ERYTHEMA MULTIFORME

This term introduces a flurry of confusion in the mind of any student of medicine. It will be the purpose of this section to attempt to dispel that confusion. Erythema multiforme as originally described by Hebra is an uncommon distinct disease of unknown cause characterized by red iris-shaped or bulls-eyelike macules, papules, or bullae confined mainly to the extremities, the face and the lips, accompanied by mild fever, malaise and arthralgia, occurring usually in children and young adults in the spring and the fall, with a duration of 2 to 4 weeks, and frequently recurrent for several years (Fig. 32).

The only relationship between Hebra's erythema multiforme and the following diseases or syndromes is the clinical appearance of the eruption.

Stevens-Johnson syndrome is a very severe and oftentimes fatal variant of erythema multiforme. It is characterized by high fever, extensive purpura, bullae, and ulcers of the mucous membranes and, after 2 to 3 days, ulcers of the skin. Eye involvement can result in blindness.

Erythema Multiforme Bullosum. This is a severe, chronic, bullous disease of adults. (See p. 164.)

Erythema Multiformelike Drug Erup-

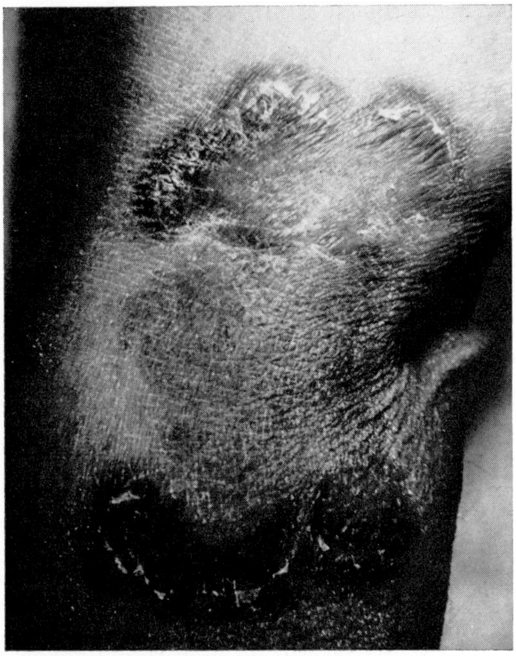

Fig. 33. Erythema perstans.
Chronic lesions on elbow.
(Patient of Drs. L. Grayson and H. Shair.)

tion. Frequently due to phenacetin, quinine, penicillin, mercury, arsenic, Butazolidin, barbiturates, Tridione, Dilantin, sulfonamides and antitoxins. (See p. 55.)

Erythema Multiformelike Eruption. This eruption is seen with rheumatic fever, pneumonia, meningitis, measles, pregnancy, cancer, following deep x-ray therapy, and as an allergic reaction to foods.

Erythema perstans group of diseases (Fig. 33). There are over a dozen clinical entities in this group with impossible-to-remember names. (See Dictionary-Index under "Erythema perstans.") All have varying sized erythematous patches, papules or plaques with a definite red border and a less active center forming circles, half circles, groups of circles, and linear bands. Multiple causes have been ascribed, including tickbites, allergic reactions, fungus, bacterial, virus and spirochetal infections, and internal cancer. The duration of and the response to therapy varies with each individual case.

Reiter's Syndrome. This is a triad of conjunctivitis, urethritis and, most important, arthritis, predominantly in males, which lasts approximately 6 months.

Behçet's syndrome consists of a triad of genital, oral and ophthalmic ulcerations seen most commonly in males; it can last for years with recurrences.

Differential Diagnosis of Hebra's Erythema Multiforme. *Urticaria* (clinically, it may resemble erythema multiforme, but hives are associated with only mild systemic symptoms; it can occur in any age group; iris lesions are unusual; usually it can be attributed to penicillin or other drug therapy; responds rapidly but often not completely to antihistamine therapy, p. 67).

Treatment. Child, aged 12, has bullseyelike lesions on hands, arms and feet, erosions of the lips and mucous membranes of the mouth, malaise and temperature of 101° orally. He had a similar eruption last spring.

1. Order bed rest and increased oral fluid intake.
2. Aspirin, 300 mg. #30
   Sig: 2 tablets q.i.d.
3. Tetracycline capsules, 250 mg. #20
   Sig: 1 capsule q.i.d.

For severe cases, such as the Stevens-Johnson form, intensive corticosteroid therapy with intravenous infusions, gamma globulin and other supportive measures will be indicated.

ERYTHEMA NODOSUM

Erythema nodosum is an uncommon reaction pattern seen mainly on the anterior tibial areas of the legs which appears as erythematous nodules in successive crops preceded by fever, malaise and arthralgia.

Primary Lesions. See bilateral red, tender, rather well-circumscribed nodules, mainly on the pretibial surface of the legs but also on the arms and the body. Later, the flat lesions may become raised, confluent and purpuric. Only a few lesions develop at one time.

Secondary Lesions. They never suppurate or form ulcers.

Course. The lesions last several weeks, but the duration can be affected by therapy directed to the cause if it is known. Relapses are related to the cause.

Etiology. Careful clinical and laboratory examination is necessary to determine the cause of this toxic reaction pattern. The following tests should be performed: complete blood count, sedimentation rate, urinalysis, serologic test for syphilis, chest roentgenogram, and specific skin tests as indicated. The causes of erythema nodosum are streptococcal infection (rheumatic fever, pharyngitis, scarlet fever, arthritis), fungus infection (coccidioidomycosis, *Trichophyton* infection), lymphogranuloma venereum, syphilis, chancroid, drugs (sulfonamides, iodides, bromides) and rarely tuberculosis.

Age and Sex Incidence. Predominantly in adolescent and young females.

Laboratory Findings. Histopathologic examination will reveal a nonspecific but characteristically localized inflammatory infiltrate in the subcutaneous tissue and in and around the veins.

Differential Diagnosis

Erythema induratum (this is a chronic tuberculid of young women that occurs on the posterior calf area and often suppurates; biopsy shows a tuberculoid infiltrate, usually with caseation).

Periarteritis nodosa (a rare, fatal arteritis, most often in males; 25% of cases show painful subcutaneous nodules and purpura mainly of the lower extremities).

Nodular vasculitis (chronic painful nodules of the calves of middle-aged women which rarely ulcerate, recur commonly, biopsy is of value, may be a variant of erythema nodosum).

Superficial thrombophlebitis migrans of Buerger's disease (an early venous change of Buerger's disease commonly seen in males, with painful nodules of the anterior tibial area, biopsy is of value).

Nodular panniculitis or *Weber-Christian disease* (mainly in obese middle-aged women; see tender, indurated, subcutaneous nodules, and plaques, usually on the thighs and the buttocks, each crop preceded by fever and malaise, leaves residual atrophy and hyperpigmentation).

Treatment

1. Treat the cause if possible.
2. Rest, local heat and aspirin are valuable. The eruption is self-limited if the cause can be eliminated.

STASIS DERMATITIS

This is a common condition due to impaired venous circulation in the legs of older patients. Almost all cases are associated with varicose veins, and since the tendency to develop varicosities is a familial characteristic, stasis dermatitis is also familial (Fig. 32).

Primary Lesions. Early cases of stasis dermatitis begin as a red, scaly, pruritic patch that rapidly becomes vesicular and crusted, due to scratching and subsequent secondary infection. The bacterial infection is responsible for the spread of the patch and the chronicity of the eruption. Edema of the affected ankle area results in a further decrease in circulation and, consequently, more infection. The lesions may be unilateral or bilateral.

Secondary Lesions. Three secondary conditions can arise from untreated stasis dermatitis:

1. *Hyperpigmentation* is quite inevitable following the healing of simple or severe stasis dermatitis of the legs. This increase in pigmentation is slow to dis-

appear and in many elderly patients it never does.

2. *Stasis ulcers* (p. 104) can occur as the result of edema, deeper bacterial infection, or improper care of the primary dermatitis.

3. *Infectious eczematoid dermatitis* (p. 105) may develop on the legs, the arms and even the entire body, either slowly or as an explosive rapidly spreading eruption.

Course. The rapidity of healing depends on the age of the patient and other factors listed under "etiology." In elderly patients who have untreated varicose veins, stasis dermatitis can persist for years with remissions and exacerbations. If a patient in the 40-to-50 age group develops stasis dermatitis the prognosis is particularly bad for future recurrences and possible ulcers unless the varicosities are removed.

Etiology. Poor venous circulation due to the sluggish blood flow in tortuous dilated varicose veins is the primary cause. If the factors of obesity, lack of proper rest or care of the legs, pruritus, secondary infection, low protein diet and old age are added to the circulation problem, the result can be a chronic, disabling disease.

Differential Diagnosis

Contact dermatitis (history important, especially regarding nylon hose, new socks, contact with ragweed, high-top shoes, etc., see no venous insufficiency, p. 42).

Neurodermatitis (thickened, dry, very pruritic patch, see no venous insufficiency, p. 62).

Treatment. Laborer, age 55, has scaly, reddish, slightly edematous, excoriated dermatitis on medial aspect of left ankle and leg of 6-weeks duration.

1. Prescribe rest and elevation of the leg as much as possible by lying in bed. The foot of the bed should be elevated 4 inches by placing 2 bricks under the legs. Sitting in a chair with the leg propped on a stool is of very little value.

2. Boric acid wet packs

Sig: 1 tablespoon of boric acid crystals to 1 quart of warm water. Apply cloths wet with this solution for 30 minutes twice a day.

3. An antibiotic-corticosteroid ointment q.s. 15.0

Sig: Apply to leg t.i.d.

4. Surgical removal of varicose veins. This should be strongly recommended, particularly in younger patients, to prevent recurrences and eventual irreversible changes, including ulcers.

For the more *severe case* of stasis dermatitis with oozing, cellulitis, and 3 plus pitting edema, the following treatment should be ordered in addition:

1. Hospitalization or enforced bed rest at home for the purpose of (A) applying the boric acid wet packs for longer periods of time, and (B) strict rest and elevation of the leg.

2. A course of an oral antibiotic

3. Ace Elastic Bandage, 3 inches wide, No. 8

After the patient is dismissed from the hospital and will be on his feet, give instructions for the correct application of this bandage to the leg before arising in the morning. This helps to reduce the edema that could cause a relapse of the dermatitis.

Seborrheic Dermatitis, Acne and Rosacea

CHAPTER **10**

SEBORRHEIC DERMATITIS
(Plates 8 and 9)

SEBORRHEIC DERMATITIS or dandruff is exceedingly common on the scalp but less common on the other areas of predilection: ears, face, sternal area, axillae and pubic area. It is well to consider seborrheic dermatitis as a "condition" of the skin and not as a "disease." It occurs as part of the "acne-seborrhea complex," most commonly seen in the brown-eyed brunette who has a family history of these conditions. Dandruff is spoken of as oily or dry, but it is all basically oily. If dandruff scales are pressed between two pieces of tissue paper, an oily residue is expressed, leaving its mark on the tissue.

Certain misconceptions that have arisen concerning this common dermatosis need to be corrected. Seborrheic dermatitis cannot be cured, but remissions for varying amounts of time do occur naturally or as the result of treatment. Seborrheic dermatitis does not cause permanent hair loss or baldness unless it becomes grossly infected. Seborrheic dermatitis is not infectious or contagious. The cause, contrary to magazine ads, is unknown.

Primary Lesions. Redness and scaling appear in varying degrees. The scale may be of the so-called "dry" type or of the "greasy" type (Fig. 34).

Secondary Lesions. Rarely seen are excoriations from severe itching and secondary bacterial infection. Neurodermatitis with lichenification can follow a chronic itching and scratching habit.

Course. Exacerbations and remissions are common, depending on the season, treatment, age and general health of the individual. Since this is a condition of the skin and not a disease, a true "cure" is impossible.

Seasonal Incidence. This condition is worse in colder weather, presumably due to lower indoor humidity and lack of summer sunlight.

Differential Diagnosis

SCALP LESIONS:

Psoriasis: sharply defined, whitish, dry, scaly patches, typical psoriasis lesions on elbows, knees, nails or elsewhere (p. 83)

Neurodermatitis: usually a single patch on the posterior scalp area or around the ears, intense itching, excoriation, and thickening of the skin (p. 62)

Tinea Capitis: usually in a child, see broken-off hairs with or without pustular reaction. Fluoresces under Wood's light. Culture is positive (p. 144)

Atopic Eczema: usually infants or chil-

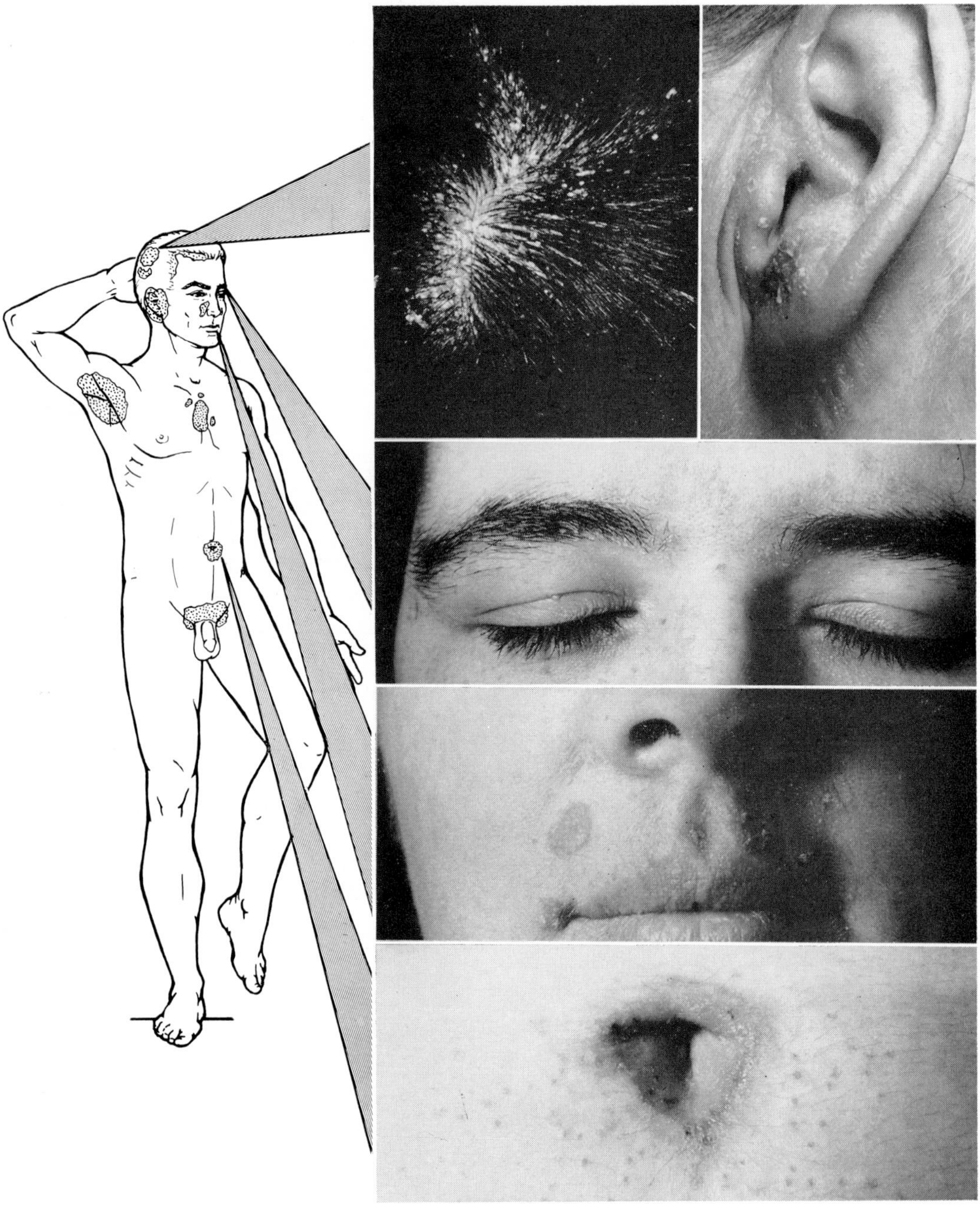

Fig. 34. Seborrheic dermatitis.

dren, diffuse dry scaliness; eczema also on face, arms and legs (p. 51)

FACE LESIONS:

Acute Disseminated Lupus Erythematosus: faint reddish, slightly scaly "butterfly" eruption, aggravated by sunlight, with fever, malaise, positive L. E. cell test (p. 174)

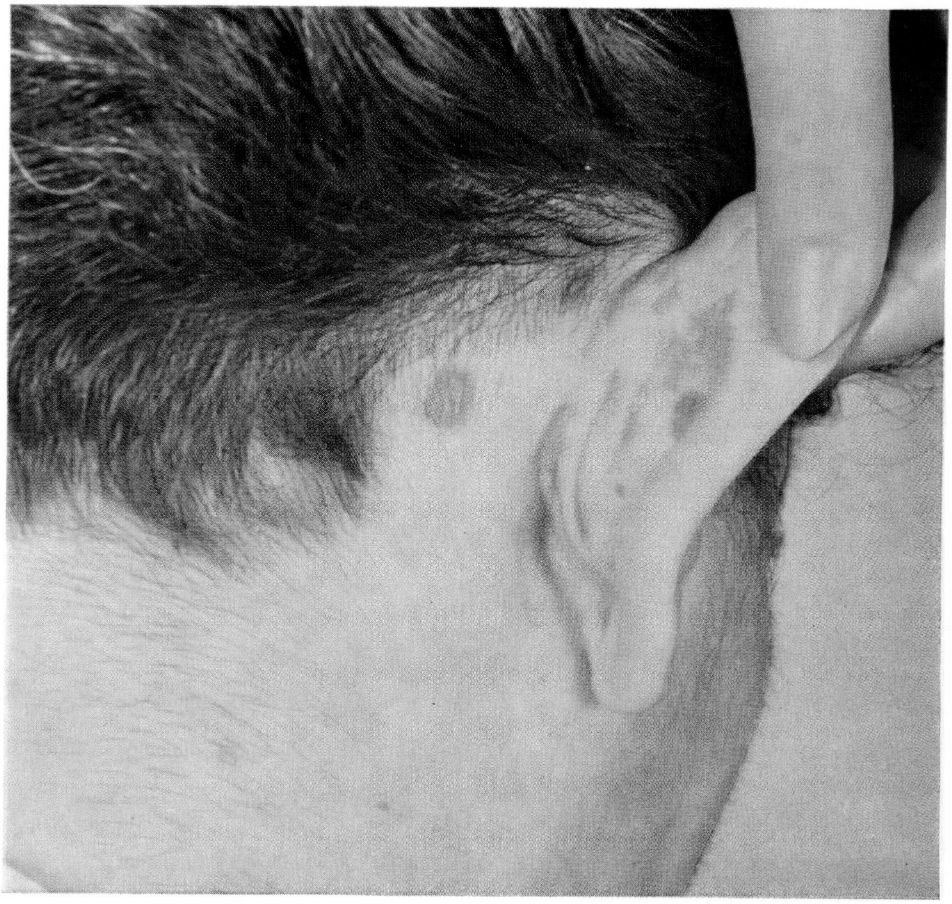

Plate 8. Seborrheic dermatitis behind the ear and at the border of the scalp.
(*Smith, Kline & French Laboratories*)

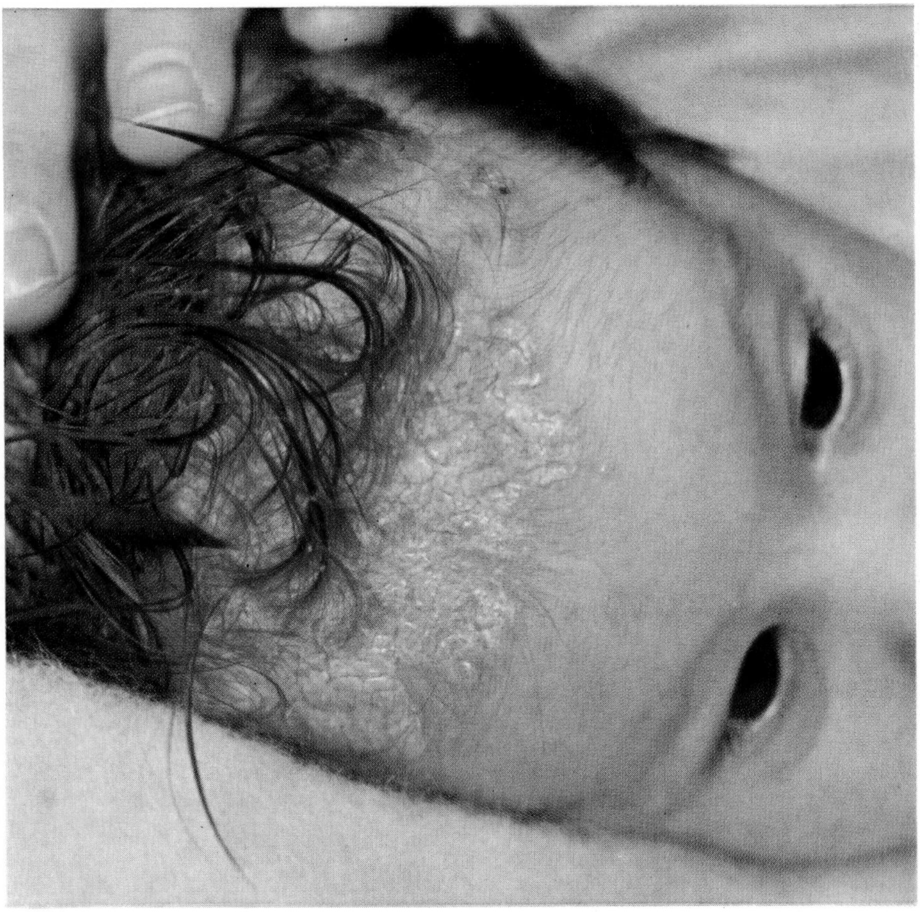

Plate 9. Seborrheic dermatitis of infancy.

This is one of the causes of "cradle cap."
(Smith, Kline & French Laboratories)

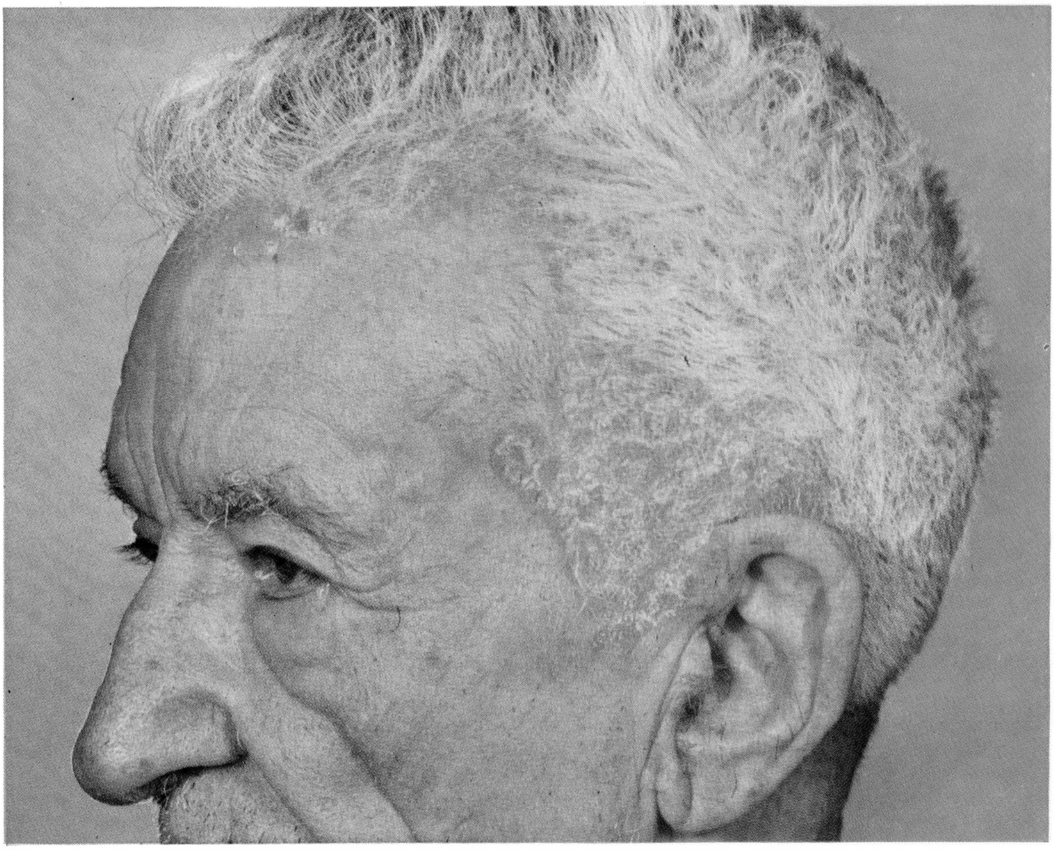

Plate 10. Psoriasis of the border of the scalp.

Psoriasis in this location is often difficult to distinguish from seborrheic dermatitis.

(Smith, Kline & French Laboratories)

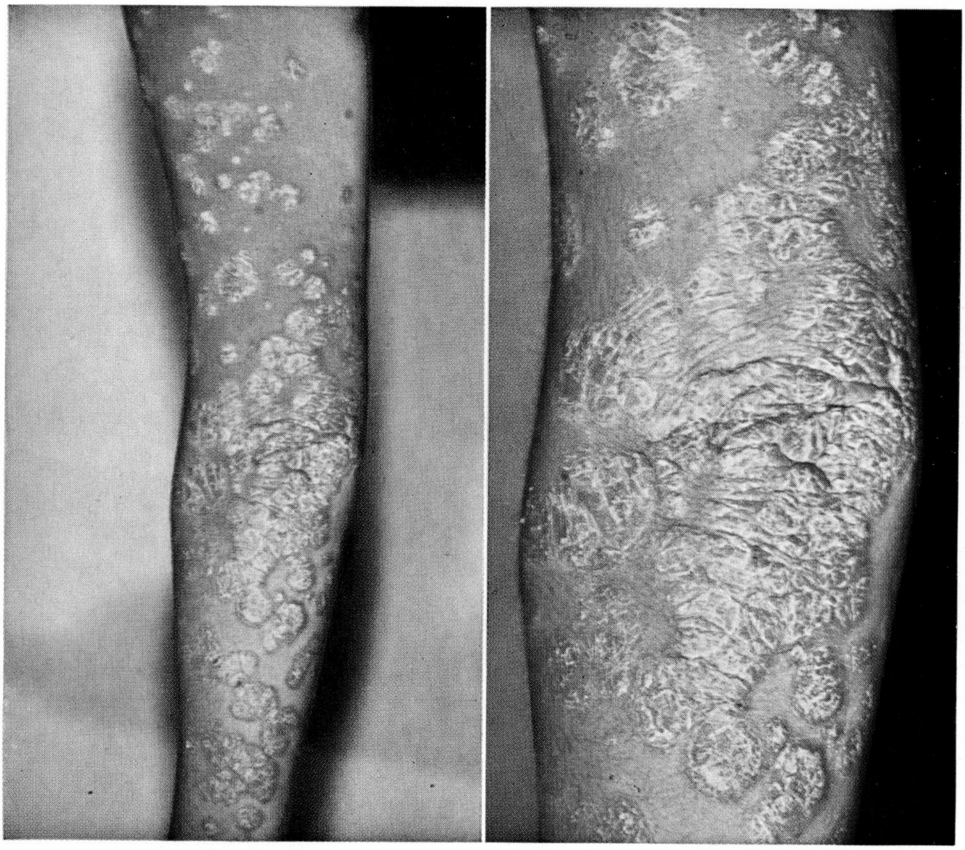

Plate 11. Psoriasis of a 17-year-old girl.

Moderately extensive psoriasis in classic distribution on elbows, back and knees. (K.U.M.C.)
(Roche Laboratories)

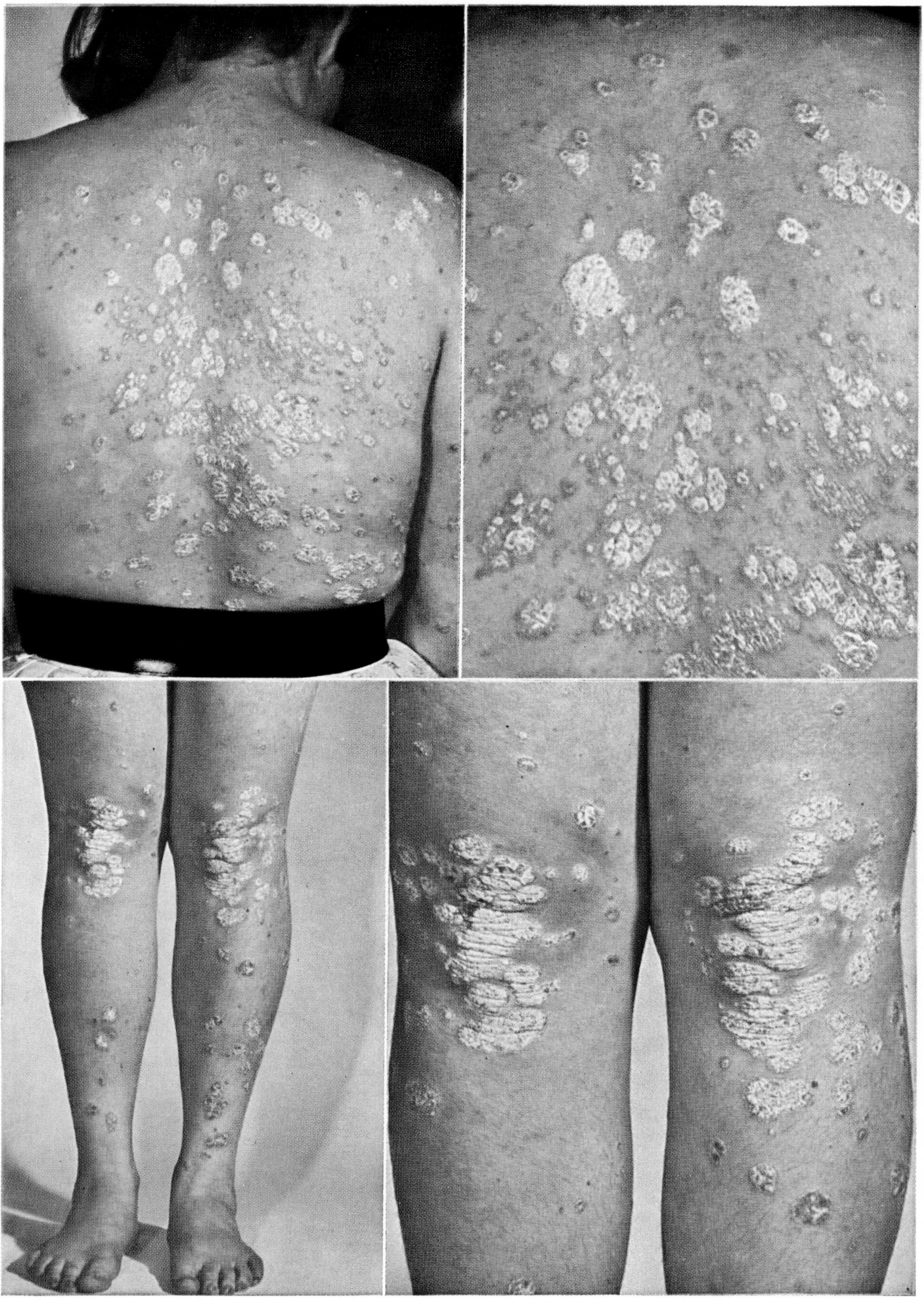

Plate 11 (*Continued*)

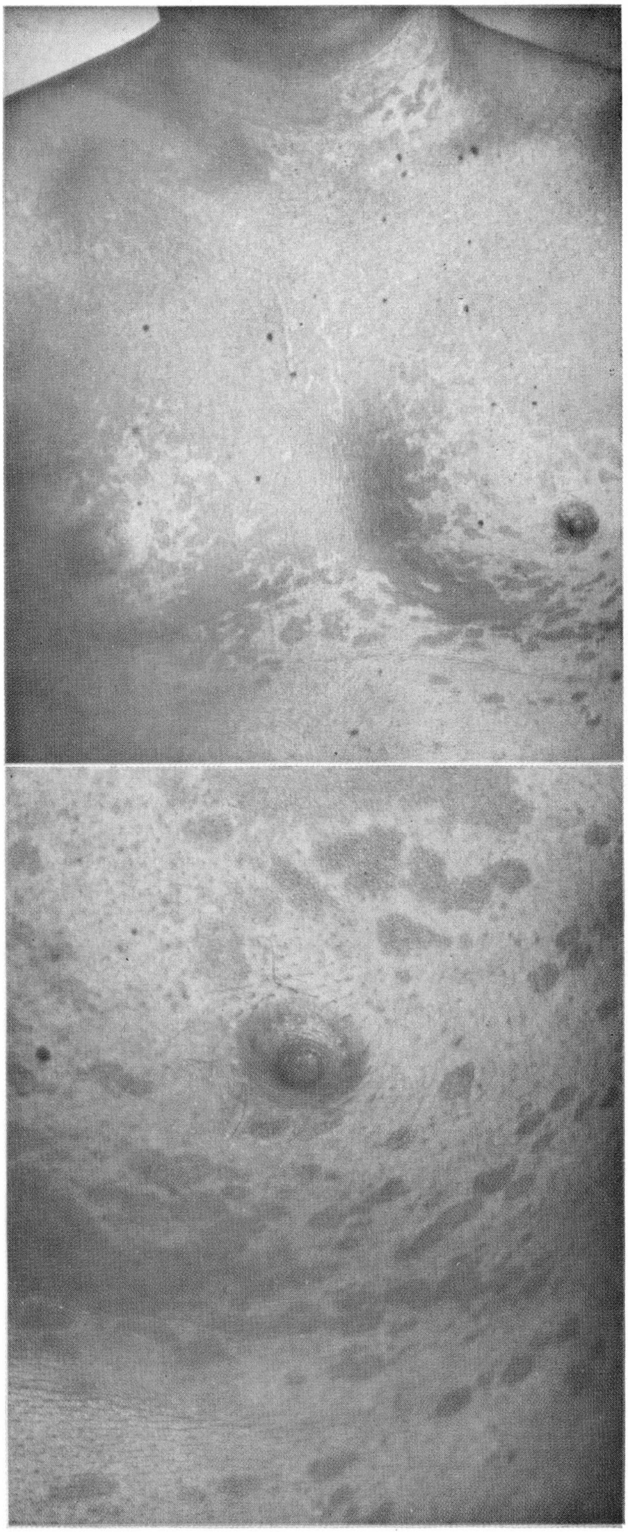

Plate 12. Tinea versicolor on the chest.

The dark areas of the skin are infected with the fungus. (K.U.M.C.)
(*Sandoz Pharmaceuticals*)

Plate 13. Lichen planus on the wrist and the dorsum of the hand in a Negro.

Note the violaceous color of the papules and the linear Koebner phenomenon on the dorsum of the hand.
(*E. R. Squibb & Sons*)

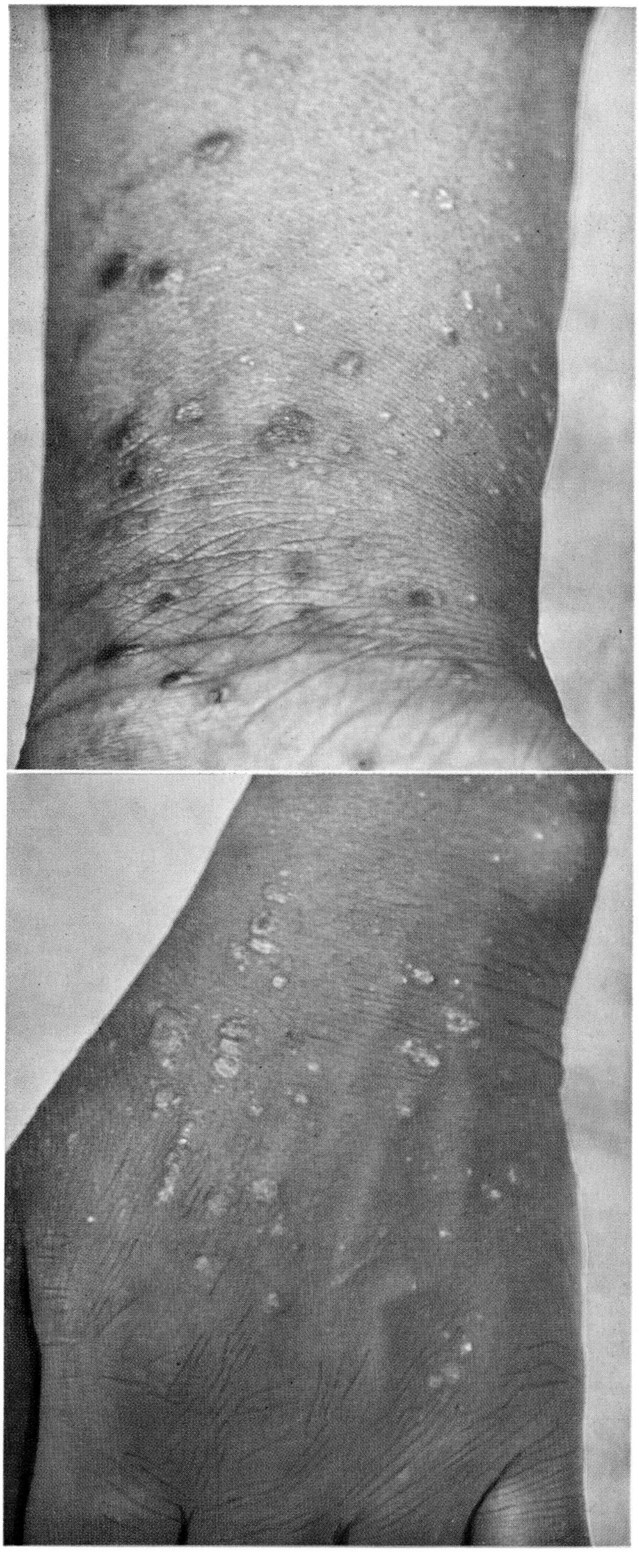

Chronic Discoid Lupus Erythematosus: sharply defined, red, scaly, atrophic areas with large follicular openings, resistant to local therapy (p. 172)

BODY LESIONS:

Tinea Corporis (p. 143)

Psoriasis (p. 83)

Pityriasis Rosea (p. 87)

Tinea Versicolor (p. 90)

Treatment. Young man with recurrent, red, scaly lesions at border of scalp and forehead, and diffuse, mild, whitish scaling throughout scalp.

1. Selsun Suspension 120.0
   Sig: Shampoo hair with 3 applications, leaving last application on for 5 minutes before rinsing off with hot water. Repeat shampoo twice a week for 2 weeks, then weekly. Use no other soap. Refill prescription p.r.n.

The only major complaint about Selsun Suspension is that it often results in increased oiliness of the hair. It is nontoxic unless taken internally, and even then it would be regurgitated because of the soap base. Reports of hair loss following its use have not been substantiated. For the occasional patient not benefited by Selsun Suspension, a newer shampoo can be prescribed which is more acceptable cosmetically but slightly less effective for dandruff —Capsebon Suspension. The directions for use are the same.

2. Pragmatar Ointment 15.0
   Sig: Apply to scalp lesions nightly for 1 to 2 weeks and to any recurrences not controlled by Selsun Suspension.

Pragmatar is also excellent for seborrheic dermatitis occurring on other locations of the body.

3. Vitamin B_{12}. For resistant cases give 500 mcg. subcutaneously once a week.

ACNE

Acne vulgaris is a very common skin condition of adolescents and young adults. It is characterized by any combination of comedones (blackheads), pustules, cysts and scarring of varying severity (Figs. 35 and 36).

Primary Lesions. Comedones, papules, pustules and, in severe cases, cysts.

Secondary Lesions. Pits and scars in severe cases. Excoriations of the papules are seen in some adolescents but most often they appear as part of the acne of women in their twenties and thirties.

Distribution. Face, neck and less commonly on the back, the chest and the arms.

Course. Begins at ages of 9 to 12 or later and lasts with new outbreaks for months or years. Subsides in the majority of cases by the age of 18 to 19, but occasional flare-ups may occur for years. The residual scarring varies with severity of the case and the response to treatment.

Subjective Complaint. Tenderness of the large pustules, itching rarely. Emotional upset is common as a result of the unattractive appearance.

Etiology. These factors are important: heredity, hormonal balance, diet, cleanliness and general health.

Season. Most cases are better during the summer.

Contagiousness. None.

Differential Diagnosis

Drug eruption: history of ingestion of iodides, bromides, Tridione, or testosterone and ACTH by injection (p. 55)

Contact dermatitis from industrial oils (p. 47)

Adenoma sebaceum: rare, see papular lesions, associated with epilepsy and mental deficiency

Treatment

FIRST VISIT of 14-year-old patient with moderate amount of facial blackheads and pustules:

1. Acne diet and instructions regarding skin care (see sheet that can be given to

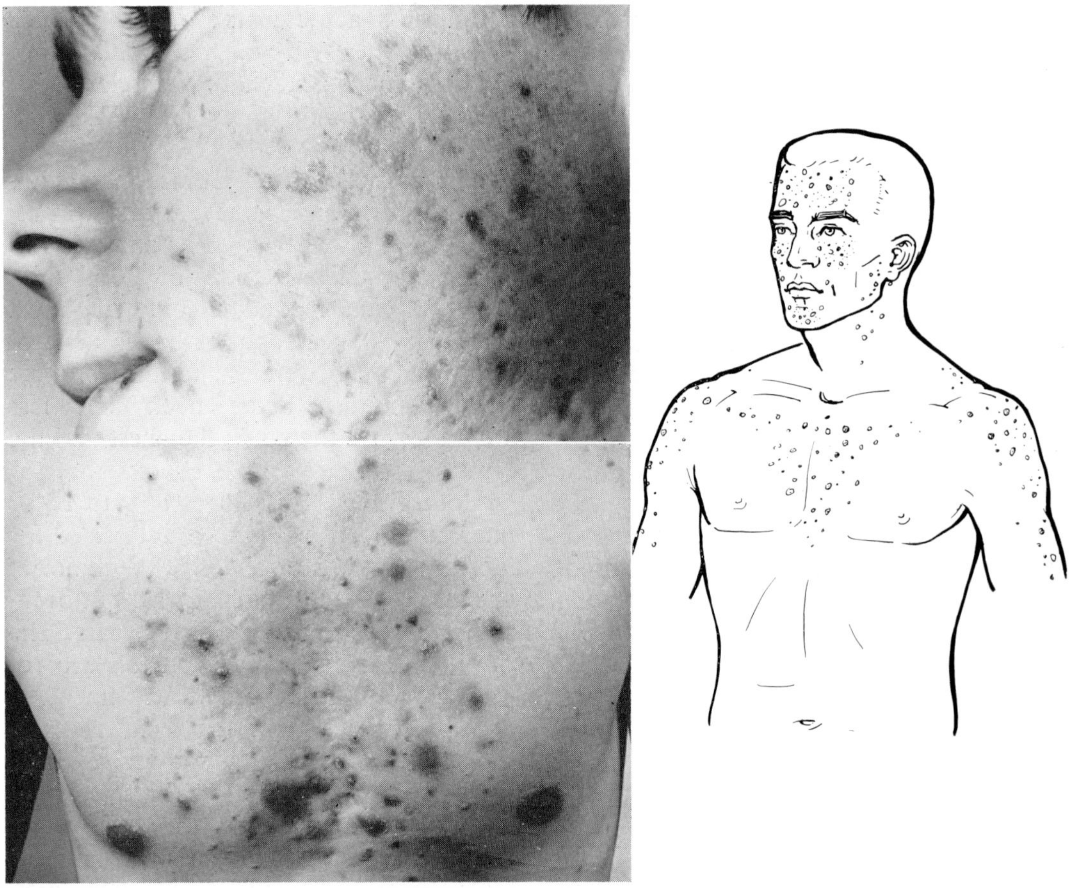

Fig. 35. Acne of face and chest.

patient, "What You Should Know About Acne," page 78). Stress the fact to the patient and the parent that not one factor but several factors (heredity, hormones, diet, cleanliness and general health) are important in clearing up acne.

2. Dial soap. The affected areas should be washed twice a day with a washcloth and this soap.

3. Sulfur, ppt. 6%
Resorcinol 4%
Colored alcoholic shake lotion
q.s. 60.0
Sig: Apply locally b.i.d. with fingers. (Boys may object to the powdery look and, if so, should use the lotion at night only.)

Proprietary substitutions for the above lotion include Resulin lotion (Almay) and Liquimat (Texas Pharmacal).

4. Remove the blackheads with a comedone extractor in the office.

Subsequent Visits. Ultraviolet therapy with increasing suberythema doses once or twice a week. Treat both sides of the face. This is especially indicated for those patients with mild but persistent acne, or those with severe acne but under the age of 16.

Treatment for a Severe Case of Cystic Acne

1. Tetracycline, or similar antibiotic, 250 mg. #20

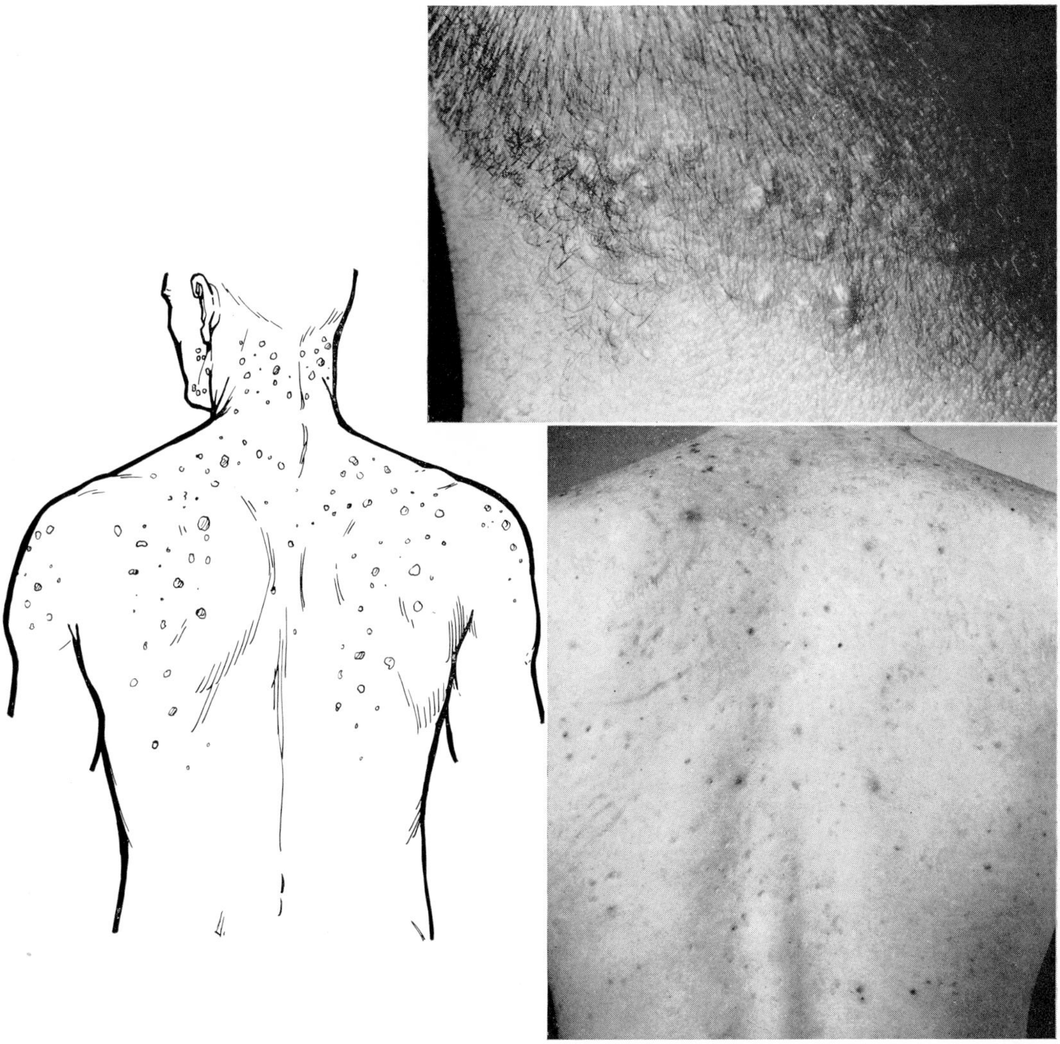

Fig. 36. Acne of neck and back.

Sig: 1 capsule q.i.d. for 4 days then 1 b.i.d. Following a good response, which may necessitate treatment for several weeks, the 125 mg. capsule can be used b.i.d., particularly if a potentiated tetracycline is prescribed.

This is an expensive form of therapy, but it becomes a necessity to prevent scarring in moderate or severe cystic acne cases.

2. Diethylstilbestrol (Enseals)
0.25 mg. #30

Sig: *Females:* 1 tablet a day for 10 days before and during the menstrual period. Take for 3 to 4 cycles. May temporarily alter the menstrual cycle. *Males:* 1 tablet a day. For very severe cystic acne the initial dose can be 1 mg. a day for 1 to 2 weeks, then decreased. A dose of 0.25 mg. a day can be safely continued for 1 to 2 months or until the breasts become tender.

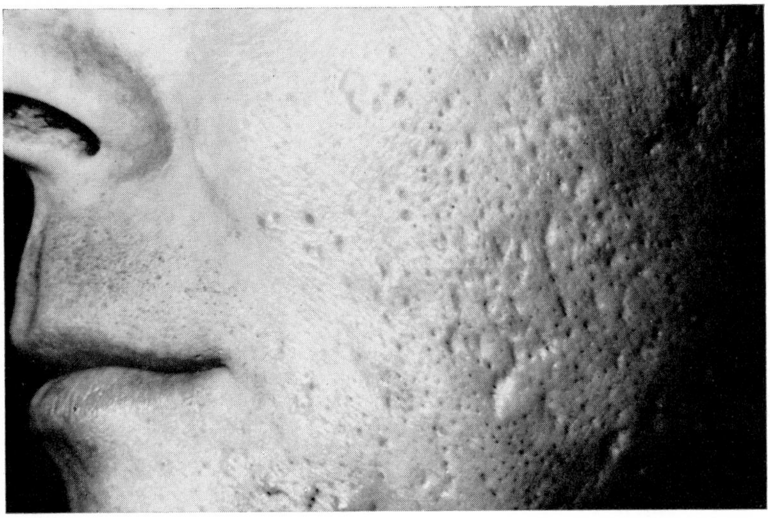

Fig. 37. Residual scarring from severe facial acne.

3. X-ray Therapy. This can be given after the age of 16 (younger in severe cases) and offers the best chance for lasting improvement of acne. This therapy should be administered only by a dermatologist or a radiologist. The usual treatment would consist of 75 r of unfiltered superficial x-ray given to both sides of the face (or to the back and the chest if needed) for 8 to 12 weekly treatments. The half-value layer of most superficial x-ray machines is 0.9 to 1.0 mm. of aluminum. Given in this manner, a total dose of 1,000 to 1,200 r is known to be safe. Further x-ray therapy must not be given to the area treated at *any time* in the future.

4. Other Treatments:

A. Vitamin A (water-soluble natural Aqua-sol A or water-soluble synthetic Stabil A) 50,000 U.

Sig: 1 capsule t.i.d. for 2 to 3 months.

B. Staphylococcus Toxoid (Merck Sharp & Dohme)

Sig: 0.1 cc. (Dilution 1) subcutaneously and increased by 0.1 cc. at weekly intervals up to 1.0 cc.

5. The residual scarring of severe acne (Fig. 37) can be lessened by surgical dermabrasion, using a rapidly rotating wire brush or diamond fraise. This procedure is being done by many dermatologists and plastic surgeons.

What You Should Know About Acne

Acne is a disorder in which the oil glands of the skin are overactive. It usually involves the face and, frequently, the chest and the back, for these areas are the richest in oil glands. When an oil gland opening becomes plugged, a blackhead is formed and irritates the skin in exactly the same way as any other foreign body, such as a sliver of wood. This irritation takes the form of red pimples or deep, painful cysts. These infections destroy the tissues and, when healed, may result in permanent scars.

The tendency to develop acne may run in families, especially those in which one or both parents have an oily skin. Acne is occasionally associated with glandular disturbances, such as menstrual disorders, and usually is made worse by nervous tension, overwork, lack of sleep, and dietary indiscretions. Any or all of these factors may exaggerate the tendency of the oily skin to develop acne.

Because acne is so common, is not contagious and does not cause loss of time from school or work, many people tend to ignore it or regard it as a necessary part of growing up. Actually, the old statement, "You'll be all right when you're married," has little or no significance. Marriage itself has no relationship to acne, except that ordinarily by the time a person is ready to get married, he or she usually is past the acne age and would have become well anyway.

Reasons for Treating Acne

There are at least two very important reasons for seeking medical care for acne. The first is to prevent the scarring mentioned previously. Once scarring has occurred, it is permanent in character. Then a patient must go through the rest of his life being embarrassed and annoyed by the scars, even though active pimples are no longer present. This scarring may vary from tiny little pits, which are frequently mistaken for "enlarged pores," to deep, large, disfiguring pockmarks.

The second reason for starting active treatment for acne, even without scarring, is that the condition may become the source of much psychological disturbance to a patient. Even though the acne may appear to others to be very mild and inconspicuous, it may seem very noticeable to the patient and lead to embarrassment, worry and nervousness.

Treatment Measures to Be Carried Out by the Patient

Cleansing Measures: Your face is to be washed twice a day with soap and a washcloth. The doctor may suggest a particular soap for use. Do not use any face cream, cold cream, cleansing cream, nourishing cream, or any other kind of grease on the face. This includes the avoidance of so-called "pancake" lotions which may contain oil, grease, or wax. Acne is caused by excessive oiliness of the skin, and every effort will be made to make it dry. Use of greases and creams increases the oiliness. You may think your face is dry because of the flakes on it, but these are actually flakes of dried oil. Later, when the treatment begins to take effect, your skin will actually become dry, even to the point where it is chapped and tender, especially around the mouth and the sides of the chin. When this point is reached, you will be advised as to suitable corrective measures for this temporary dryness. If the skin becomes red and uncomfortable between office visits, the applied remedy may be discontinued for one or two nights.

Girls may use face powder, dry rouge (not cream rouge), lipstick, but no face creams. Boys with acne should shave as regularly as necessary, and should not use oils, greases, pomades, or *hair tonics* except those which may be prescribed by the physician. Hair should be dressed only with water. Many cases of acne are associated with oily hair and dandruff and, for these cases, suitable local scalp applications and shampoos will be prescribed by the physician.

Plenty of rest is important, and you should have at least 8 hours of sleep each night. Violent exercise should be avoided, since increased perspiration is usually accompanied by increased activity of the oil glands. For this reason it is important to avoid *excessive* exposure to the sun and sunburn. You may think that there is temporary improvement following a suntan, because of its disguising effects, but, in the long run, prolonged sun exposure tends to make acne worse. If you go to the beach, do not use suntan oils or greases.

Diet: Do not eat any of the following foods:

1. *Chocolate:* including chocolate candy, chocolate ice cream, chocolate cake, chocolate nuts, chocolate sodas, cocoa and *cola* drinks. Hard candy (not chocolate) and soft drinks, other than the cola drinks, are all right in small or moderate amounts.
2. *Seafoods:* avoid shrimp, lobster, oysters, crab, and any food taken from the ocean. Fresh water fish is permitted.
3. *Iodized salt, nerve and headache medicines* (such as Bromo Seltzer), *certain cough remedies and tonics.* Look at the package of salt in the kitchen. If it is iodized, throw it away. Use plain, non-iodized salt both for cooking and on the table.
4. *Nuts:* especially peanuts and peanut butter.
5. *Milk Products:* no more than 1 glass of milk daily, preferably skimmed milk with the cream poured off. Reduce the use of sweet and sour cream, whipped cream, butter, rich creamy cheeses and ice cream. Avoid sharp cheeses, but cottage cheese is permitted.
6. *Avoid an excess of any sweets and fats,* especially French fried potatoes.
7. *Spicy Foods:* reduce as much as possible the use of spicy sauces, Worcestershire, chili, catsup, spicy smoked meats and delicatessen products.

The following of this diet does not mean that you should starve yourself. Eat plenty of lean meats, fresh and cooked vegetables, fruits (and their juices) and all breads. *Overweight patients* should lose 2 pounds weekly by reducing their total intake of the foods that are permitted. Bowel habits should be regular; for this reason, a diet rich in fresh fruits and vegetables is helpful. Drink plenty of water (6 to 8 glasses) daily, especially on arising each morning, and laxatives will not be necessary. *Do not take any laxatives or any other medicine internally without the knowledge of the physician.*

Medical Treatment of Acne

In addition to the prescribed treatment you will apply yourself, there are several aspects of the treatment of acne that must be carried out by the doctor or the nurse.

One important method of treatment is the proper removal of blackheads. *This is part of the doctor's job and should not be done by the patient.* Pimples which have pus in them and are ready to open should be opened by the doctor or the nurse. This is done with surgical instruments which are designed for the purpose and do not damage tissue or cause scars. Picking pimples by the patient can cause scarring and should be avoided completely. When the blackheads are removed and the pustules opened in the doctor's office, the skin heals faster, and scarring is minimized.

Another important method of treatment of acne is x-ray therapy. A series of 8 to 12 x-ray treatments properly given by a competent dermatologist will reduce the overactivity of the oil glands. There are several misconceptions about x-rays which some people have. *As given in acne, x-rays never cause sterility.* Sterility can be produced by giving large amounts of x-ray to the sex glands, but that is not done in treating acne. *X-rays do not cause the scars* that result from the more severe cases of acne. When acne is cleared up, the scars which were previously present or developing, but were not noticed among the pimples, will become more noticeable. Acne leaves scars in exactly the same way that chickenpox does, that is, by destroying tissue. X-rays, by their healing action, actually prevent scarring or minimize what otherwise would be more severe scarring. You may have a flare-up of your acne after several x-ray treatments, but this is temporary and will soon subside.

Ultraviolet light and other medicines, including some taken internally, may be prescribed by the doctor.

Conclusion

Do not become discouraged! Treatment is effective in at least 95 per cent of all cases. It may be several weeks (4 to 6) before noticeable improvement appears. There may be occasional mild flare-ups, but, eventually, you will improve, and you and your friends will notice the difference. You can be sure that your doctor is doing everything in his power to give you a clear, healthy complexion. Your co-operation, patience and understanding will help.

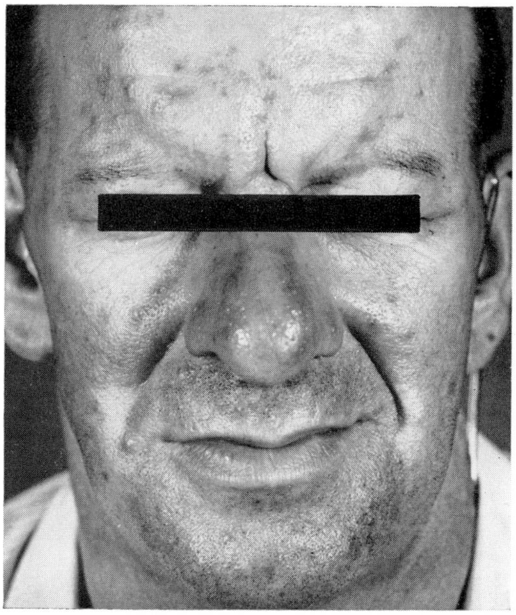

Fig. 38. Rosacea.

ROSACEA

An uncommon pustular eruption of the butterfly area of the face in adults of the 40 and 50 age group (Fig. 38).

Primary Lesions. Diffuse redness, papules, pustules, and later dilated venules, mainly of the nose, the cheeks and the forehead.

Secondary Lesions. Severe long-standing cases eventuate in the bulbous greasy, hypertrophic nose characteristic of *rhinophyma.*

Course. The pustules are recurrent and difficult to heal. Rosacea keratitis of the eye is rare but can be very serious.

Etiology. Several factors influence the disease: (1) hereditary factor of oily skin and, usually, brunette complexion; (2) some patients have no free hydrochloric acid in the stomach; (3) excess ingestion of alcoholic beverages, hot drinks and acne-producing foods.

Differential Diagnosis

Boils: usually only one large lesion, can be recurrent but may occur sporadically; an early case of rosacea may look like small boils (p. 100)

Iodide or Bromide Drug Eruption: clinically similar but drug eruption usually is more widespread; history positive for drug (p. 55)

Seborrheic Dermatitis: pustules uncommon, red and scaly, in scalp also (p. 73)

Rosacealike Tuberculid of Lewandowsky: rare; biopsy helpful.

Treatment

First Visit of a 44-year-old male with redness and pustules on the butterfly area of the face.

1. Prescribe avoidance of these foods: chocolate, nuts, cheese, cokes, iodized salt, seafood, alcohol, spices and very hot drinks.
2. Dial soap
   Sig: Use as face cleanser with a washcloth twice a day.
3. Sulfur, ppt. 6%
   Resorcinol 4%
   Colored alcoholic shake lotion q.s. 60.0
   Sig: Apply to face h.s.

4. Allbee capsules (or other Vitamin B medication) #50
   Sig: 1 capsule t.i.d., a.c.

SUBSEQUENT VISIT

1. Acidulin capsules (oral hydrochloric acid) #50
   Sig: 1 capsule t.i.d., a.c.
2. Kynex or Madribon tablets #30
   Sig: 2 tablets stat and then 1 b.i.d., later decreased to 1 a day. (This sulfonamide therapy is quite effective in stopping pustule formation. Watch for agranulocytosis, which is a rare toxic effect of any sulfa medication. If preferred, an oral antibiotic can be prescribed.)
3. X-ray therapy as given for acne by a dermatologist or a radiologist is indicated in severe cases.

Papulosquamous Dermatoses

CHAPTER 11

THIS classic group of skin eruptions includes several specific entities that predominantly affect the chest and the back with clinically similar macular, papular and scaly lesions (see Fig. 12). The commonest diseases in the group are psoriasis, pityriasis rosea, tinea versicolor, lichen planus, seborrheic dermatitis, secondary syphilis and drug eruptions. The last three conditions will be considered elsewhere in the book. To be complete with regard to the differential diagnoses of this group, the following rarer diseases can also be included: parapsoriasis, lichen nitidus and pityriasis rubra pilaris.

PSORIASIS
(Plates 1E, 10 and 11)

Psoriasis is a common, chronically recurring, papulosquamous disease, characterized by varying sized whitish scaly patches seen most commonly on the elbows, the knees and the scalp (Figs. 39, 40).

Primary Lesions. Erythematous, papulosquamous lesions vary in shapes and sizes from drop size to large circinate areas which can become generalized. The scale is usually thick and silvery and bleeds from minute points when it is removed by the fingernail.

Secondary Lesions. Unusual, but can see excoriations, thickening (lichenification), or oozing.

Distribution. Most commonly on the scalp, the elbows and the knees but can involve any area of the body, including the nails.

Course. Notoriously chronic and recurrent. However, severe cases have been known to clear up and not recur.

Etiology. Unknown. Approximately 30% of patients with psoriasis have a family history of the disease.

Subjective Complaints. Fortunately, only 30% of patients with psoriasis itch.

Season. Worse in winter usually, probably because of low winter indoor humidity and relative lack of sunlight.

Age Group. Any age but unusual in children.

Contagiousness. None.

Related to Employment. Psoriatic lesions can develop or flare up in areas of skin injury (Koebner phenomenon).

Laboratory Findings. Microscopic section is characteristic in typical cases.

Differential Diagnosis

Tinea Corporis: single lesion usually with healing in center, scraping and culture positive for fungi (p. 143)

Seborrheic Dermatitis: lesions more greasy, occur in hairy areas, scalp lesions are often impossible to differentiate from psoriasis (p. 73)

Pityriasis Rosea: "herald" patch, acute onset (p. 87)

Atopic Eczema: patches on flexural surfaces, allergic history (p. 51)

Secondary or Tertiary Syphilis: can be psoriasiform; blood serology positive; local therapy is of little value (p. 113)

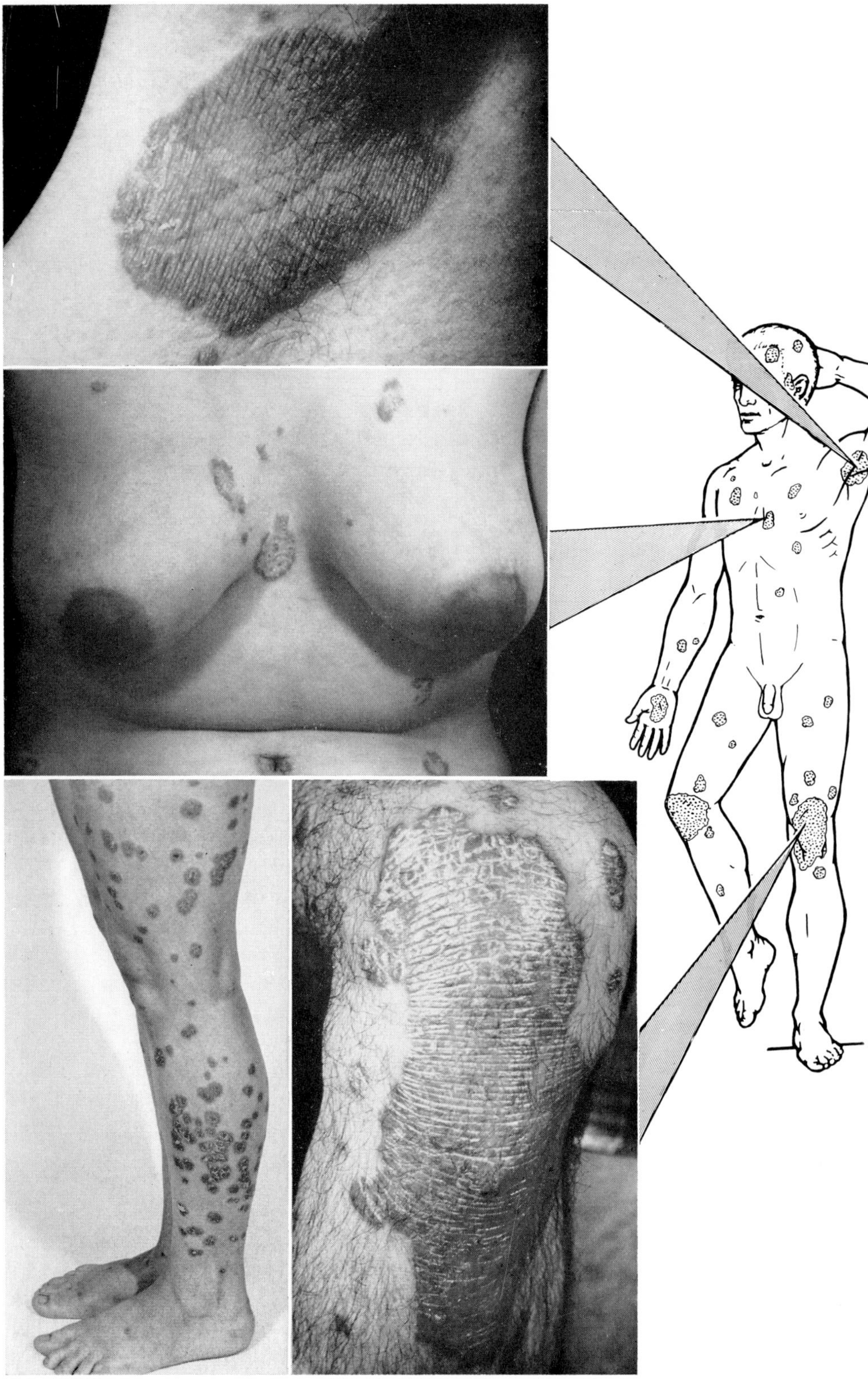

Fig. 39. Psoriasis.

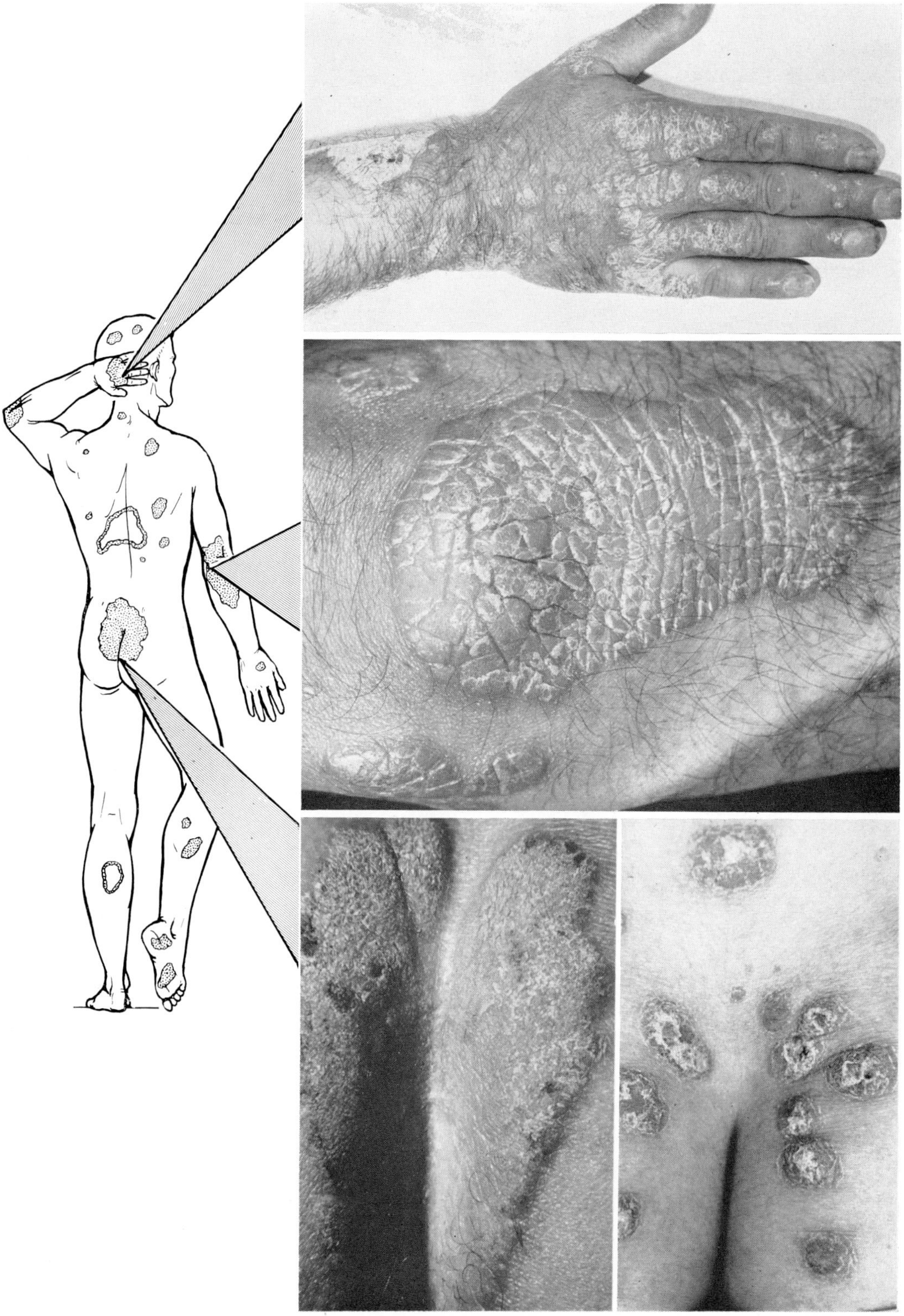

Fig. 40. Psoriasis.

Lichen Planus: lesions violaceous, small papules, very little scaling (p. 92).

A single lesion of psoriasis may resemble *neurodermatitis.*

Psoriasis of nails is similar to *tinea of nails.*

Treatment

FIRST VISIT OF PATIENT WITH RED SCALY LESIONS ON SCALP AND ELBOWS ONLY

1. *For body lesions*
   Coal tar solution 5%
   Sulfur, ppt. 5%
   White petrolatum q.s. 30.0
   Sig: Apply locally b.i.d. to body lesions.
2. *For scalp lesions*
   Pragmatar ointment 15.0
   Sig: Apply to scalp lesions b.i.d. (Can use the ingredients of salve No. 1 in a water washable base such as Unibase, Neobase, etc.).
3. Selsun suspension 120.0
   Sig: Shampoo scalp twice a week as long as salve is used in scalp. Use without any other soap. (Useful in relieving itching.)

SUBSEQUENT VISITS OF LOCALIZED CASE

1. For body lesions, gradually increase the strength of the medicines in the above salve (No. 1) to 10% and add salicyclic acid 4 to 10%.

2. Or stop above salve and use:
   Ammoniated mercury 5 to 10%
   White petrolatum q.s. 30.0

(A salve containing both sulfur and ammoniated mercury will cause a black discoloration of the skin.)

3. X-ray therapy can be given to localized areas by a dermatologist or a radiologist. If a lesion does not respond after 4 to 6 treatments of weekly doses of 75 r unfiltered, the lesion is not likely to respond to further x-ray therapy.

FIRST VISIT OF PATIENT WITH PSORIASIS ON 65% OF THE BODY SURFACE

1. Coal tar solution 120.0
   Sig: 2 tablespoons to the bath tub with 6 to 8 inches of warm water. Soak for 15 minutes once a day. Soap may be used unless there is a lot of itching.
2. Prescribe a mild body salve:
   Coal tar solution 3%
   White petrolatum q.s. 120.0
   Sig: Apply locally b.i.d.
   Increase the concentration slowly.
3. Methischol or Lipotropic capsules #100
   Sig: 2 capsules t.i.d., a.c.

Given to correct a possible fat metabolism error.

4. Crude liver injection (2 mcg. of vitamin B_{12} per cc.)
   Sig: Give 2 cc. intramuscularly once or twice a week for 6 to 8 injections.

5. Ultraviolet therapy in increasing suberythema doses once or twice a week. This can be used following a daily thin application of a tar salve.

SUBSEQUENT VISITS OF RATHER GENERALIZED CASE

1. Increase the concentrations of medicines used locally or use:
   Chrysarobin 0.1%
   White petrolatum q.s. 30.0
   Sig: Apply locally b.i.d. Avoid getting salve near the eyes.

The concentration of the chrysarobin can be increased cautiously, as necessary.

2. Low fat diet is thought by some to be helpful.

3. Systemic corticosteroids are of very little value except for triamcinolone (Aristocort or Kenacort). If conjunctive local therapy is not effective, relapses are the rule after corticosteroid therapy and may be difficult to handle. This is not a recommended form of therapy.

PITYRIASIS ROSEA

Pityriasis rosea is a moderately common papulosquamous eruption, mainly of the trunk of young adults, mildly pruritic, occurring most often in the spring and the fall (Figs. 41, 42).

Primary Lesions. Papulosquamous, oval erythematous discrete lesions. A larger "herald patch" resembling a patch of "ringworm" may precede the general rash by 2 to 10 days.

Secondary Lesions. Excoriations, rarely. The effects of overtreatment contact dermatitis are commonly seen.

Distribution. Chest and trunk mainly, along the lines of cleavage. In atypical cases the lesions are seen in the axillae and the groin only. Face lesions are rare for adults but are rather commonly seen in children and Negroes.

Course. Following the development of the "herald patch," new generalized lesions continue to appear for 2 to 3 weeks. The entire rash commonly disappears within 6 weeks. Recurrences are rare.

Subjective Complaints. Itching varies from none to severe.

Etiology. Unknown.

Season. Spring and fall "epidemics" are common.

Age Group. Young adults mainly.

Contagiousness. None.

Differential Diagnosis

Tinea Versicolor: lesions tannish and irregularly shaped, fungi seen on scraping (p. 90)

Drug Eruption: no "herald patch," positive drug history for bismuth or sulfa (p. 55)

Secondary Syphilis: no itching (99% true), history or presence of genital lesions, positive blood serology (p. 113)

Psoriasis: also usually on elbows, knees and scalp; lesions have whitish scale (p. 83)

Seborrheic Dermatitis: greasy, irregular scaly lesions on sternal and other hairy areas (p. 73)

Lichen Planus: lesions more papular, violaceous colored, on mucous membranes of cheeks (p. 92)

Parapsoriasis: rare, very chronic.

If the pityriasis rosealike rash does not itch, obtain a blood serologic test for syphilis.

Treatment

FIRST VISIT

1. Reassure the patient that he does not have a "blood disease," that the eruption is not contagious, and that it would be rare to get it again. (Active treatment is preferred to saying, "Go home, it will disappear in six weeks." There are 3 reasons for this: (1) treatment *may* shorten the duration of the disease; (2) the usual itching must be alleviated; and (3) if you do not treat these patients they might go to someone else less qualified. If the eruption does not itch and the patient is reassured of the mild nature of the disease, then no treatment is necessary.)
2. Starch bath.
   Sig: Use ½ box (small) of Linit starch to the tub containing 6 to 8 inches of lukewarm water. Bathe for 10 to 15 minutes every day or every other day. Avoid soap as much as possible to reduce any itching.
3. Nonalcoholic white shake lotion q.s. 120.0
   Sig: Apply b.i.d. locally to affected areas.
4. If there is itching, prescribe an antihistamine drug such as:
   Temaril tablets, 2.5 mg. #30
   Sig: 1 tablet a.c. and h.s.
5. Ultraviolet therapy in increasing suberythema doses once or twice a week

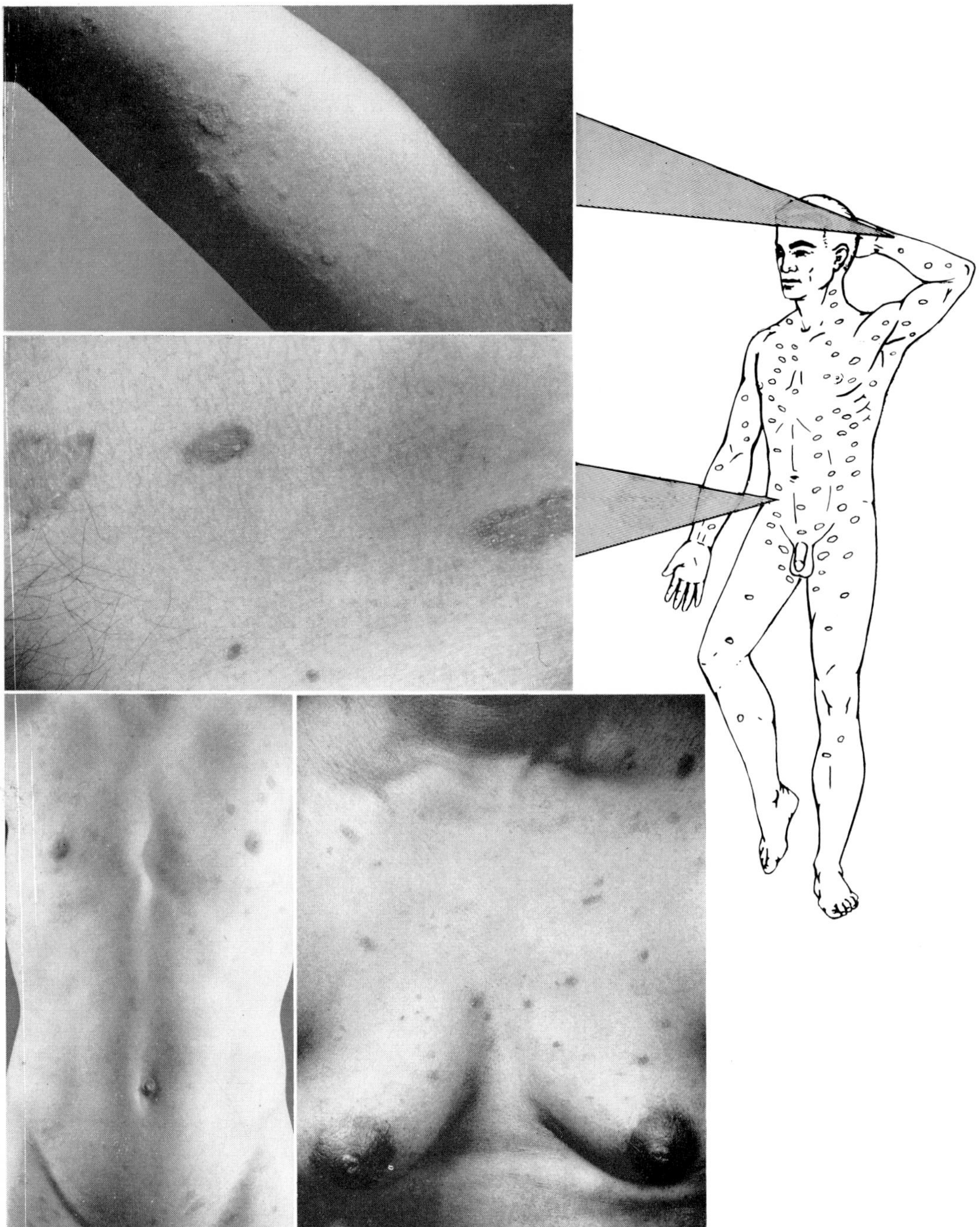

Fig. 41. Pityriasis rosea.

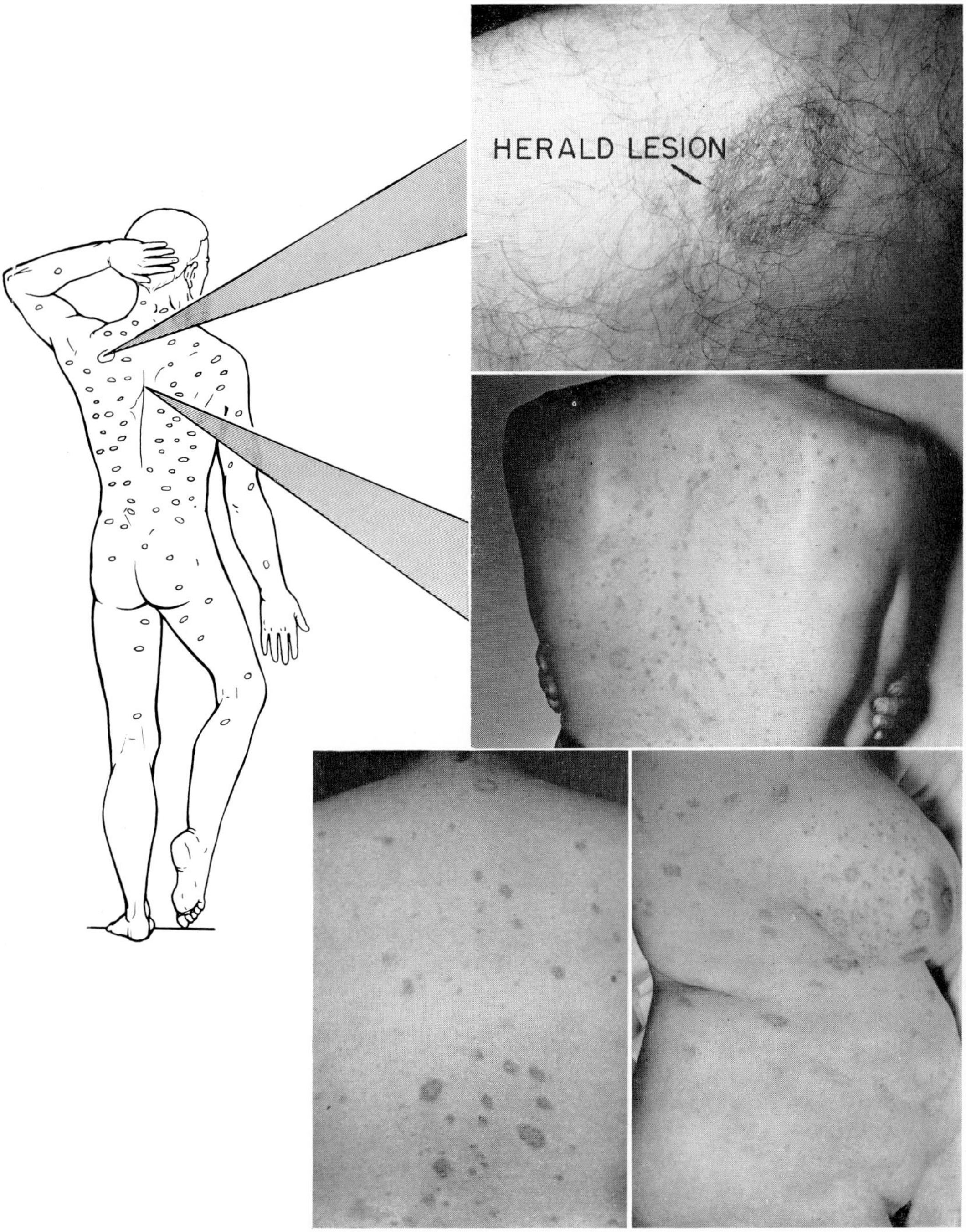

Fig. 42. Pityriasis rosea.

may be given. The entire body is treated with 2 front and 2 back exposures.

Subsequent Visits

1. If the skin becomes too dry from the starch bath and the sulfur lotion, stop the lotion or alternate it with the following:

White petrolatum 60.0
Sig: Apply b.i.d. locally to dry areas.

2. Continue the ultraviolet treatments.

Severely Pruritic Cases (in addition to the above)

Prednisolone, 5 mg. or other corticosteroid #24
Sig: 1 tablet q.i.d. for 3 days, then 1 t.i.d. for 4 days, then 1 b.i.d. for 1 to 2 weeks, as symptom of itching demands.

TINEA VERSICOLOR
(Plate 12)

This is a moderately common skin eruption with characteristics of tannish colored, irregularly shaped, scaly patches causing no discomfort, usually located on the upper chest and back. It is caused by a fungus. (See p. 136.)

Primary Lesions. Papulosquamous or maculosquamous, tan and irregularly shaped (Fig. 43).

Secondary Lesions. Relative depigmentation due to the fact that the involved skin does not tan when exposed to sunlight. This cosmetic defect, obvious in the summer, often brings the patient to the office.

Distribution. Upper part of chest, back, neck and arms. Rarely on face or generalized.

Course. The eruption can persist for years unnoticed. Correct treatment is readily effective but, if treatment is not thorough, the tinea can recur.

Etiology. A fungus, *Malassezia furfur*.

Contagiousness. Rare.

Laboratory Findings. A scraping of the scale placed on a microscope slide, covered with a 20% solution of potassium hydroxide and a cover slip will show the fungus. Under the low power of the microscope very thin mycelial filaments are seen. Diagnostic grapelike clusters of spores are seen best with the high-power lens. This fungus never has been grown satisfactorily on culture media.

Differential Diagnosis

Pityriasis Rosea: acute onset, lesions oval-shaped with definite border (p. 87)

Seborrheic Dermatitis: greasy scales in hairy areas mainly (p. 73)

Mild Psoriasis: see thicker scaly lesions on trunk and elsewhere (p. 83)

Secondary Syphilis: more widely distributed and rarely only scaly (p. 113)

Treatment

First Visit

1. Bathe thoroughly every night with Fostex Cake Soap and then apply household white vinegar to the involved areas with a cotton ball soaked in the solution. Let this dry on the skin.

2. Then treat the area thoroughly with 20% Sodium Thiosulfate Solution applied with soaked cotton balls.

3. Treatment should be continued for 7 to 10 days after apparent "cure," or the tinea will recur.

Subsequent Visits

1. These are usually not necessary except to check on the progress of the treatment. Rarely, a stronger antifungal medicine is necessary, such as:

A. Sulfur 6%
Resorcinol 4%
Colored alcoholic shake lotion q.s. 120.0

B. Salundek ointment q.s. 60.0

2. Depigmented spots may remain after the tinea is cured and, if desired, these can be tanned by gradual exposure to the sunlight or ultraviolet light.

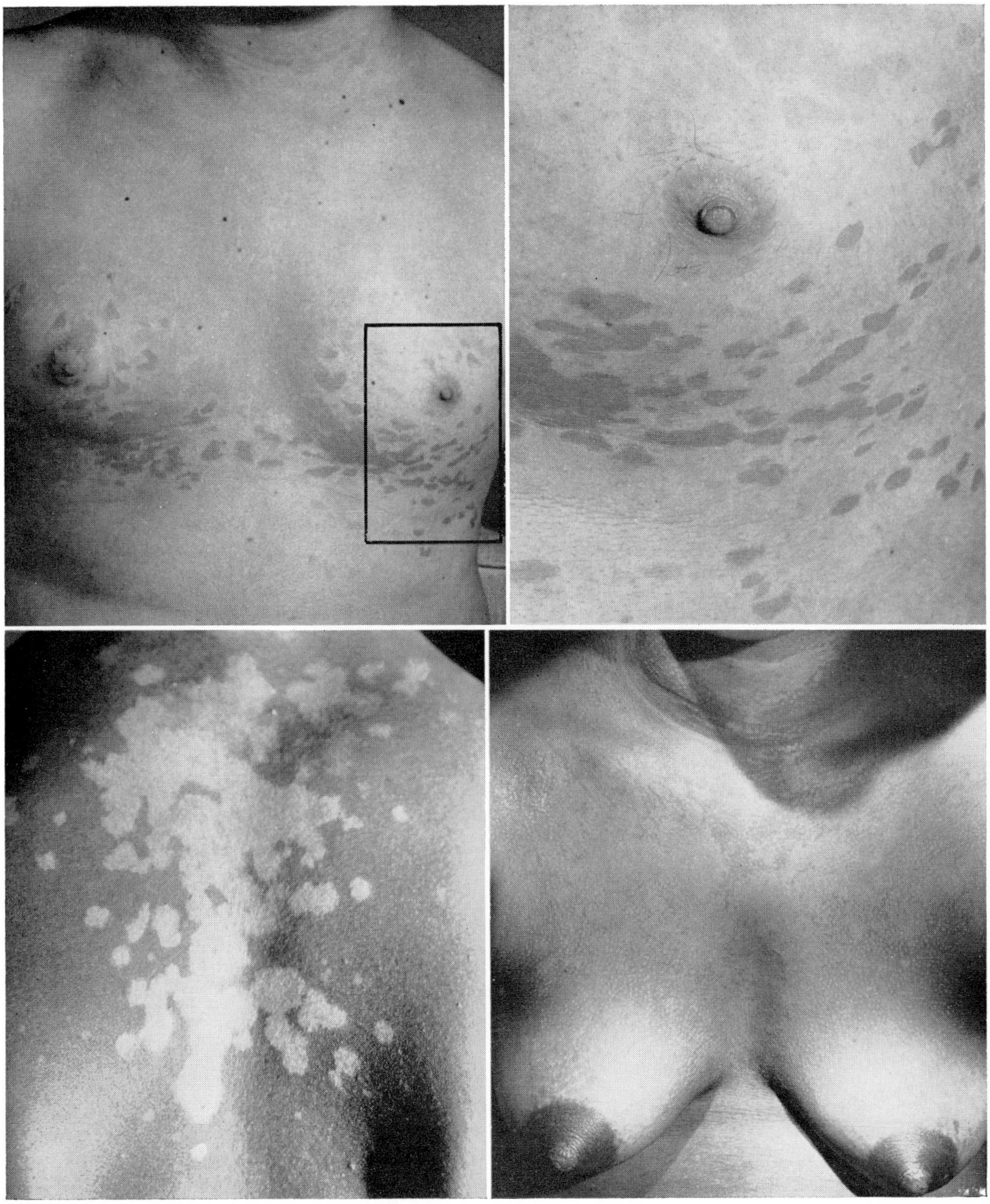

Fig. 43. Tinea versicolor.
Lower photographs are of Negro patients.

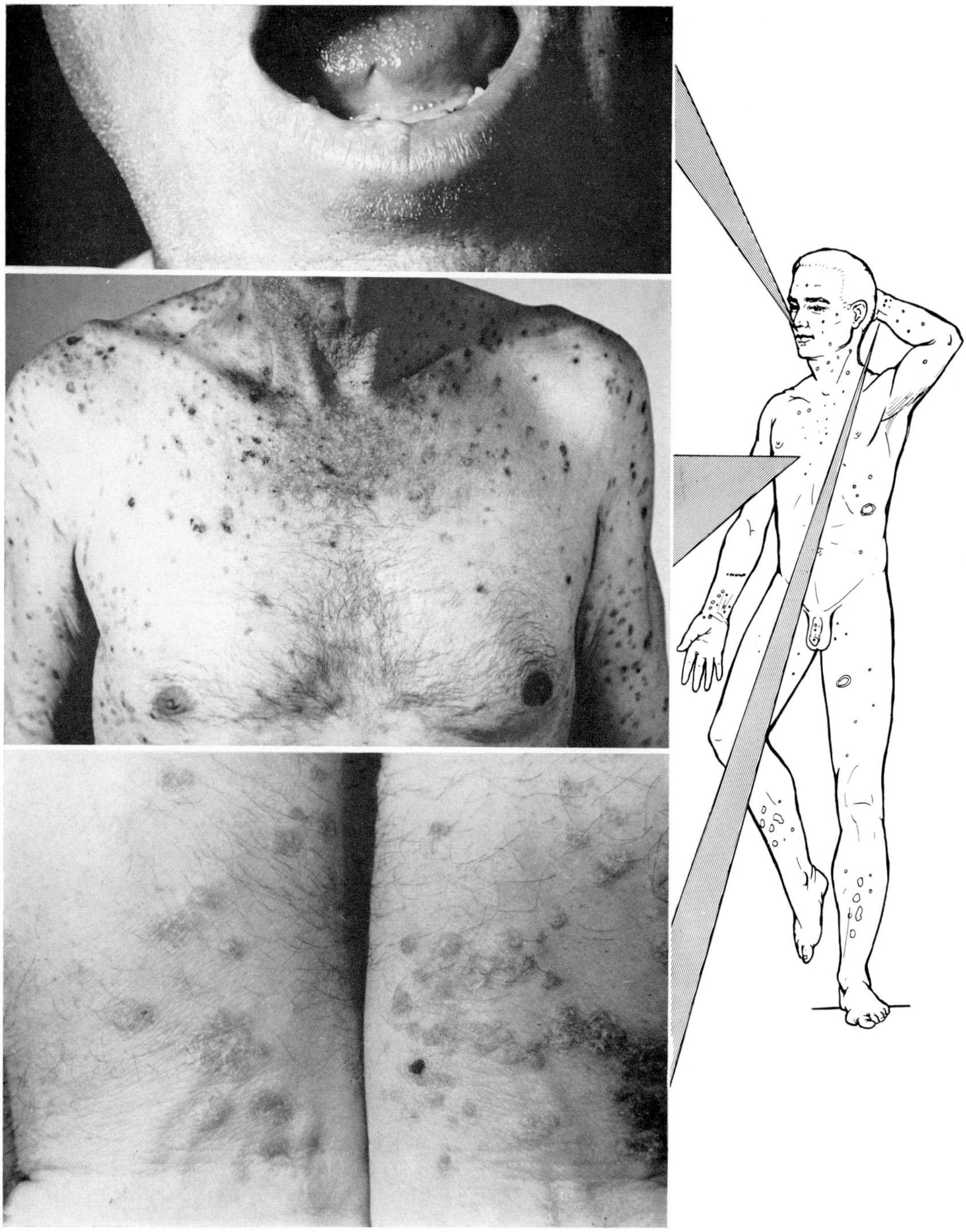

Fig. 44. Lichen planus.

LICHEN PLANUS
(Plate 1B and 13)

Lichen planus is an uncommon, chronic, pruritic disease characterized by violaceous colored, flat-topped papules usually seen on the wrists and the legs. Mucous membrane lesions on the cheeks or lips are whitish (Figs. 44, 45, 46).

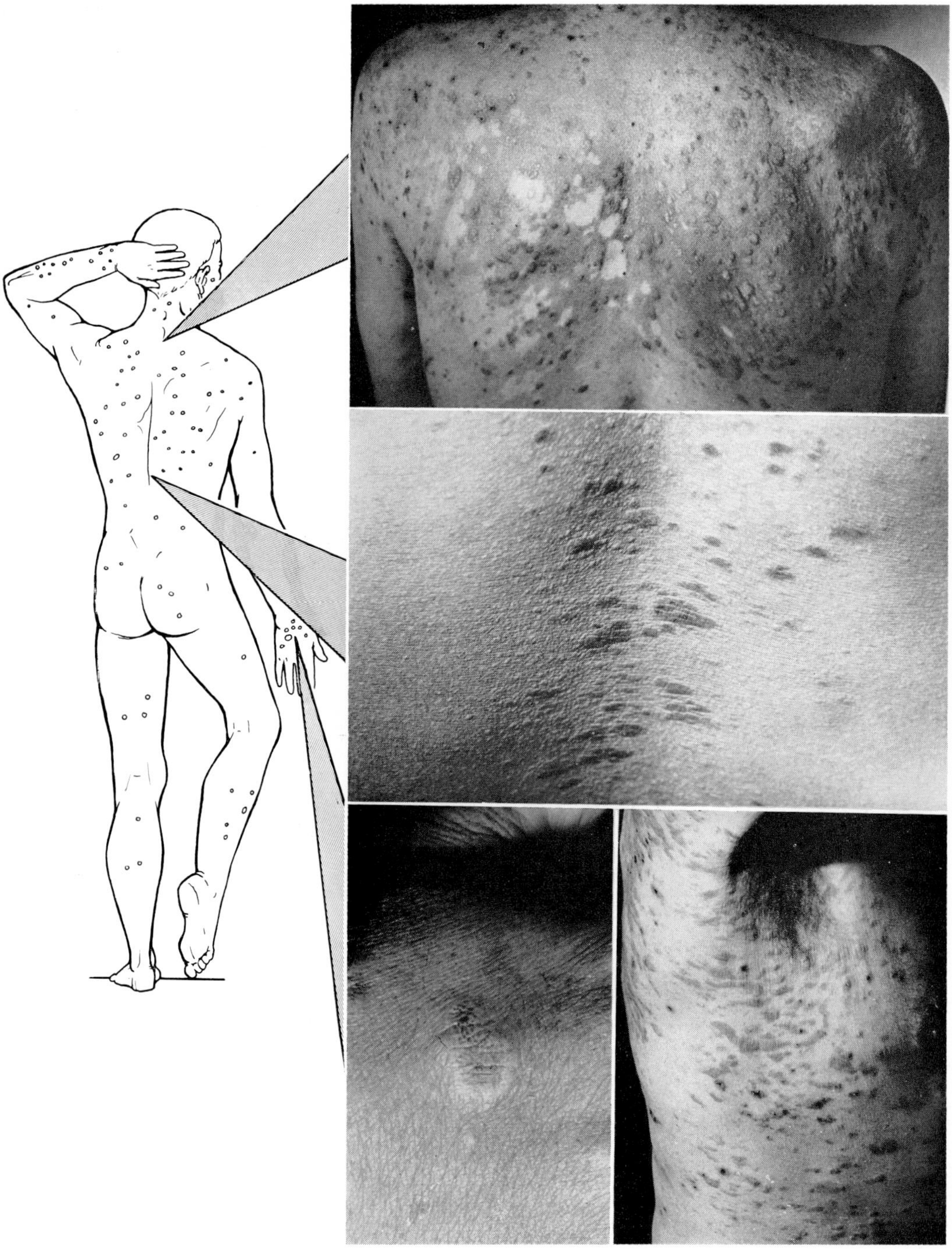

Fig. 45. Lichen planus.

Primary Lesions. Flat-topped, violaceous colored papules and papulosquamous lesions. Uncommonly, the lesions may assume a ring-shaped configuration. On the mucous membranes the lesions appear as a whitish lacy network.

Secondary Lesions. Excoriations and, on the legs, thick scaly lichenified patches.

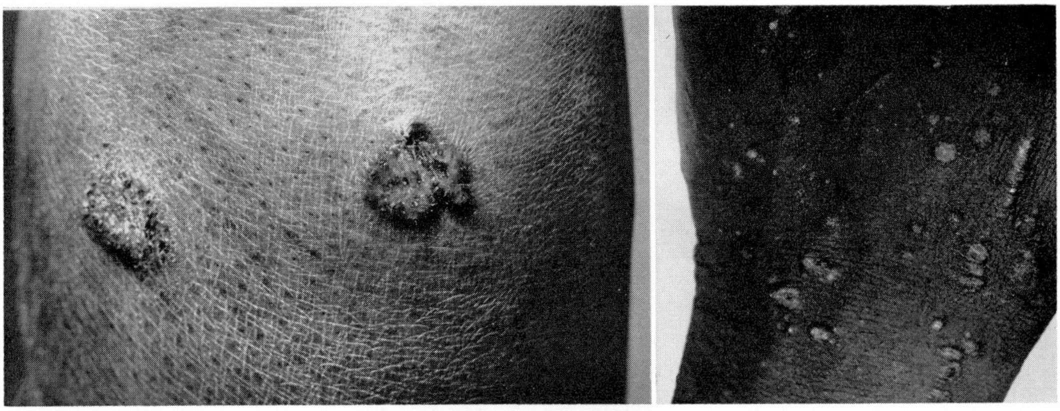

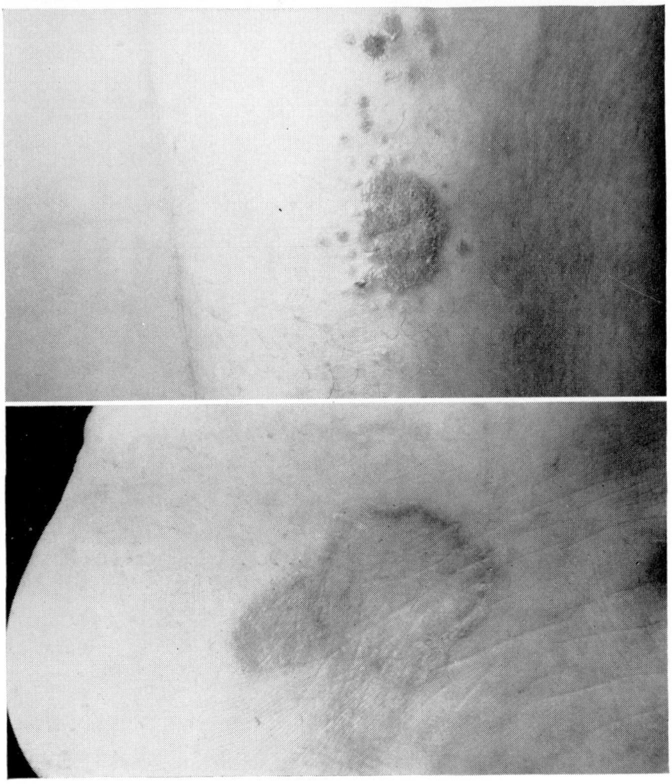

(*Top, left*) Nodular form on arm of Negro. This resembled sarcoidosis clinically. (K.U.M.C.)

(*Top, right*) On dorsum of hand showing Koebner phenomenon. (K.U.M.C.)

(*Center*) Hypertrophic form on anterior tibial area of leg.

(*Bottom*) Annular form on ankle. Clinically this resembled tinea.

Fig. 46. Lichen planus variations.

Distribution. Most commonly on the flexural aspects of the wrists and the ankles, the penis and the oral mucous membranes, but can be anywhere on the body or become generalized.

Course. Rather sudden outbreak with chronic course averaging 9 months' duration. Some cases last several years. No effect on the general health except for itching. Recurrences are moderately common.

Etiology. Unknown. Rather frequently associated with nervous or emotional upsets.

Subjective Complaints. Itching varies from mild to severe.

Contagiousness. None.

Related to Employment. As in psoriasis, the lichen planus lesions can develop in scratches or skin injuries (Koebner phenomenon).

Laboratory Findings. Microscopic section is quite characteristic.

Differential Diagnosis

Secondary Syphilis: no itching, blood serology positive (p. 113)

Drug Eruption: history of taking atabrine, arsenic or gold (p. 55)

Psoriasis: lesions more scaly, whitish, on knees and elbows (p. 83)

Pityriasis Rosea: "herald" patch, on trunk mainly (p. 87)

Lichen planus on leg may resemble *neurodermatitis* (usually one patch only, intensely pruritic, no mucous membrane lesions, p. 92).

Treatment

First visit of case with generalized papular eruption and moderate itching.

1. Assure the patient that the disease it not contagious, is not a blood disease and is chronic but not serious.
2. Avoid excess bathing with soap.
3. Menthol ¼ %
   Alcoholic white shake lotion q.s. 120.0
   Sig: Apply locally b.i.d.
4. Bistrimate tablets #50
   Sig: 1 tablet t.i.d., a.c. (Causes blackish stools and bismuth line on gums if continued for a long period; check urine occasionally for albuminuria.)

Subsequent Visits

1. Bismuth cevitamate, 2 cc. I.M., once a week for 6 to 8 weeks. (Watch for bismuth gum line and diarrhea.)
2. Add phenol 0.5%, camphor 2%, or coal tar solution 5% to the lotion prescribed on the first visit.
3. Meprobamate, 200 mg. #40
   Sig: 1 tablet q.i.d. (For relief of tension and itching.)
4. It is important in some resistant cases to rule out a focus of infection in teeth, tonsils, gallbladder, genito-urinary system, etc.
5. Corticosteroids orally are of definite value for temporarily relieving the acute cases that have severe itching or a generalized eruption.
6. If necessary, have the patient consult a dermatologist to corroborate your diagnosis, reassure the patient and suggest further therapy.

Dermatologic Bacteriology

CHAPTER 12

Bacteria exist on the skin as normal nonpathogenic resident flora, or as pathogenic organisms. The pathogenic bacteria cause primary, secondary and systemic infections. For clinical purposes it is justifiable to divide the problem of bacterial infection into these 3 classifications.

CLASSIFICATIONS

1. **Primary Bacterial Infections**
   A. Impetigo
   B. Ecthyma
   C. Folliculitis
      a. Superficial folliculitis
      b. Folliculitis of the scalp
         Superficial—acne necrotica miliaris
         Deep—folliculitis decalvans
      c. Folliculitis of the beard
      d. Stye
   D. Furuncle
   E. Carbuncle
   F. Sweat gland infections
   G. Erysipelas
2. **Secondary Bacterial Infections**
   A. Cutaneous diseases with secondary infection
   B. Infected ulcers
   C. Infectious eczematoid dermatitis
   D. Bacterial intertrigo
3. **Systemic Bacterial Infections**
   A. Scarlet fever
   B. Granuloma inguinale
   C. Chancroid
   D. Mycobacterial infections
      a. Tuberculosis of the skin
      b. Leprosy
   E. Sarcoidosis

PRIMARY BACTERIAL INFECTIONS (PYODERMAS)

The commonest causative agents of the primary skin infections are the coagulase-positive micrococci (staphylococci) and the beta hemolytic streptococci. Superficial or deep bacterial lesions can be produced by these organisms.

In managing the pyodermas certain *general principles of treatment* must be initiated.

1. *Improve the Bathing Habits.* More frequent bathing and the use of a bacteriocidal soap, such as Dial soap, is indicated. Any pustules or crusts should be removed during the bathing to facilitate penetration of the local medications.

2. *General Isolation Procedures.* Clothing and bedding should be changed frequently and cleaned. The patient should have a separate towel and wash cloth.

3. *Diet.* For patients with persistent or chronic bacterial infections these foods should be restricted: chocolate, nuts, cokes and cheeses (see Acne Instruction Sheet, p. 78). The patient should be questioned regarding ingestion of drugs which can cause lesions that mimic pyodermas, such as iodides and bromides.

4. *Diabetes.* Rule out diabetes by history and laboratory examination in chronic skin infections, particularly recurrent boils.

Impetigo

(Plate 1G and 14)

Impetigo is a very common superficial

bacterial infection seen most often in children. This is the "infantigo" every mother respects. (Figs 47A and B.)

Primary Lesions. They vary from small vesicles to large bullae that rupture and discharge a honey-colored serous liquid. New lesions can develop rapidly in a matter of hours.

Secondary Lesions. Crusts form from the discharge and appear to be lightly stuck on the skin surface. When removed, a superficial erosion remains which may be the only evidence of the disease. In debilitated infants the bullae may coalesce to form an exfoliative type of infection called *Ritter's disease* or *pemphigus neonatorum*.

Distribution. Most commonly on the face but may be anywhere.

Contagiousness. It is not unusual to see brothers or sisters of the patient and, rarely, the parents similarly infected.

Differential Diagnosis

Contact Dermatitis Due to Poison Ivy: see linear blisters, does not spread as rapidly, itches (p. 42)

Tinea of Smooth Skin: fewer lesions, spreads slowly, small vesicles in annular configuration which is an unusual form for impetigo, fungi found on scraping (p. 143).

Treatment

1. Outline the general principles of treatment. Emphasize the removal of the crusts once or twice a day during the bathing with Dial soap.

2. Sulfur, ppt. 4%
   Neo-Polycin or other antibiotic ointment q.s. 15.0
   Sig: Apply t.i.d. locally. (The addition of sulfur enhances the effectiveness of the antibiotic preparation.)

3. Advise the mother to continue the treatment for 3 days after the lesions apparently have disappeared.

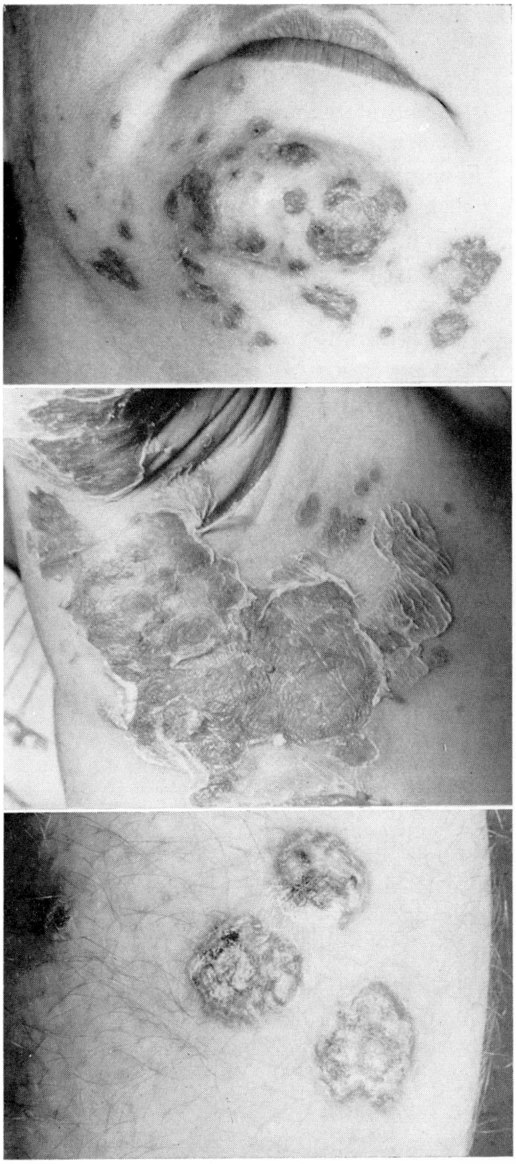

Fig. 47. Primary bacterial infections.
(*A, top*) Impetigo on the chin.
(*B, center*) Bullous impetigo of axilla and lateral chest wall of infant.
(*C, bottom*) Ecthyma on the thigh.

ECTHYMA

Ecthyma is another superficial bacterial infection but it is seen less commonly than impetigo and is deeper than impetigo. It is usually caused by beta hemolytic streptococci and occurs on the buttocks and the thighs of children. (Fig. 47C.)

Primary Lesion. Vesicle or vesicopustule that rapidly changes into the secondary lesion.

Secondary Lesion. This is a piled-up crust 1 to 3 cm. in diameter overlying a superficial erosion or ulcer. In neglected cases scarring can occur as a result of extension of the infection into the corium.

Distribution. Most commonly seen on the posterior aspect of the thighs and the buttocks, from which areas it can spread. Ecthyma commonly follows the scratching of chigger bites.

Age Group. Mainly seen in children.

Contagiousness. Ecthyma is rarely found in other members of the family.

Differential Diagnosis

Psoriasis: unusual in children, see whitish firmly attached scaly lesion, also in scalp, on knees and elbows (p. 83)

Impetigo: much smaller crusted lesions, not as deep (p. 96).

Treatment

1. Outline the general principles of treatment listed on p. 96. The crusts must be removed daily. Response to therapy is slower than with impetigo, but the treatment is the same for both conditions.

2. Systemic antibiotics. Commonly with extensive ecthyma in children, but only rarely with impetigo, there is a low-grade fever and evidence of bacterial infection in other organs, such as the kidney. If so, give penicillin by injection (600,000 units a day for 3 to 4 days) or one of the tetracycline syrups orally (125 mg. q.i.d. for 4 or more days).

Folliculitis

This is a very common pyogenic infection of the hair follicles, usually caused by coagulase-positive staphylococci. Seldom does a patient consult the doctor for a single outbreak of folliculitis. The physician is consulted because of recurrent and chronic pustular lesions. The patient realizes that the present acute episode will clear up with the help of nature, but seeks the medicine and the advice that will prevent recurrences. For this reason the *general principles of treatment* listed on p. 96, particularly the diet and the diabetes investigation, are important. Some physicians feel that a focus of infection in the teeth, the tonsils, the gallbladder or the genito-urinary tract should be ruled out when pyodermas are recurrent.

The folliculitis may invade only the superficial part of the hair follicle or it may extend down to the hair bulb. Many variously named clinical entities based upon the location and the chronicity of the lesions have been carried down through the years. A few of these entities bear presentation here, but the majority are defined in the Dictionary-Index.

Superficial Folliculitis

Most commonly seen on the arms, the face and the buttocks of children and adults with the "acne-seborrhea complex." The physician is rarely consulted for this minor problem; but if he is, a history of excessive use of hair oils, bath oils, or suntan oils, can often be obtained. These agents should be avoided.

Folliculitis of the Scalp

A *superficial form* has the appelation, *acne necrotica miliaris*. This is an annoying, pruritic, chronic, recurrent folliculitis of the scalp in adults. The scratching of the crusted lesions occupies the patient's evening hours.

Treatment of superficial folliculitis of the scalp

1. General principles
2. Selsun suspension 120.0
   Sig: Shampoo twice a week as directed on the label. Use no other shampoo or rinse.
3. Sulfur, ppt. 5%
   Coal tar solution 5%

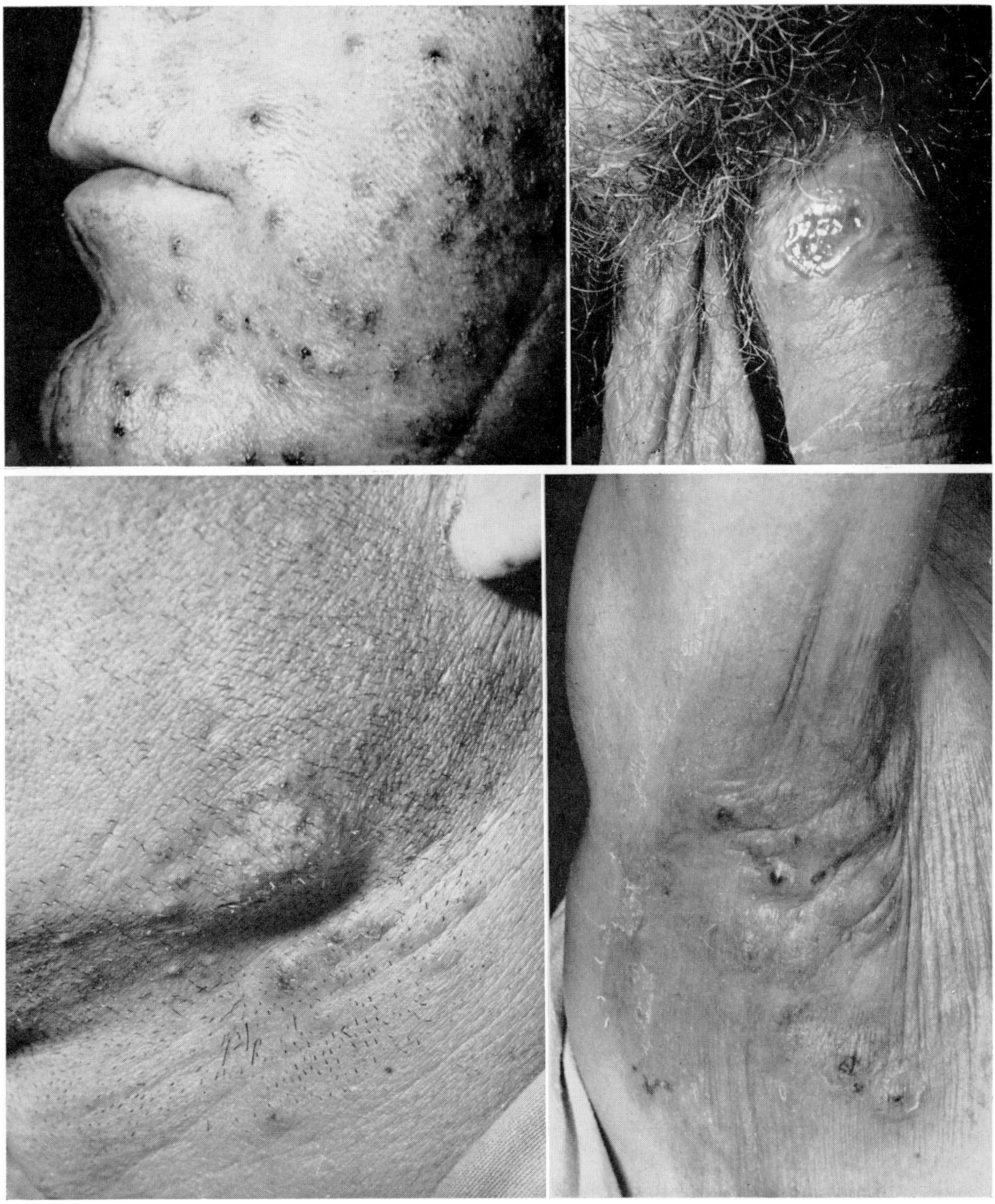

Fig. 48. Primary bacterial infections.

(*A, top, left*) Folliculitis of the face.
(*B, top, right*) Furuncle of the penis.
(*C, bottom, left*) Folliculitis of the face.
(*D, bottom, right*) Chronic sweat gland infection of the axilla. (K.C.G.H.)

Neo-Magnacort or other antibiotic-corticosteroid ointment q.s. 15.0
Sig: Apply to scalp h.s.

4. Staphylococcus toxoid (Merck Sharp & Dohme), Dilution 1

Give 0.1 cc. subcutaneously and increase by 0.1 cc. every 4 to 7 days until 1.0 cc. is given. This form of therapy works for some cases, apparently from a nonspecific protein action stimulating the adrenal cortex.

The *deep form* of scalp folliculitis is called *folliculitis decalvans*. This is a chronic, slowly progressive folliculitis with an active border and scarred atrophic center. The end-result after years of progression is patchy, scarred areas of alopecia, with eventual burning out of the infection.

Differential Diagnosis of deep form of folliculitis

Chronic Discoid Lupus Erythematosus: see redness, enlarged hair follicles (p. 172)

Alopecia Cicatrisata: rare, no evidence of infection (p. 191)

Tinea of the Scalp: it is important to culture the hair for fungi in any chronic infection of the scalp; *T. tonsurans* group can cause a similar clinical picture (p. 144).

Treatment of the deep form of scalp folliculitis is very disappointing. Follow the routine for the superficial form of folliculitis and give oral antibiotics.

Folliculitis of the Beard

This is the familiar "barber's itch" which in the days prior to the antibiotics was very resistant to therapy. This bacterial infection of the hair follicles is spread rather rapidly by shaving, but after treatment is begun, shaving should be continued (Fig. 48A and C).

Differential Diagnosis

Contact Dermatitis due to Shaving Lotions: history of new lotion applied, general redness of the area with some vesicles (p. 42)

Tinea of the Beard: very slowly spreading infection, hairs broken off, a deeper nodular type of inflammation is usually seen, culture of hair produces fungi (p. 147)

Ingrown Beard Hairs: see hair circling back into the skin with resultant chronic infection, a hereditary trait, especially in Negroes. Close shaving aggravates the condition. Local antibiotics rarely help, but locally applied depilatories do help.

Treatment of folliculitis of the beard

1. General principles, stressing the use of Dial soap for washing of the face.
2. Shaving instructions:

A. Change the razor blade daily or sterilize the head of the electric razor by placing it in 70% alcohol for 1 hour.

B. Apply the following salve very lightly to the face before shaving and again after shaving.

3. Neo-Polycin or other antibiotic ointment q.s. 15.0
Sig: Apply to face before shaving, after shaving and at bedtime.

Stye (Hordeolum)

A stye is a deep folliculitis of the stiff eyelid hairs. A single lesion is treated with hot packs of 1% boric acid solution and an ophthalmic antibiotic ointment. Recurrent lesions may be linked with the blepharitis of seborrheic dermatitis (dandruff). For this type, Selsun Suspension scalp shampoos are indicated.

Furuncle
(Plate 16)

A furuncle or boil is a more extensive infection of the hair follicle, usually due to the staphylococcus (Fig. 48 B). A boil can occur in any individual at any age, but certain predisposing factors account for most outbreaks. An important factor is the "acne-seborrhea complex" (oily skin, dark complexion, and history of acne and dandruff). Other factors include poor hygiene, diet rich in sugars and fats, diabetes, local skin trauma from friction of clothing, and maceration in obese individuals. One boil usually does not bring the patient to the doctor, but recurrent boils do.

Differential Diagnosis

SINGLE LESION: *primary chancre-type diseases* (see list in Dictionary-Index)

MULTIPLE LESIONS: *drug eruption from iodides or bromides* (p. 58).

Treatment. A young male has had recurrent boils for 6 months. He does not have diabetes, is not obese, is taking no drugs and bathes daily. He now has a large boil on his buttock.

1. Boric acid solution hot packs.
   Sig: 1 tablespoon of boric acid crystals to 1 quart of hot water. Apply hot wet packs for 30 minutes twice a day.
2. Incision and drainage. This should be done only on "ripe" lesions where a necrotic white area appears at the top of the nodule. Drains are not necessary unless the lesion has extended deep enough to form a fluctuant *abscess.*
3. Penicillin injection 600,000 U.
   Sig: Administer intramuscularly in hip daily for 2 to 4 days unless patient gives a history of penicillin sensitivity. (Other antibiotics could be substituted and used orally.)
4. To prevent recurrences:
   A. General principles of treatment, stressing diet and use of Dial soap.
   B. Rule out focus of infection in teeth, tonsils, genito-urinary tract, etc.
   C. Staphylococcus Toxoid injections as outlined under folliculitis of the scalp (p. 100) may be of value.
   D. Sulfonamide or oral antibiotic therapy. Over a long period this can be effective in breaking the cycle of infections. Check the white blood count at intervals during sulfa therapy.

CARBUNCLE
(Plates 15 and 18)

A carbuncle is an extensive infection of several adjoining hair follicles which drains with multiple openings onto the skin surface. Fatal cases were not unusual in the preantibiotic days. A common location for a carbuncle is the posterior neck region. Large, ugly, crisscross scars in this area in an older patient demonstrate the outdated treatment for this disease, namely, multiple, bold incisions. Since a carbuncle is in reality a multiple furuncle, the same etiologic factors apply. Recurrences are uncommon.

Treatment. The same as for a boil (p. 100) but with greater emphasis on systemic antibiotic therapy and physical rest.

SWEAT GLAND INFECTIONS
(Plate 17)

Primary *eccrine* sweat gland or duct infections are very rare. However prickly heat, a sweat retention disease, very frequently develops secondary bacterial infection.

Primary *apocrine* gland infection is rather common. Two types of infection exist:

Apocrinitis denotes infection of a single apocrine gland, usually in the axilla, and commonly associated with a change in deodorant. It responds to the therapy listed under furuncles (p. 100). In addition, a shake lotion containing a powdered antibiotic aids in keeping the area dry.

The second form of apocrine gland infection is *hidradenitis suppurativa* (Fig. 48 D). This chronic, recurring, pyogenic infection is characterized by the development of multiple nodules, abscesses, draining sinuses and eventual hypertrophic bands of scars. The most common location is in the axillae, but it can also occur in the groin, the perianal and the suprapubic regions. It does not occur before puberty. Etiologically, there appears to be a hereditary tendency in these patients toward occlusion of the follicular orifice and subsequent retention of the

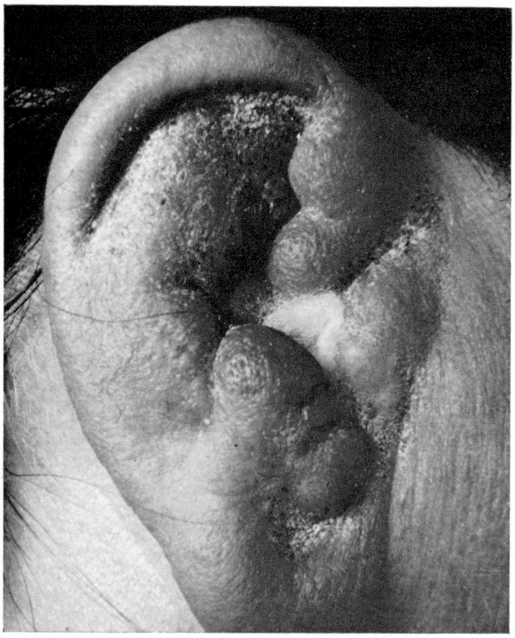

Fig. 49. Elephantiasis nostras of ear.
(Patient of Dr. M. Feldaker.)

secretory products. Two other diseases are related to hidradenitis suppurativa and may be present in the same patient: a severe form of acne called *acne conglobata* and *dissecting cellulitis of the scalp.*

Treatment of hidradenitis suppurativa: The management of these cases is difficult and preferably should be in the hands of a dermatologist. In addition to the general principles mentioned above, one should use hot packs locally and an oral antibiotic, such as oxytetracycline (Terramycin) 250 mg. q.i.d., for several weeks. Plastic surgery is indicated in severe cases.

Erysipelas

Erysipelas is an uncommon beta hemolytic streptococcus infection of the subcutaneous tissue that produces a characteristic type of cellulitis with fever and malaise. Recurrences are frequent.

Primary Lesion. A red, warm, raised, brawny, sharply bordered plaque that enlarges peripherally. Vesicles and bullae may form on the surface of the plaque. Usually a pre-existing skin wound or pyoderma will be found that initiated the acute infection. Multiple lesions of erysipelas are rare.

Distribution. Most commonly on the face and around the ears (following earpiercing), but no area is exempt.

Course. Untreated cases last for 2 to 3 weeks, but when treated with antibiotics the response is rapid. Recurrences are common in the same location and may lead to lymphedema of that area which eventually can become irreversible. The lip, the cheek and the legs are particularly prone to this chronic change which is called *elephantiasis nostras* (Fig. 49).

Subjective Complaints. Fever and general malaise can precede the development of the skin lesion and persist until therapy is instituted. Pain at the site of the infection can be severe.

Differential Diagnosis

Cellulitis: lacks sharp border; recurrences are rare.

Contact Dermatitis: sharp border absent; fever and malaise absent; eruption is predominantly vesicular (p. 42).

Treatment

1. Bed rest, and therapy directed toward reducing the fever. If patient is hospitalized, semi-isolation procedures should be initiated.
2. Penicillin 600,000 U.
   Give intramuscularly daily until temperature is normal for 48 hours.
3. Local cool wet dressings as necessary for comfort.

SECONDARY BACTERIAL INFECTIONS

Secondary infection develops as a complicating factor upon a pre-existing skin disease. The invasion of an injured skin surface with pathogenic streptococci or

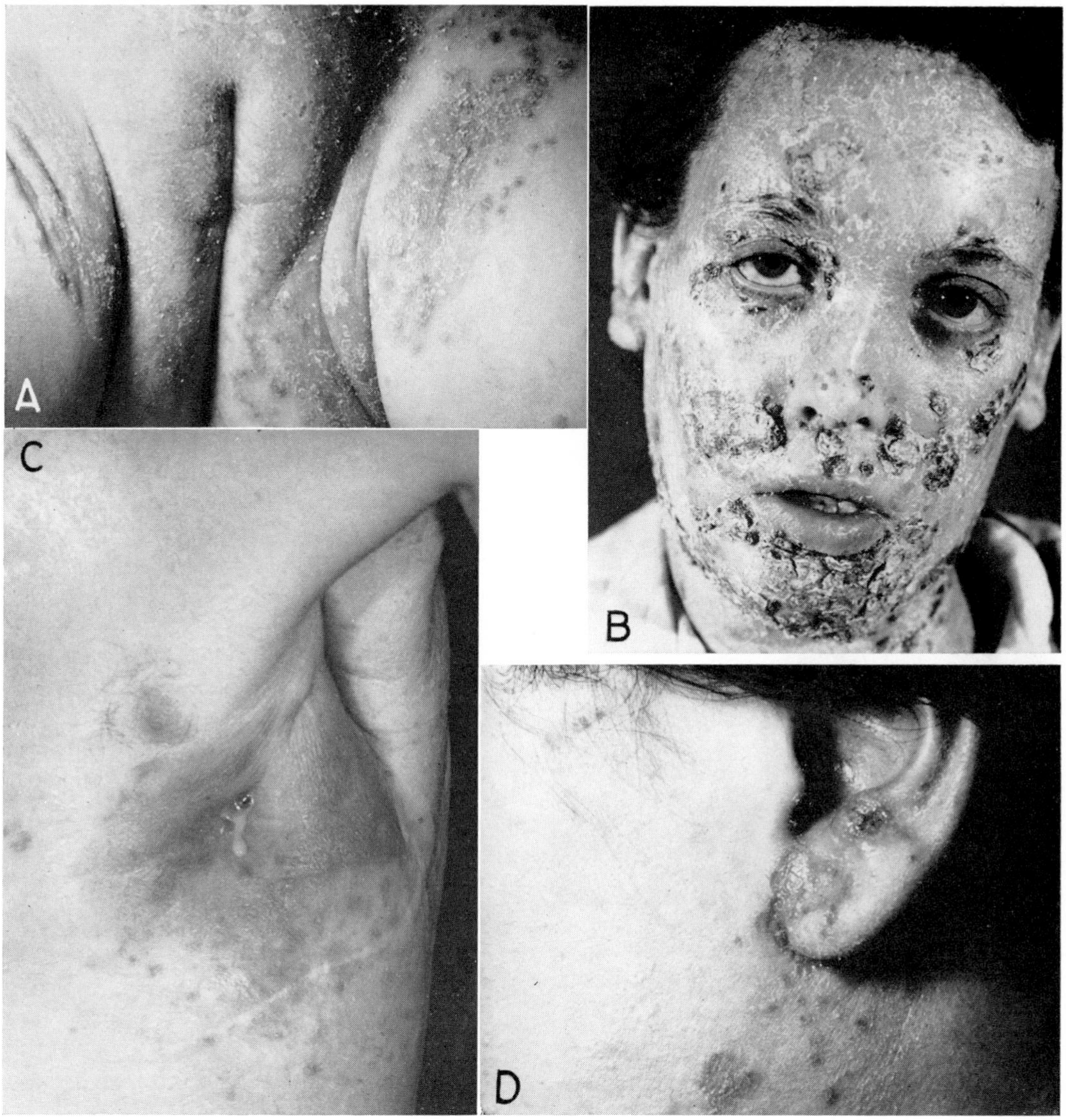

Fig. 50. Secondary bacterial infections.

A. Bacterial intertrigo of infant.
B. Atopic eczema with marked secondary bacterial infection.
C. Infectious eczematoid dermatitis secondary to empyema sinus.
D. Infectious eczematoid dermatitis secondary to external otitis.

staphylococci is enhanced in skin conditions that are oozing and of long duration.

Cutaneous Diseases with Secondary Infection

Failure in the treatment of many common skin diseases can be attributed to the physician's not recognizing the presence of secondary bacterial infection. Any type of skin lesion, such as hand dermatitis, poison ivy dermatitis, atopic eczema, chigger bites, fungus infection, traumatic

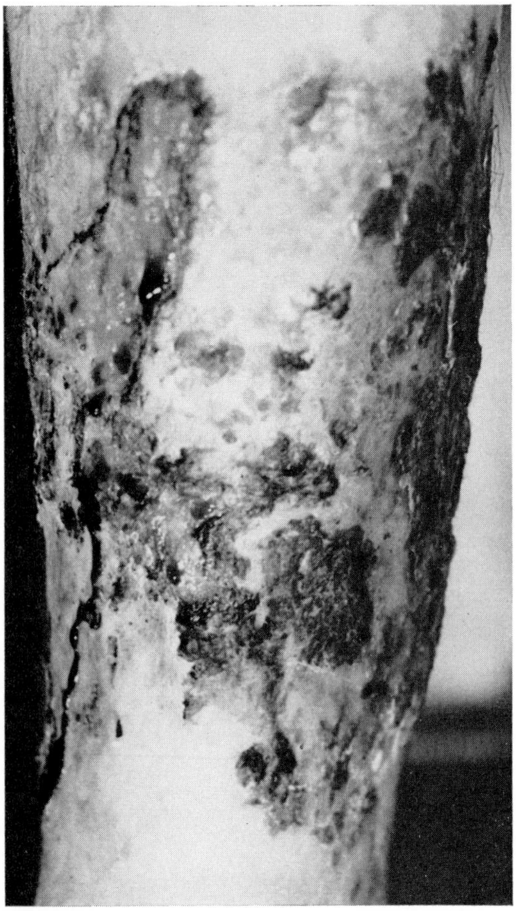

Fig. 51. Pyoderma gangrenosum of leg of patient with ulcerative colitis.
(*K.C.G.H.*)

abrasion, etc., can become secondarily infected (Fig. 50 B).

The treatment is simple. Add an antibacterial agent to the treatment you would ordinarily use for the dermatosis in question. For example, a secondary bacterial infection of contact dermatitis due to poison ivy would be treated by the addition of an antibiotic, such as chlortetracycline (Aureomycin) powder, 1% to 3%, to the antipruritic lotion or salve.

Infected Ulcers

Ulcers are deep skin infections due to injury or disease which invade the subcutaneous tissue and on healing leave scars. Ulcers can be divided into primary and secondary ulcers, but all become secondarily infected with bacteria.

Primary ulcers result from the following causes: gangrene due to pathogenic streptococci, staphylococci and Clostridium species, syphilis, chancroid, tuberculosis, diphtheria, fungi, leprosy, anthrax, cancer and lymphoblastomas.

Secondary ulcers can be related to the following diseases: vascular (arteriosclerosis, thromboangiitis obliterans, Raynaud's phenomenon, phlebitis, thrombosis); neurologic (spinal cord injury with bedsores or decubiti, CNS syphilis, spina bifida, poliomyelitis, syringomyelia); diabetes; trauma; ulcerative colitis (Fig. 51); allergic local anaphylaxis, and other conditions. Finally, there is a group of secondary ulcers called phagedenic ulcers, variously described under many different names, that arise in diseased skin or on the apparently normal skin of debilitated individuals. These ulcers undermine the skin in large areas, are notoriously chronic and are resistant to therapy.

Treatment

1. For primary ulcers specific therapy is indicated, if available. The response to therapy is usually quite rapid.
2. For secondary ulcers appropriate therapy should be directed toward the primary disease. The response to therapy is usually quite slow.
3. The basic rules of local therapy for ulcers can be illustrated best by outlining the management of a patient with a *stasis leg ulcer* (see Stasis Dermatitis, p. 71).

A. Rest of the affected area. If rest in bed is not feasible, then an Ace Elastic Bandage, 3 inches wide, should be worn. This bandage is applied over the local medication and before getting out of bed in the morning. A more permanent support is a modification of Unna's boot (Dome-Paste Bandage or Gelocast). This boot can be applied for a week or more at a time, if secondary infection is under control.

B. Elevation of the affected extremity. This should be carried out in bed and can be accomplished by placing two bricks, flat surface down, under both feet of the bed. (Arteriosclerotic leg ulcers should not be elevated.)

C. Boric acid wet packs

Sig: 1 tablespoon of boric acid crystals to 1 quart of warm water. Apply wet dressings of gauze or sheeting for 30 minutes 3 times a day.

D. If débridement is necessary, this can be accomplished by enzymes, such as Varidase jelly or Tryptar ointment, applied twice a day and covered with gauze.

E.	Gentian violet	1%
	Distilled water, q.s.	15.0

Sig: Apply to ulcer b.i.d. with applicator.

A liquid is usually better tolerated on ulcers than a salve. If the gentian violet solution becomes too drying, the following salve can be used alternately for short periods of time:

F. Neosporin or other antibiotic ointment, q.s. 15.0

Sig: Apply to ulcer and surrounding skin b.i.d.

The best treatment for one ulcer, does not necessarily work for another ulcer. Many other local medications are available and valuable.

Infectious Eczematoid Dermatitis

This term is more often used incorrectly than correctly. Infectious eczematoid dermatitis is an uncommon disease characterized by the development of an acute eruption around an infected exudative primary site, such as a draining ear, mastitis, a boil or a seeping ulcer (Fig. 50 C and D). Widespread eczematous lesions can develop at a distant site from the primary infection, presumably due to autoinoculation.

Primary Lesions. Vesicles and pustules in circumscribed plaques that spread peripherally from an infected central source. Central healing usually does not occur as with ringworm infection

Secondary Lesions. Crusting, oozing and scaling predominate in widespread cases.

Distribution. Mild cases may be confined to a small area around the exudative primary infection, but widespread cases can cover the entire body, obscuring the initial cause.

Course. This depends on the extent of the eruption. Chronic cases respond poorly to therapy. Recurrences are common even after the primary source is healed.

Subjective Complaints. Itching is usually mild.

Etiology. Coagulase-positive staphylococci are frequently isolated.

Contagiousness. In spite of the strong autoinoculation factor, passage of the infective material to another individual rarely elicits a reaction.

Differential Diagnosis

Contact Dermatitis With Secondary Infection: no history or finding of primary exudative infection; have history of contact with poison ivy, new clothes, cosmetics, or dishwater; responds faster to therapy (p. 103).

Nummular Eczema: no primary infected source, see coin-shaped lesions, on extremities, clinical differentiation of some cases can be difficult (p. 54).

Seborrheic Dermatitis: no primary infected source; see seborrhea-acne complex with greasy, scaly eruption in hairy areas (p. 73).

Treatment. Case of an 8-year-old boy with draining otitis media and pustular, crusted dermatitis on side of face, neck and scalp.

1. Treat the primary source, the ear infection in this case.
2. Boric acid wet packs.

Sig: 1 tablespoon of boric acid to 1 quart of warm water. Apply wet sheeting or gauze to area for 20 minutes t.i.d.

3. Neosporin or other antibiotic ointment q.s. 15.0

Sig: Apply t.i.d. locally, after the wet packs are removed.

A widespread case might require hospitalization, potassium permanganate baths, oral antibiotics and corticosteroid therapy.

Bacterial Intertrigo

The occurrence of friction, heat and moisture in areas where two opposing skin surfaces contact each other will lead to a secondary bacterial or fungus infection. Bacterial intertrigo concerns us here (Fig. 50 A).

Primary Lesion. Redness from friction and heat of opposing surfaces, and maceration from inability of the sweat to evaporate freely, leads to an eroded patch of dermatitis.

Secondary Lesion. The bacterial infection may become severe enough to result in fissures and cellulitis.

Distribution. Inframammary region, axillae, umbilicus, pubic, crural, genital and perianal areas, and between the toes.

Course. In certain individuals it tends to recur each summer.

Etiology. The factors of obesity, diabetes, prolonged contact with urine, feces and menstrual discharges predispose to the development of intertrigo.

Differential Diagnosis

Monilial intertrigo: see scaling at border of erosion, presence of surrounding small satellite lesions; scraping and culture reveals *C. albicans* (p. 150).

Tinea: see scaly or papulovesicular border, scraping and culture positive for fungi (p. 141).

Seborrheic Dermatitis: greasy red scaly areas, also seen in scalp; bacterial intertrigo may co-exist with seborrheic dermatitis (p. 73).

Treatment. Case of 2-month-old baby with red, pustular dermatitis in diaper area, axillae and folds of neck.

1. Bathe child once a day in lukewarm water with Dial soap. Dry affected areas thoroughly.
2. The diapers should be double-rinsed to remove all soap.
3. Change diapers as frequently as possible and apply a powder each time, such as:

   Talc, unscented 45.0

   Sig: Place in powder can.

4. Sulfur, ppt. 2%

   Nonalcoholic white shake lotion q.s. 90.0

   Sig: Apply to affected areas t.i.d.

SYSTEMIC BACTERIAL INFECTIONS

Scarlet Fever

Scarlet fever is a moderately common streptococcal infection characterized by a sore throat, high fever and a scarlet rash that avoids the circumoral area. The eruption develops after a day of rapidly rising fever, headache, sore throat and various other symptoms. The rash begins first on the neck and the chest but rapidly spreads over the entire body, except for the area around the mouth. Close examination of the pale scarlet eruption reveals it to be made up of diffuse pinhead sized or larger macules. In untreated cases the rash reaches its peak on the 4th day, and scaling commences around the 7th day and continues for a week or two. The "strawberry tongue" is seen at the height of the eruption.

The presence of petechiae on the body is a grave prognostic sign. Complications are numerous and common in untreated cases. Nephritis, in mild or severe form, is a serious complication.

The Dick test is a seldom-used diagnostic test. A positive red reaction to the injected toxin supposedly indicates a susceptibility to scarlet fever due to lack of antitoxin.

Fig. 52. Systemic bacterial infections.

A. Granuloma inguinale of the crural area.
B. Chancroid of the penis.
C. Papulonecrotic tuberculid of the leg.
D. Sarcoidosis on the neck.

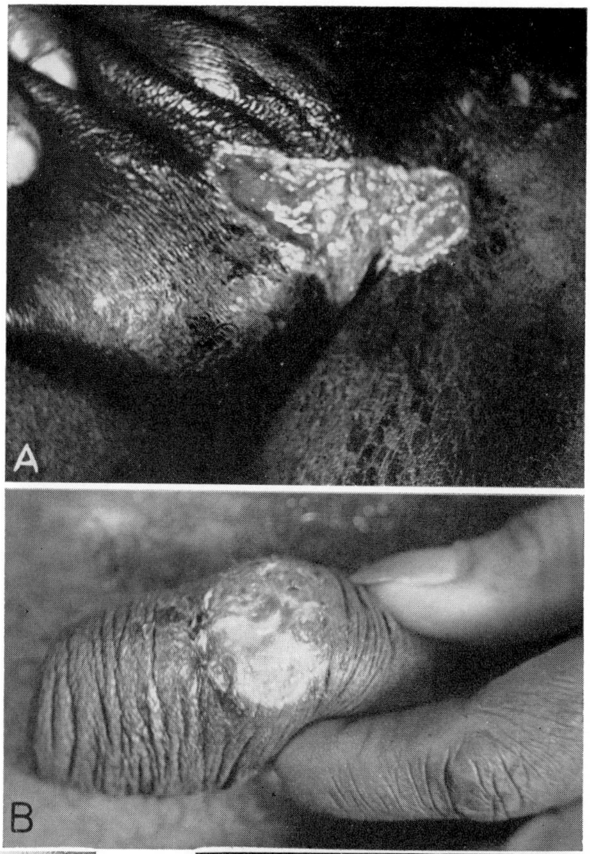

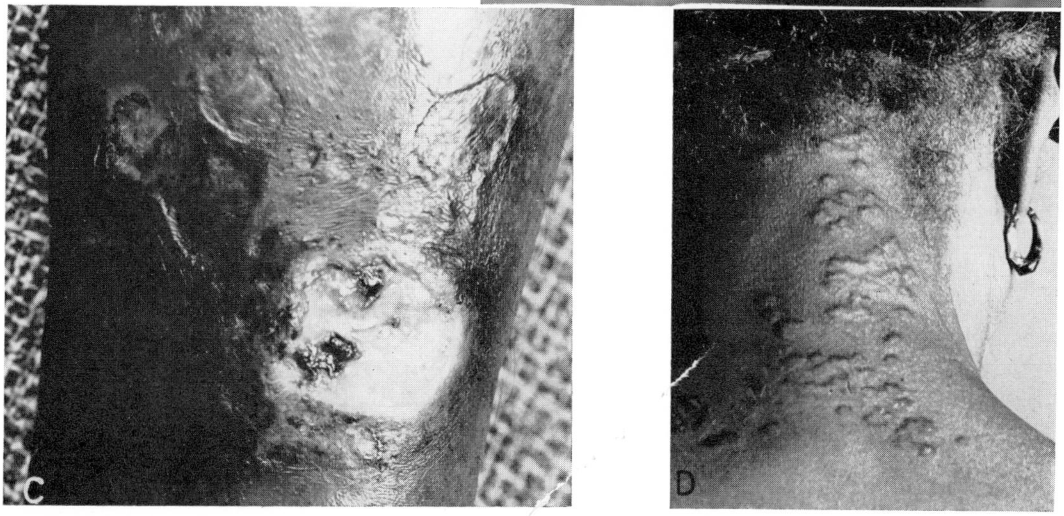

Differential Diagnosis

Measles: see early rash on face and forehead, larger macular rash, running eyes, and cough (p. 132).

Drug Eruption: see lack of high fever and other constitutional signs; atropine and quinine can cause eruption clinically similar to scarlet fever (p. 55).

Treatment. Penicillin by injection is the therapy of choice. Complications should be watched for and should be treated early.

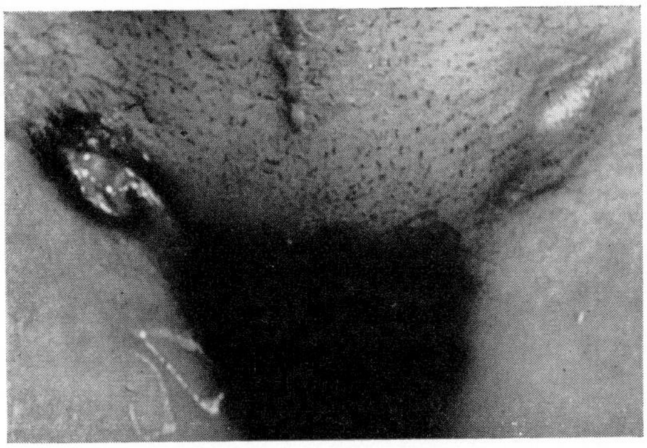

Fig. 53. Chancroid, showing inguinal lymph node involvement in a Negro female.

Granuloma Inguinale

Prior to the use of streptomycin this disease was one of the most chronic and resistant afflictions of man. Formerly, it was a rather common disease in the South, particularly among Negroes. Granuloma inguinale should be considered a venereal disease, although other factors may have to be present to initiate infection. (Fig. 52 A.)

Primary Lesion. An irregularly shaped, bright-red, velvety appearing, flat ulcer with rolled border.

Secondary Lesions. Scarring may lead to complications similar to those seen with lymphogranuloma venereum. A prickle cell epithelioma can develop in old, chronic lesions.

Distribution. Genital lesions are most common on the penis, the scrotum, the labia, the cervix or the inguinal region.

Course. Without therapy, the granuloma grows slowly and persists for years, causing marked scarring and mutilation. Under modern therapy, healing is rather rapid, but recurrences are not unusual.

Etiology. Granuloma inguinale is due to *Donovania granulomatis,* which can be cultured on special media.

Laboratory Findings. Scrapings of the lesion reveal Donovan bodies, which are dark-staining, intracytoplasmic, cigar-shaped bacilli, found in large macrophages. The material for the smear can be obtained best by snipping off a piece of the lesion with a small scissors and rubbing the tissue on several slides. Wright or Giemsa stains can be used.

Differential Diagnosis

Of a small lesion, consider *granuloma pyogenicum:* history of injury usually, short duration; rarely on genitalia; no Donovan bodies (p. 228).

Primary Syphilis: short duration, inguinal adenopathy, serology may be positive, find spirochetes (p. 112).

Chancroid: short duration, lesion small, not red and velvety, no Donovan bodies (see below).

Prickle Cell Epithelioma: more indurated lesion with nodules, may co-exist with granuloma inguinale, biopsy specific.

Treatment. Dihydrostreptomycin, 4 Gm. daily for 1 to 2 weeks, or oxytetracycline (Terramycin) 1 to 2 Gm. a day for 2 to 4 weeks.

Chancroid

Chancroid is a venereal disease with a very short incubation period of 1 to 5 days. It is caused by *Hemophilus ducreyi* (Fig. 52 B).

Primary Lesion. A small, superficial or deep erosion with surrounding redness and edema. Multiple genital or distant lesions can be produced by autoinoculation.

Secondary Lesions. Deep, destructive ulcers form in chronic cases which may lead to gangrene. Marked regional adenopathy, usually unilateral, is common and eventually suppurates in untreated cases (Fig. 53).

Course. Without therapy most cases heal within 1 to 2 weeks. In rare cases, severe, local destruction and draining lymph nodes (buboes) result. Early therapy is quite effective.

Laboratory Findings. The organisms arranged in "schools of fish" can often be demonstrated in smears of clean lesions.

The Ducrey skin test is positive within 2 weeks after the appearance of the primary lesion and remains positive for life.

Differential Diagnosis

SYPHILIS *must be considered in any patient with a penile lesion. It can be ruled out only by darkfield examination or blood serology tests.*

Primary or Secondary Syphilis Genital Lesions: longer incubation period, more induration, *Treponema pallidum* found on darkfield examination, serology positive in late primary and secondary stage (p. 112).

Herpes Simplex Progenitalis: recurrent multiple blisters or erosions, mild inguinal adenopathy (p. 121).

Lymphogranuloma Venereum: rarely see primary lesion; Frei test positive (p. 131).

Granuloma Inguinale: chronic, red velvety plaque; Donovan bodies seen on tissue smear (p. 108).

Treatment. Triple sulfonamides, 2 to 4 Gm. daily for 7 days, or tetracycline 1 Gm. daily for 10 to 15 days. A fluctuant bubo never should be incised but aspirated with a large needle.

Tuberculosis
(Plate 2 B)

Skin tuberculosis is rare in the United States. However, a text on dermatology would not be complete without some consideration of this infection. For this purpose the commonest tuberculous infection, lupus vulgaris, will be discussed. A classification of skin tuberculosis is presented in the Dictionary-Index (Fig. 52 C).

Lupus vulgaris is a chronic, granulomatous disease characterized by the development of nodules, ulcers and plaques arranged in any conceivable configuration. Scarring in the center of active lesions or at the edge in severe, untreated cases leads to atrophy and contraction resulting in mutilating changes.

Distribution. Facial involvement is most common.

Course. Often slow and progressive in spite of therapy.

Laboratory Findings. The histopathology shows typical tubercle formation with epithelioid cells, giant cells and a peripheral zone of lymphocytes. The organism, *Mycobacterium tuberculosis,* is not abundant in the lesions. The 48-hour tuberculin test is usually positive.

Differential Diagnosis. Other granulomas are to be ruled out by appropriate studies, such as *syphilis, leprosy, sarcoidosis, deep fungus disease* and *neoplasms.*

Treatment

1. Dihydrostreptomycin, 1 Gm. intramuscularly 2 or 3 times a week for several months. Can be given alone or with Isoniazid.
2. Isonicotinic acid hydrazide (Isoniazid), 150 to 300 mg. orally daily for adults for several months.
3. Para-aminosalicylic acid, 16 to 20 Gm. a day combined with Isoniazid or streptomycin.

Leprosy

Leprosy is to be considered in the differential diagnosis of any skin granulomas. It is endemic in the southern part of the United States and in semitropical and tropical areas the world over.

The Sixth International Congress of Leprology held in 1953 attempted to clarify the classification of leprosy. The Congress recommended that two definite types of leprosy should be recognized: lepromatous and tuberculoid. In addition, there are cases that cannot presently be classified into these two categories but eventually develop either lepromatous or tuberculoid leprosy.

Lepromatous leprosy is the malignant form which represents minimal resistance to the disease with a negative lepromin reaction, characteristic histology, infil-

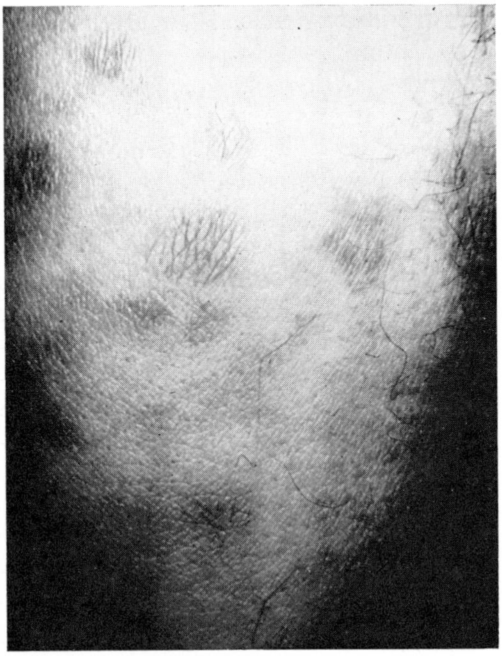

Fig. 54. Tuberculoid leprosy.
Macular erythematous lesions on the arm.

trated cutaneous lesions with ill-defined borders, and progression to death from tuberculosis and secondary amyloidosis.

Tuberculoid leprosy is generally benign in its course because of considerable resistance to the disease on the part of the host. This is manifested by a positive lepromin test, histology not diagnostic, cutaneous lesions frequently erythematous with elevated borders, and minimal effect of the disease on the general health (Fig. 54).

Early lesions of the lepromatous type include reddish macules with an indefinite border, nasal obstruction and nosebleeds. Erythema-nodosumlike lesions occur commonly. The tuberculoid type of leprosy is diagnosed early by the presence of an area of skin with impaired sensation, polyneuritis, and skin lesions with a sharp border and central atrophy.

Etiology. Due to *Mycobacterium leprae* (Hansen's bacillus).

Contagiousness. The source of infection is thought to be from patients with the lepromatous form. Infectiousness is of a low order.

Laboratory Findings. The bacilli are usually uncovered in the lepromatous type but seldom in the tuberculoid type. Smears should be obtained from the tissue exposed by a small incision made into the corium through an infiltrated lesion.

The lepromin reaction, a delayed reaction test similar to the tuberculin test, is of value in differentiating the lepromatous form from the tuberculoid form of leprosy as stated above. False-positive reactions do occur.

Biologic false-positive tests for syphilis are common in patients with the lepromatous type of leprosy.

Differential Diagnosis. Consider any of the granulomatous diseases such as *syphilis, tuberculosis, sarcoidosis,* and *deep fungus infections.*

Treatment. The sulfones are more effective than any other form of therapy. Diaminodiphenyl sulfone (DDS) and Diasone are used predominantly.

Sarcoidosis

Sarcoidosis is a moderately common systemic granulomatous disease of unknown cause that affects skin, lungs, lymph nodes, liver, spleen, bones and eyes. Any one of these organs or all of them may be involved with sarcoid granulomas. Lymphadenopathy is the commonest single finding. Negroes are affected more commonly than Caucasians (Fig. 52 D).

Only the skin manifestations of sarcoidosis will be discussed.

Primary Lesions. The superficial lesions consist of reddish papules, nodules and plaques which may be multiple or solitary, and of varying size and configuration. Annular forms of skin sarcoidosis are common. These superficial lesions usually involve the face, the shoulders and the arms. Subcutaneous nodular forms and telangiectatic lesions are more rare.

Secondary Lesions. Central healing can result in atrophy and scarring.

Course. Most cases of sarcoidosis run a chronic but benign course with remissions and exacerbations. Spontaneous "cure" is not unusual.

Etiology. The cause is unknown, but an infectious cause has not been ruled out completely.

Laboratory Findings. The histopathology is quite characteristic and consists of epithelioid cells surrounded by Langhans' giant cells. No acid-fast bacilli are found, and caseation necrosis is absent. The tuberculin skin test is negative, but the Kveim test using sarcoidal lymph node tissue is positive after several weeks. The total blood serum protein is high and ranges from 7.5 to 10.0 Gm. per cent due mainly to an increase in the globulin fraction.

Differential Diagnosis. The other *granulomatous diseases,* particularly *secondary or tertiary syphilis,* can be ruled out by biopsy and other appropriate studies.

Silica granulomas are histologically similar, but a history of such injury can usually be obtained.

Treatment. Time appears to cure or cause remission of most cases of sarcoidosis, but corticosteroids and calciferol are indicated for extensive cases.

Syphilology

(Plates 2A, 19, 20 and 21)

CHAPTER **13**

THE TERM "Syphilology" is being dropped from its long-term association with "Dermatology." The reason for this is simple: untreated syphilis is now seen only rarely. When I was stationed at the West Virginia State Rapid Treatment Center from 1946 to 1948 our average admittance was 30 patients a day with venereal disease. Approximately one third of these patients had infectious syphilis. In 1949 the Center was closed because of the low patient census. As a result of this dramatic and rewarding decline in the incidence of syphilis, many responsible physicians feel that we have prematurely lowered our guard, and syphilis will loom again as a formidable disease. While I do not believe this blow will come, it is still very important for all physicians to have a basic understanding of this polymorphous disease.

Our index of suspicion regarding syphilis must remain high in all fields of medicine. Syphilis is the great imitator and can mimic many other conditions. Cutaneous lesions of syphilis occur in all 3 stages of the disease.

Under what circumstances will the present-day physician be called upon to diagnose, evaluate, or manage a patient with syphilis? (1) The cutaneous manifestations may bring a patient to the office, such as a penile lesion or a rash that could be secondary syphilis. (2) A positive blood test found on a premarital examination or as part of a routine physical examination may be responsible for a patient's being seen by the physician. (3) Cardiac, central nervous system or other organ disease may be a reason for a patient's consulting a doctor.

To manage these patients properly a thorough knowledge of the natural *untreated* course of the disease is essential.

PRIMARY SYPHILIS

This first stage of acquired syphilis usually develops within 2 to 6 weeks (average 3 weeks) after exposure. The *primary chancre* most commonly occurs on the male or female genitalia, but extragenital chancres are not rare and are often misdiagnosed (Fig. 55). Without treatment the chancre heals within 1 to 4 weeks, depending on the location, the amount of secondary infection, and host resistance. The blood serologic test for syphilis (STS) may be negative in the early days of the chancre but eventually becomes positive. A spinal fluid examination during the primary stage reveals invasion of the spirochete in approximately 25% of cases. Clinically, the chancre may vary in appearance from a single small erosion to multiple indurated ulcers of the male or female genitalia. Primary syphilis commonly goes unnoticed in the female. Bilateral or unilateral regional lymphadenopathy is common. Malaise and fever may or may not be present.

Early Latent Stage

Latency, manifested by a positive serology and no other subjective or objective evidence of syphilis, may occur between the primary and the secondary stages.

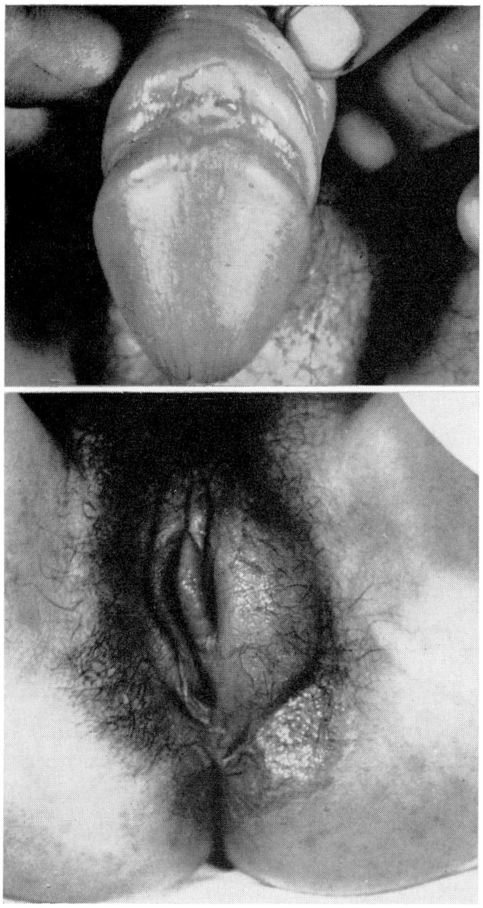

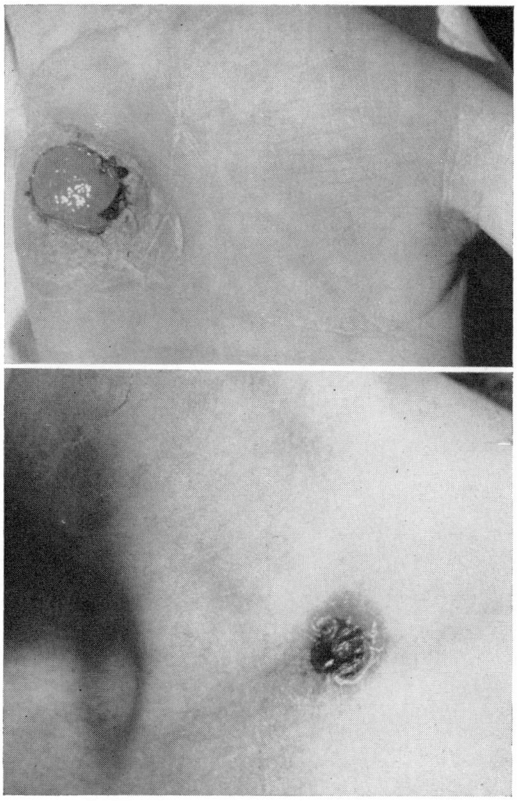

Fig. 55. Primary syphilis.

(*Left, top*) Penile chancre.
(*Left, bottom*) Vulvar chancre with edema of the labia majora.
(*Right, top*) Chancre of the palm.
(*Right, bottom*) Chancre over the clavicle.

SECONDARY SYPHILIS

Early secondary lesions (Fig. 56) may develop before the primary chancre has healed or after a latent period of a few weeks.

Late secondary lesions (Figs. 57 and 58) are more rare and usually are seen after the early secondary lesions have healed. Both types of secondary lesions contain the spirochete, *Treponema pallidum,* which can be easily seen with the darkfield microscope. The STS is positive, and approximately 30% of the cases have abnormal spinal fluid findings. Clinically, the early secondary rash can consist of macular, papular, pustular, squamous, or eroded lesions or combinations of any of these lesions. The entire body may be involved or only the palms and the soles, or the mouth, or the genitalia.

Condylomata lata is the name applied to the flat, moist, warty lesions teeming with spirochetes found in the groin and the axillae. The late secondary lesions are nodular, squamous and ulcerative and are to be distinguished from the tertiary lesions only by the time interval after the onset of infection and by the finding of the spirochete in superficial smears of serum from the lesions. Annular and semi-

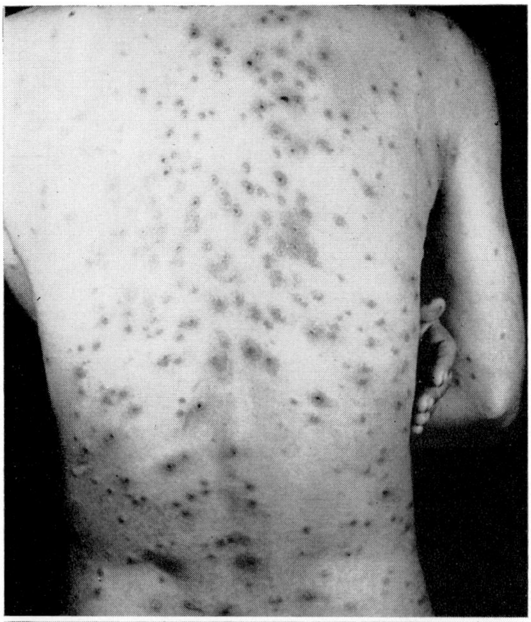

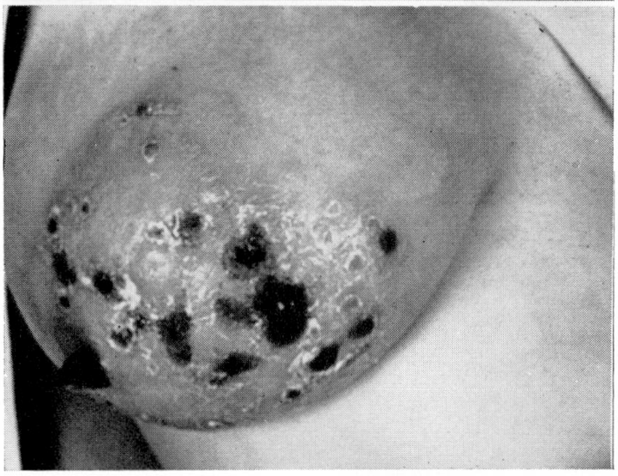

annular configurations of late secondary lesions are common. Generalized lymphadenopathy, malaise, fever and arthralgia occur in many patients with secondary syphilis.

Early Latent Stage

Following the secondary stage, many patients with untreated syphilis have only a positive STS. After 4 years of infection the patient enters the late latent stage.

Late Latent Stage

This time level of 4 years arbitrarily divides the early infectious stages from the later noninfectious stages which may or may not develop.

TERTIARY SYPHILIS

This late stage is manifested by subjective or objective involvement of any of the organs of the body, including the skin. Tertiary changes may be precocious but most often develop 5 to 20 years after the onset of the primary stage. Clinically, the skin lesions are characterized by nodular and gummatous ulcerations (Fig. 59). Solitary or multiple annular and nodular lesions are commonly seen. Subjective complaints are rare unless considerable

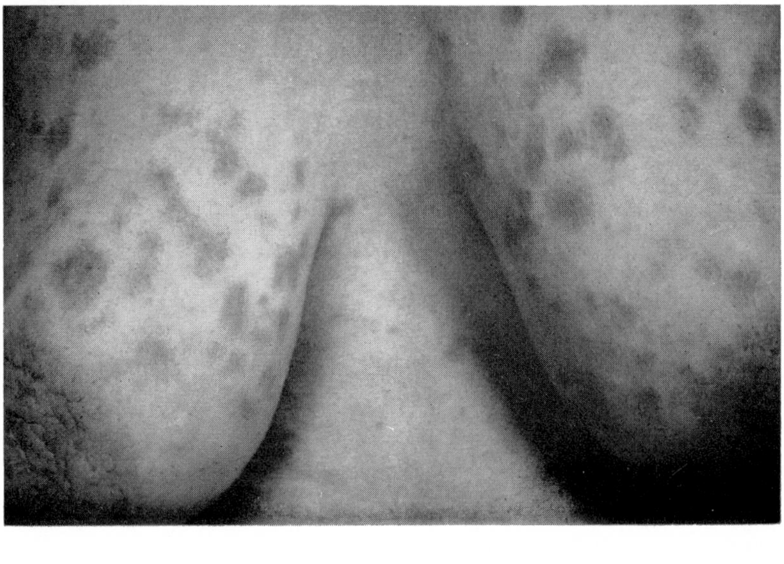

Fig. 56. Secondary syphilis.

(*Top*) Papulosquamous lesions on back.

(*Center*) Primary and secondary lesions on breast.

(*Bottom*) Macular lesions on breasts.

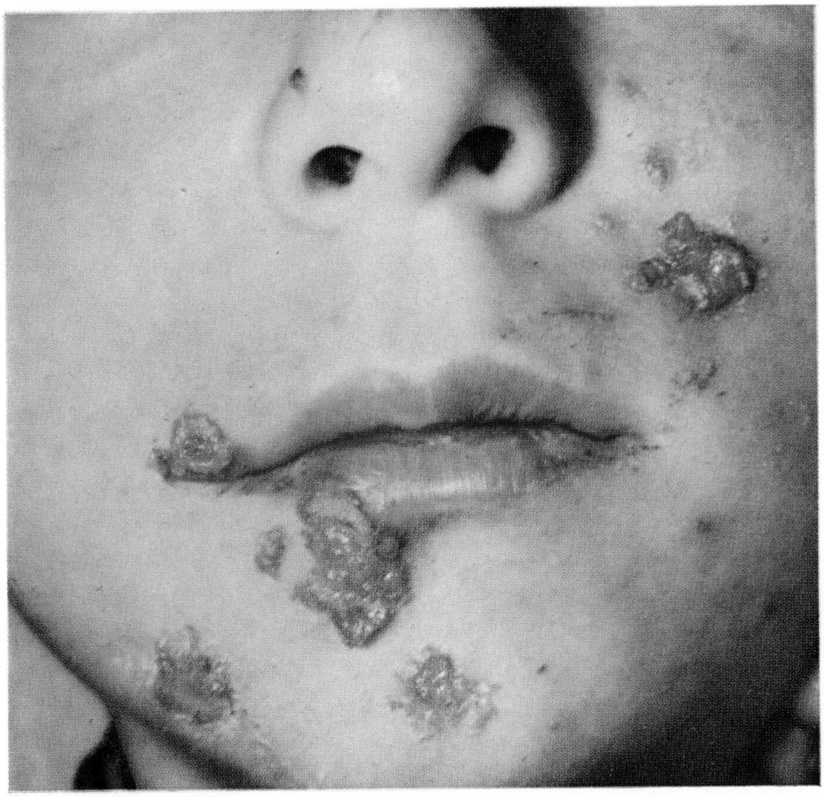

Plate 14. Impetigo of the face.

The honey-colored crusts are very typical.
(From the late Abner Kurtin: Folia Dermatologica, No. 2, Geigy Pharmaceuticals)

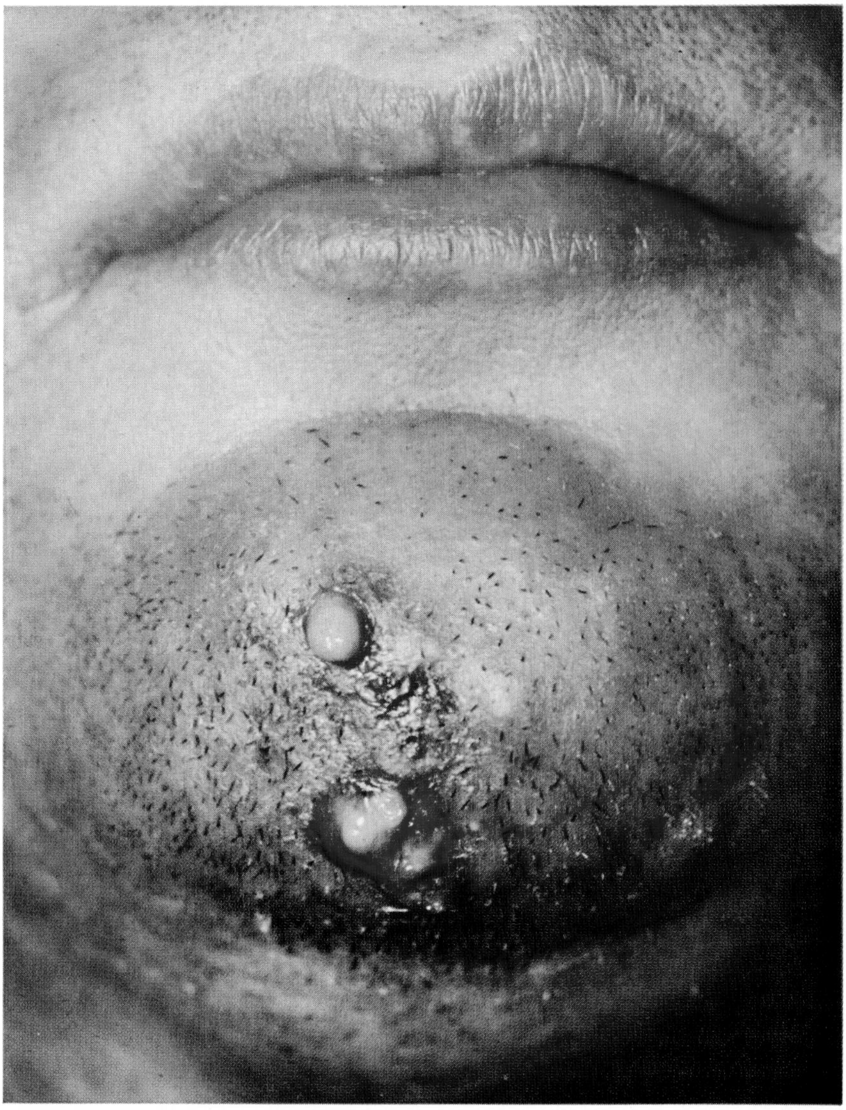

Plate 15. Carbuncle on the chin.

Notice the multiple openings.
(From the late Abner Kurtin: Folia Dermatologica, No. 2, Geigy Pharmaceuticals)

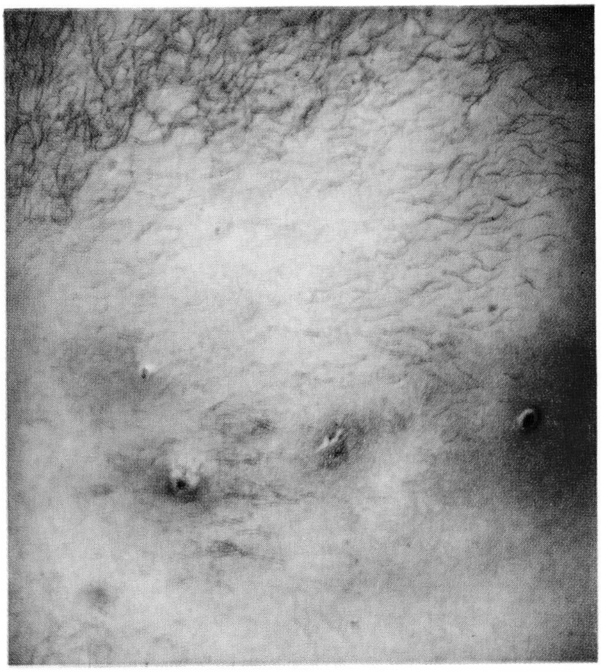

Plate 16. Multiple furuncles (boils) on the chest.

(From the late Abner Kurtin: Folia Dermatologica, No. 2, Geigy Pharmaceuticals)

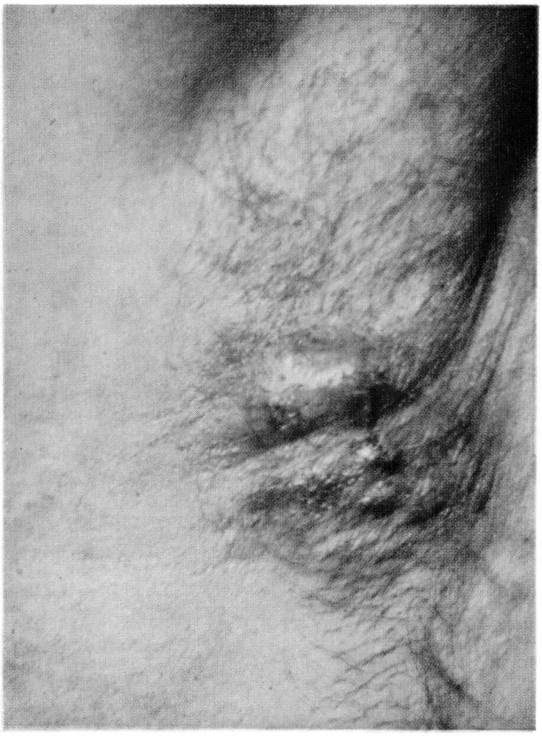

Plate 17. Sweat gland infection of the axilla (hidradenitis suppurativa).

(From the late Abner Kurtin: Folia Dermatologica, No. 2, Geigy Pharmaceuticals)

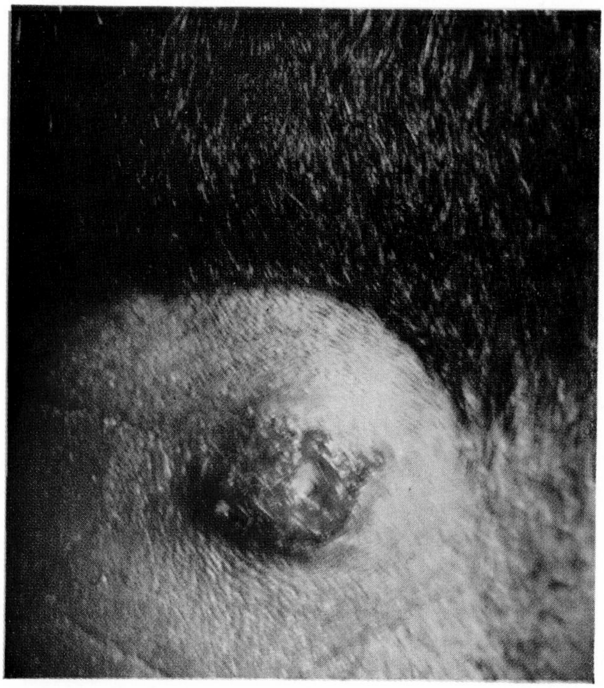

Plate 18. Carbuncle of the back of the neck.

(From J. Lamar Callaway: Folia Dermatologica, No. 4, Geigy Pharmaceuticals)

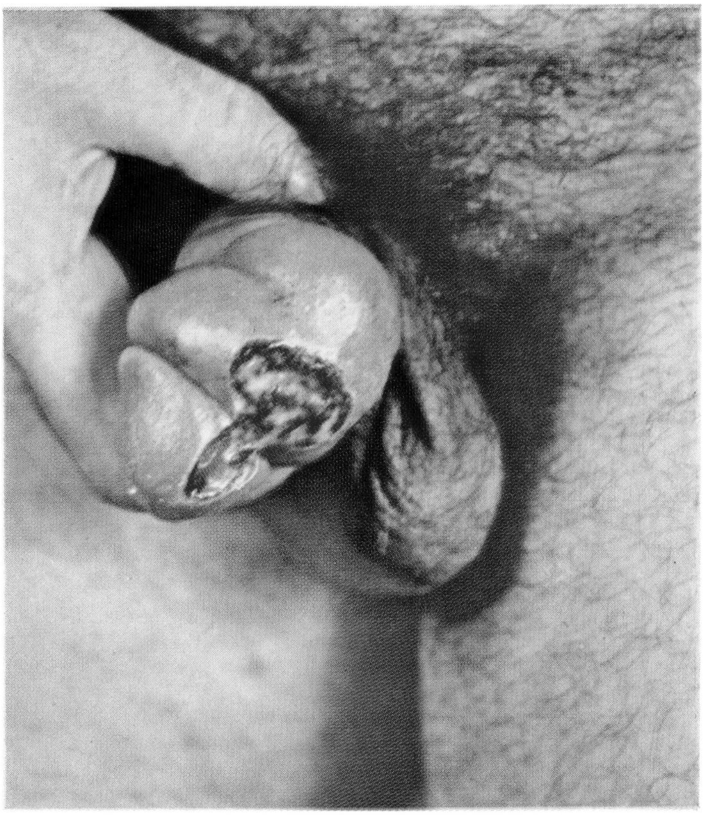

Plate 19. Primary syphilis with a chancre of the penis.

This chancre is accompanied by marked edema of the penis.
(From the late J. E. Moore and The Upjohn Company)

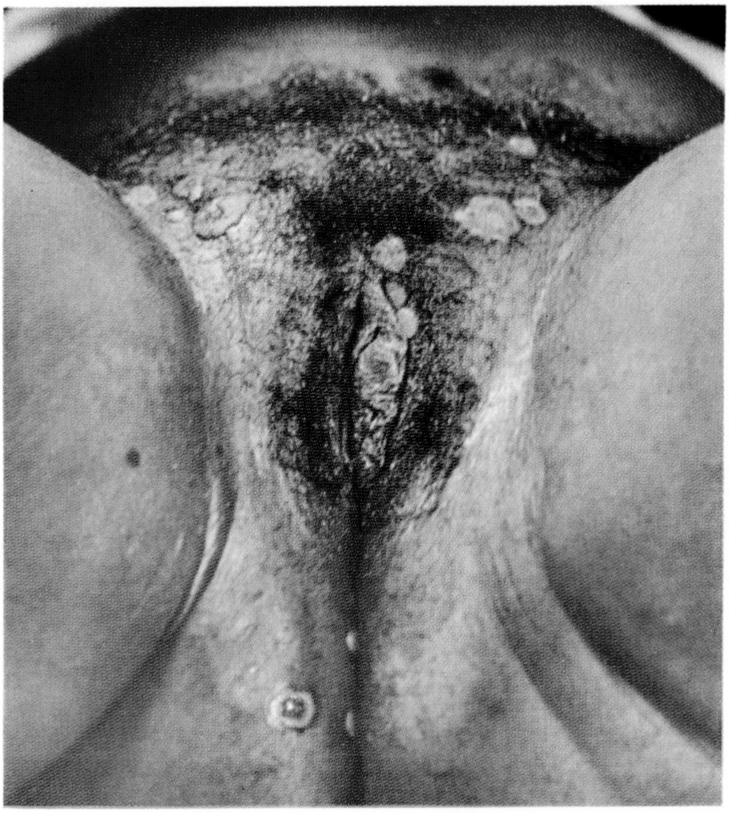

Plate 20. Secondary syphilis with condyloma lata of the vulva.

(From the late J. E. Moore and The Upjohn Company)

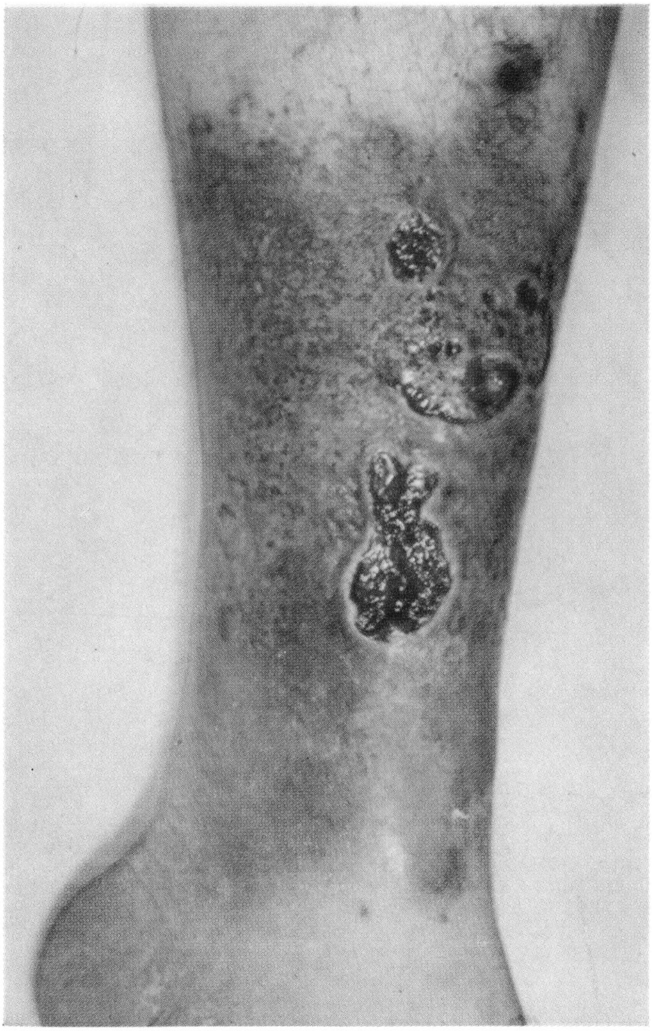

Plate 21. Tertiary syphilis with a gumma of the leg.

This resembles a stasis ulcer.

(*From the late J. E. Moore and The Upjohn Company*)

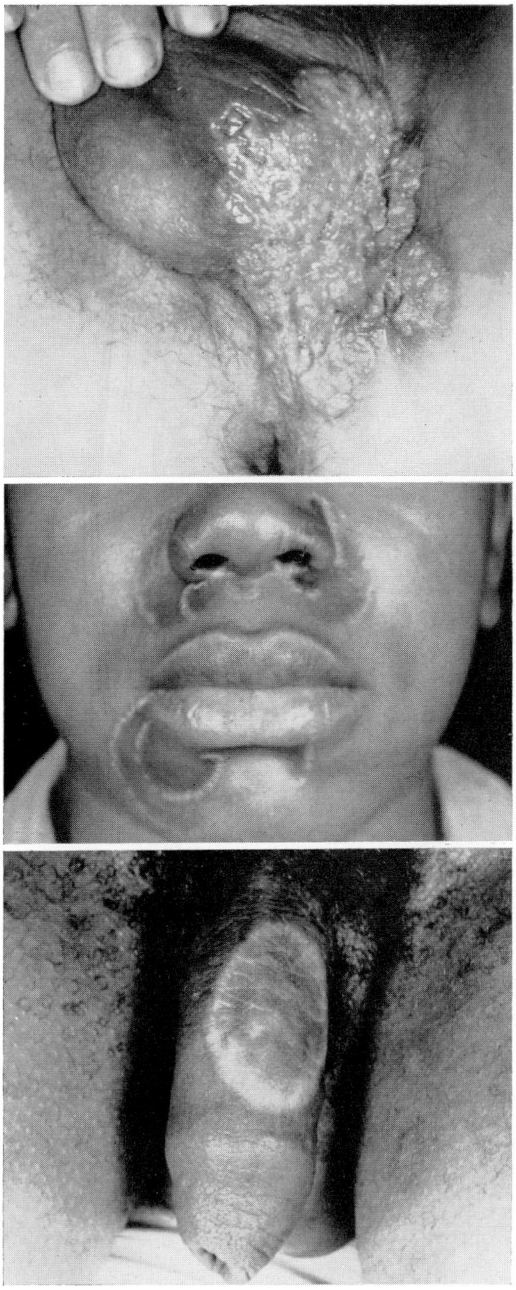

Fig. 57. Late secondary syphilis.

(*Top*) Condyloma lata of crural area.
(*Center*) Annular lesions on face of Negro.
(*Bottom*) Annular lesion on penis of Negro.

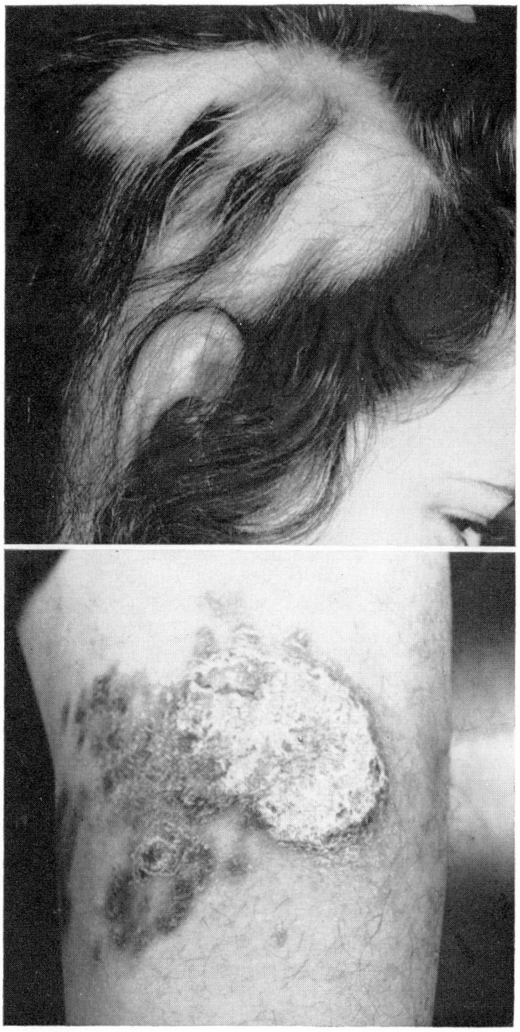

Fig. 58. Late secondary syphilis.

(*Top*) Patchy alopecia of the scalp.
(*Bottom*) Psoriatic-type lesions of the leg.

secondary bacterial infection is present in a gumma. Scarring on healing is inevitable in the majority of the tertiary skin lesions. Larger texts should be consulted for the late changes seen in the central nervous system, the cardiovascular system, the bones (Fig. 60 A), the eyes and the viscera. Approximately 15% of the patients who acquire syphilis and receive no treatment die of the disease.

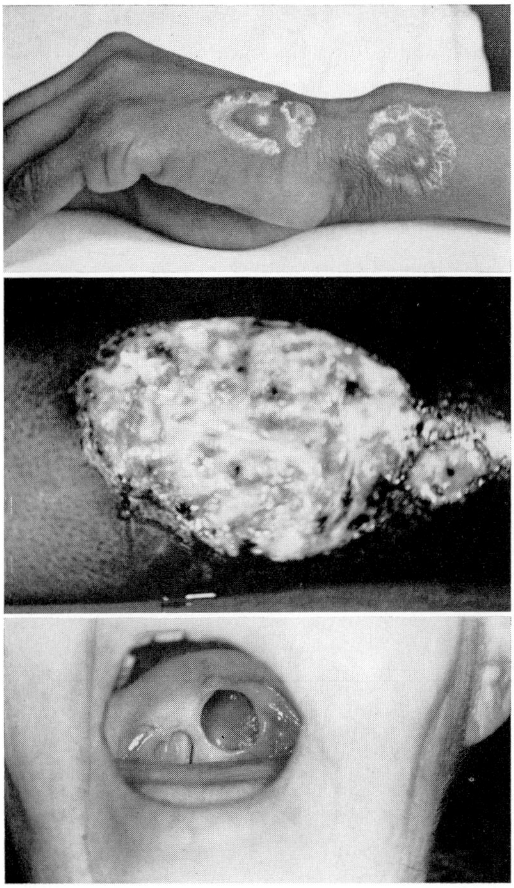

Fig. 59. Tertiary skin syphilis.
(*Top*) Annular nodular lesions on arm of Negro.
(*Center*) Gumma on leg of Negro.
(*Bottom*) Perforation of soft palate due to healed gumma.

Late Latent Stage

Another latent period may occur after natural healing of some types of benign tertiary syphilis.

CONGENITAL SYPHILIS

This is syphilis acquired in utero from an infectious mother (Fig. 60 B). The STS required of pregnant women by most states has lowered the incidence of this unfortunate disease. Stillbirths are not uncommon from mothers who are un-

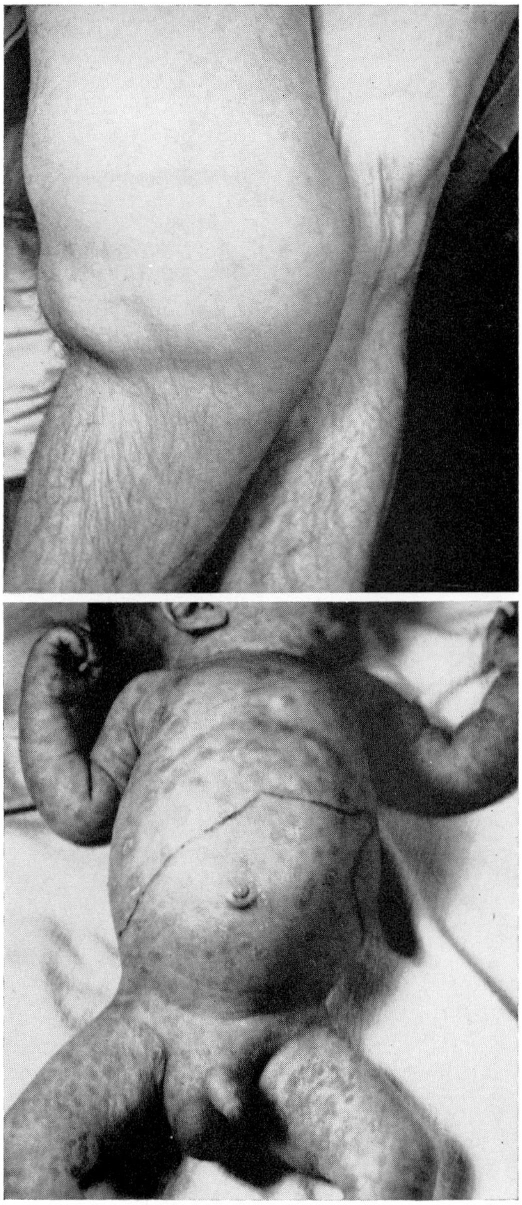

Fig. 60. Syphilis
(*Top*) Charcot knee joint of patient with tabes.
(*Bottom*) Congenital syphilis. Note skin lesions and enlarged liver and spleen.

treated. After the birth of a live infected child, the mortality rate depends on the duration of the infection, natural host resistance, and the rapidity of initiating correct treatment. Early and late lesions are seen in these children similar to those found in the adult cases of acquired syphilis.

LABORATORY FINDINGS

Darkfield Examination

The etiologic agent, *Treponema pallidum,* can be found in the serum from the primary or secondary lesions. However, a darkfield microscope is necessary, and very few doctor's offices or laboratories have this instrument. A considerable amount of experience is necessary to distinguish *T. pallidum* from other *Treponema.*

Serologic Test for Syphilis

A rather simple and readily available test is the serologic test for syphilis (STS), of which there are several modifications. The flocculation tests (VDRL, Kahn and others) are used most commonly. The complement-fixation test (Kolmer modification of Wassermann) and the *Treponema pallidum-immobilizing* antibody test (TPI test) and modifications are more difficult to perform in the laboratory and therefore are used less frequently.

When a report is received from the laboratory that the STS is positive (VDRL reactive, Kahn positive, etc.), a second blood specimen should be submitted to obtain a *quantitative* report. In some laboratories this repeat test is not necessary, since a quantitative test is run routinely on all positive blood specimens. The use of the terms "2 plus" or "4 plus" is outdated and has been replaced by the more accurate measurement of the positivity by titers. A "4 plus" specimen may be positive in a dilution of 1:2, which is only weakly positive and might be a biologic false-positive reaction, or it might be positive in a dilution of 1:32, which is strongly positive. In evaluating the response of the STS to treatment, remember that a change in titer from 1:2 to 1:4 to 1:16 to 1:32 to 1:64, or downward in the same gradations, is only a change in one tube in each instance. Thus a change from 1:2 to 1:4 is of the same magnitude as a change from 1:32 to 1:64. Quantitative tests enable the physician to (1) evaluate the efficacy of the treatment, (2) discover a relapse before it becomes infectious, (3) differentiate between a relapse and a reinfection, (4) establish a reaction as a seroresistant (Wassermann-fast) type and (5) differentiate between true and biologic false-positive serologic reactions.

Spinal Fluid Test

As has been stated, the spinal fluid is frequently positive in the primary and the secondary stages of the disease. Invasion of the central nervous system is an early manifestation, even though the perceptible clinical effects are a late manifestation. The spinal fluid should be examined at least once during the course of the disease. The best routine is to perform a spinal fluid test before treatment is initiated and repeat the test as indicated. If the spinal fluid is negative in a patient who has had syphilis for 4 years, central nervous system syphilis will not occur, and future spinal fluid tests are not necessary. If the test is positive, repeat tests should be done every 6 months for 4 years.

The following 5 tests are run on the spinal fluid:

1. **Cell Count.** The finding of 9 or more lymphocytes or polymorphonuclear leukocytes is positive. The cell count is the most labile of the tests and becomes increased early in the infection and responds fastest to therapy. Therefore, it is a good index to activity of the disease.

The cell count must be done within an hour after the fluid is withdrawn.

2. **Globulin or Pandy Test.** This qualitative protein test is positive in most cases of central nervous system syphilis.

3. **Total Protein.** When measured in mg. per cent, it normally should be below 40.

4. **Colloidal Gold.** Ten tubes are used, and in each tube the reactivity of the colloid varies from 0 to 5. A positive test shows reactivity from 2 to 5. Thus 0001111000 is negative, and 0001233321 is positive.

5. **Complement-Fixation Test.** This is the most reliable test and should be done in dilutions of 1.0, 0.5, 0.25 and 0.1 cc. This test is the last to turn positive and the slowest to return to negativity. In some cases therapy causes a decrease in the titer, but slight positivity or "fastness" can remain for the lifetime of the patient.

DIFFERENTIAL DIAGNOSIS

Primary syphilis from chancroid, herpes simplex, fusospirochetal balanitis, granuloma inguinale, and any of the primary chancre-type diseases (see index).

Secondary syphilis from any of the papulosquamous diseases, fungus diseases, drug eruption and alopecia areata.

Tertiary skin syphilis from any of the granulomatous diseases, particularly tuberculosis, leprosy, sarcoidosis, deep mycoses and lymphoblastomas.

Congenital syphilis from atopic eczema, diseases with lymphadenopathy, hepatomegaly and splenomegaly.

A true-positive syphilitic serology is to be differentiated from a biologic false-positive reaction. This serologic differentiation is accomplished best by using the *Treponema pallidum-immobilizing* antibody test or its modifications, when available, along with a good history and a thorough examination of the patient. Many patients with biologic false-positive reactions develop one of the collagen diseases at a later date.

TREATMENT

A 22-year-old married male has a 1 cm. diameter sore on his glans penis of 5 days' duration. Three weeks previously he had extramarital intercourse, and 10 days prior to this office visit he had marital intercourse.

First Visit

1. Perform a darkfield examination of the penile lesion. Treatment can be started if *Treponema pallidum* is found. If this examination is not available, then
2. Obtain a blood specimen for a serologic test for syphilis (STS).
3. While waiting for the STS report, advise the patient to soak the site in saline solution for 15 minutes twice a day. The solution is made by placing ¼ teaspoon of salt in a glass of water.
4. Advise against sexual intercourse until the reports are completed.
5. Explain to the patient the seriousness of treating him for syphilis if he does not have it. The "syphilitic" label is one he should not want if at all possible.

Second Visit

Three days later. The lesion is larger, and the STS report is "VDRL nonreactive, Kahn negative."

1. Obtain blood for a second STS.
2. Neosporin ointment 5.0
   Sig: Apply t.i.d. locally after soaking in saline solution.
3. Explain again why you are delaying therapy until a definite diagnosis is made.

Third Visit

Three days later. The sore is smaller, but the STS report is "VDRL reactive, Kahn 1:4." The diagnosis is now known to be "Primary Syphilis."

1. Reassure the patient that present-day therapy is highly successful, but he must follow your instructions closely.
2. His wife should be brought in for examination and a blood test. If the blood test is negative, it should be repeated

weekly for 1 month. However, some syphilologists believe that therapy is indicated for the marital partner in the face of a negative STS if the husband has infectious syphilis and is being treated. A single injection of 1.2 million units of a long-acting type of penicillin is used. This will prevent "ping-pong" syphilis, which is a cycle of reinfection from one marital partner to another.

3. The patient's contact should be found. The patient knows her only as "Jane," and he cannot remember over which bar she presided. Report these findings to the local Health Department.

4. A spinal fluid specimen should be obtained. (The report was returned as normal for all 5 tests.)

5. Penicillin therapy should be begun, remembering that two factors are important: (1) the dose must be adequate, and (2) the duration of effective therapy must be over a period of 10 to 14 days.

Dosage

Primary, Secondary, Early and Late Latent, and Benign Tertiary Syphilis: 600,000 or 1,200,000 units of a long-acting penicillin every 2 to 3 days for a total of 6,000,000 units.

Neurosyphilis or Cardiovascular Syphilis: A total of 9,000,000 units of a long-acting penicillin. For complicated cases, consult larger texts for therapy and care.

Congenital Syphilis: 100,000 units of penicillin per pound of body weight given twice weekly for 1 to 2 weeks. It is impractical to give smaller doses than 150,000 units in each dose. After the age of 6, or 60 pounds in weight, adult schedules should be used.

Syphilis Pearls

General

1. Any patient treated for gonorrhea should be given 1,200,000 U. of a long-acting penicillin and have a serologic test for syphilis (STS) 4 to 6 weeks later.

2. 75% of the people who acquire syphilis suffer no serious manifestations of the disease.

3. Syphilis does not cause vesicular or bullous skin lesions, except in infants with congenital infection.

Primary Stage

1. Syphilis should be ruled in or out in the diagnosis of any penile or vulvar sores.

2. Multiple primary chancres are moderately common.

Secondary Stage

1. The rash of secondary syphilis, except for the rare follicular form, does not itch.

2. Secondary syphilis should be ruled in or out in any patient with a generalized, nonpruritic rash. A high index of suspicion is necessary.

Latent Stage

The diagnosis of "latent syphilis" cannot be made for a particular patient unless spinal fluid tests have been done and are negative for syphilis.

Tertiary Stage

1. Tertiary syphilis should be considered in any patient with a chronic granuloma of the skin, particularly if it has an annular or circular configuration.

2. Invasion of the central nervous system occurs in the primary and the secondary stages of the disease. A spinal fluid test is indicated during these stages.

3. If the spinal fluid tests for syphilis are negative in a patient who has had syphilis for 4 years, central nervous system syphilis will not occur, and future spinal punctures are not necessary.

4. 20% of patients with late asymptomatic neurosyphilis have negative STS's.

Congenital Syphilis

A STS should be done on every pregnant woman to prevent congenital syphilis of the newborn.

Serology

1. The serologic test for syphilis may be negative in the early days of the primary chancre. The STS is always positive in the secondary stage.

2. A quantitative STS should be done on all syphilitic patients to evaluate the response to treatment or the development of relapse or reinfection. To label reactions as "2 plus" or "4 plus" is not now acceptable.

3. The finding of a low-titre STS in a patient not previously treated for syphilis calls for a careful evaluation to rule out a biologic false-positive reaction.

Dermatologic Virology*

CHAPTER 14

VIRUS diseases of the skin are exceedingly common. The various clinical entities are distinct, and, since we have no specific antiviral drug, the treatment varies for each entity. The following list contains the virus diseases that will be discussed. The exanthems of children will be covered in a cursory manner.

1. Herpes simplex
2. Kaposi's varicelliform eruption
3. Zoster
4. Chickenpox
5. Smallpox, vaccinia and cowpox
6. Warts
7. Molluscum contagiosum
8. Lymphogranuloma venereum
9. Exanthematous diseases: measles, German measles, roseola and erythema infectiosum.

HERPES SIMPLEX
(Plate 22 A)

Herpes simplex (fever blister) is an acute, moderately painful, viral eruption of a single group of vesicles that commonly occurs around the mouth or the genitalia (Fig. 61). The commonest type of herpes simplex is the *recurrent form* seen in adults. An uncommon *primary form* of herpes simplex affects children and young adults. In this primary form, the vesicular lesions involve the mouth and the pharynx or vaginal and vulvar areas. High fever, regional lymphadenopathy and general malaise accompany the painful sores.

The following discussion refers to the common *recurrent form* of herpes simplex.

Primary Lesions. A group of vesicles.

Secondary Lesions. Erosions and secondary bacterial infection.

Distribution. Lips, mouth, genital region of both males and females (herpes progenitalis), eye (marginal keratitis or corneal ulcer), or any body area.

Course. The vesicles last for 2 to 3 days before the tops come off. The residual erosions or crusted lesions last for another 5 to 7 days. Recurrences are common in the same area.

Etiology. Caused by a relatively large virus. Certain precipitating factors are important in producing the recurrent eruptions. These factors, which include fever, common cold, sunlight, psychic influences, stomach upsets and trauma, apparently activate a dormant phase of the virus in the cells.

Contagiousness. This can occur through intimate contact. Kaposi's varicelliform eruption is a severe example (see p. 124).

Laboratory Findings. The virus may be easily isolated from the lesions, but this is not an office procedure. A biopsy is characteristic, and neutralizing antibodies in the blood show an increasing titer.

Differential Diagnosis

OF MOUTH LESIONS

Aphthous Stomatitis: see only 1 or 2

* An excellent book on this subject has been written by Blank, H., and Rake, G.: Viral and Rickettsial Diseases of the Skin, Eye and Mucous Membranes of Man, Boston, Little, 1955.

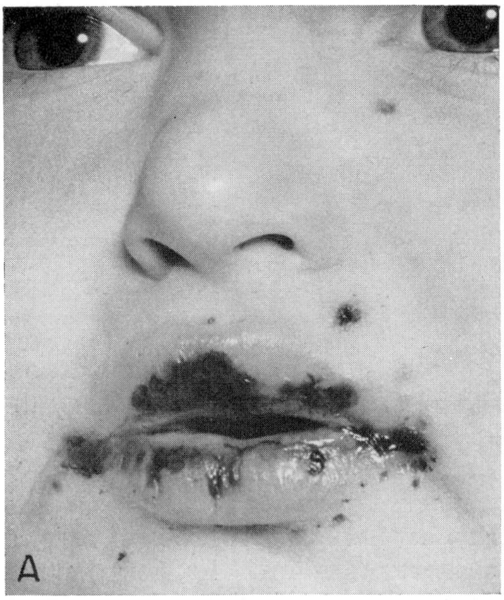

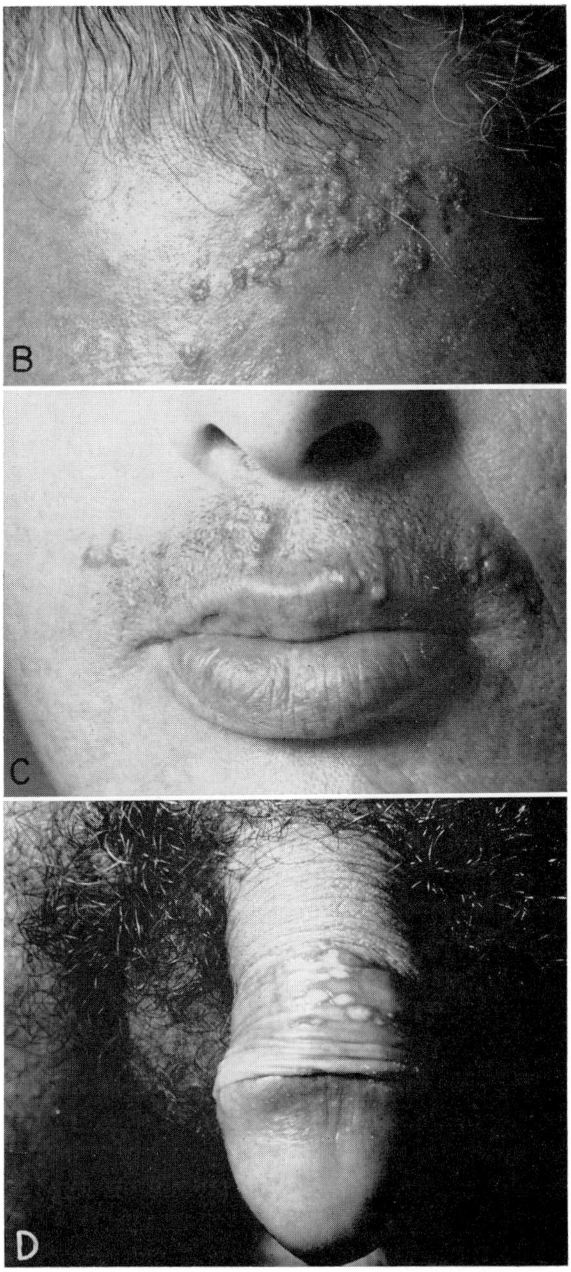

Fig. 61. Herpes simplex.

A. Primary herpes simplex gingivostomatitis of 2-year-old boy. (K.C.G.H.)
B. Recurrent herpes simplex on the forehead of an adult, initiated by a sunburn.
C. Herpes simplex in a common location on the lips, concurrent with pneumonia.
D. Herpes simplex on the penis.

painful eroded lesions, recurrent, not caused by herpes simplex virus.

OF BODY LESIONS

Zoster: see more than one group of vesicles, nerve segment distribution, not recurrent at same site, different virus (p. 124).

Tinea of Body: early vesicular case can be clinically indistinguishable from herpes, later see central healing in tinea, fungus grown from scraping or culture (p. 143).

OF GENITAL LESIONS

Primary Syphilis: can be clinically

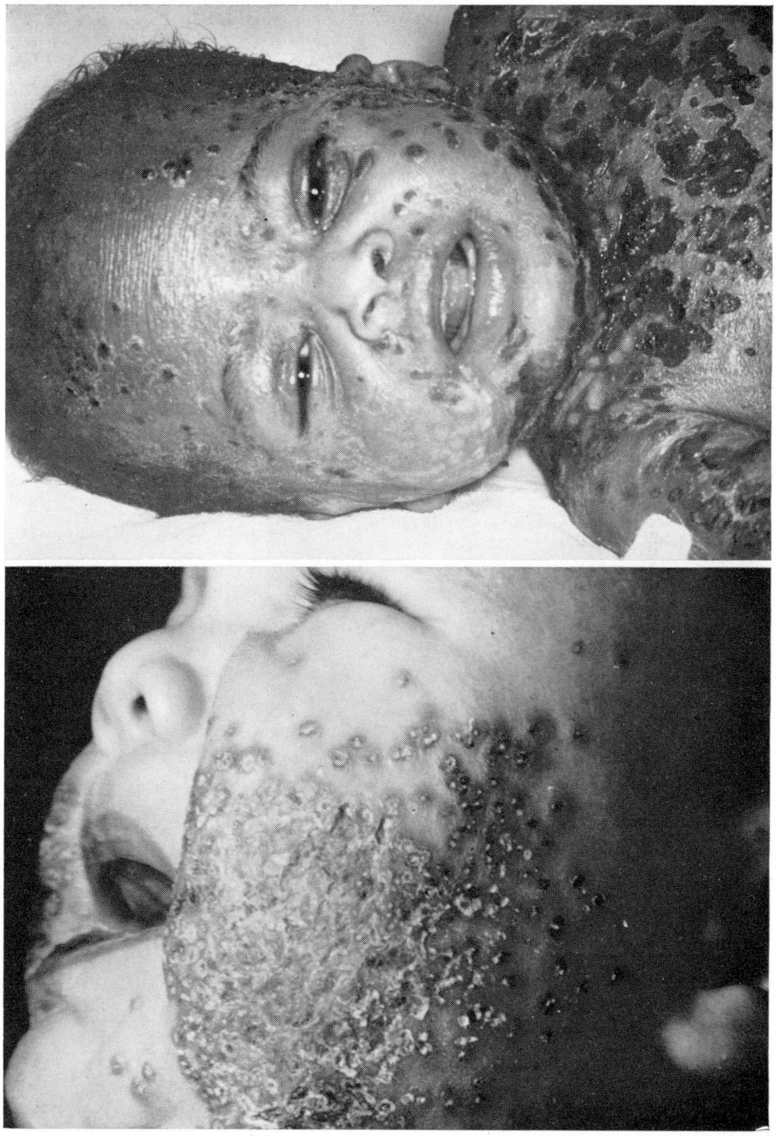

Fig. 62. Kaposi's varicelliform eruption.

(*Top*) In a 6-month-old Negro girl with atopic eczema following accidental inoculation with the vaccinia virus. (K.U.M.C.)
(*Bottom*) In a child with atopic eczema inoculated with the herpes simplex virus.

similar to herpes simplex, history of illicit or extramarital intercourse, not recurrent usually, darkfield examination is definitely indicated and would be positive, but this test is rarely available (p. 112).

Treatment. Young woman with fever blisters on lower lip that have recurred every 2 or 3 months for the past 2 years.

1. Inform the patient that no specific treatment is available to shorten the natural course of the infection.

2. Neo-Polycin or other antibiotic ointment, q.s. 5.0
   Sig: Apply locally t.i.d.

This benefits by relieving the pain and the inflammation.

3. Smallpox vaccination
   Sig: Repeat once a week for 6 weeks. If a "take" occurs, delay the next vaccination until it heals.

The benefit of this therapy is presumably due to a nonspecific protein effect.

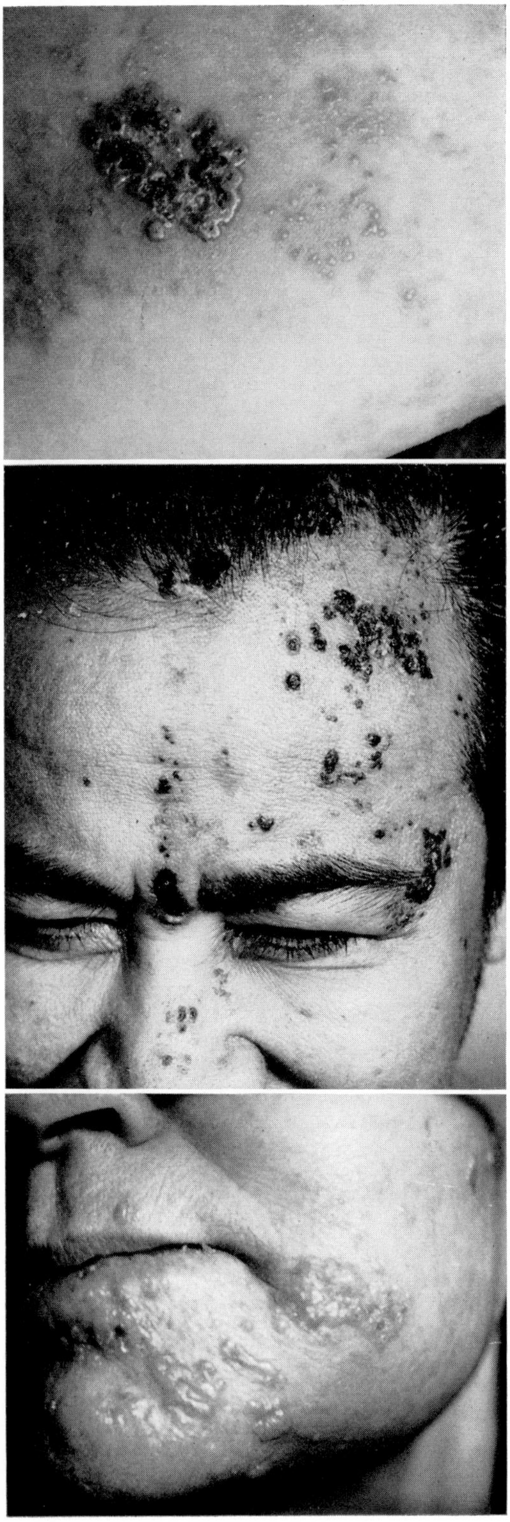

Fig. 63. Zoster.

(*Top*) Grouped vesicles of zoster on the thigh of a 21-month-old child.
(*Center*) Zoster of the ophthalmic branch of the trigeminal nerve. Note sharp mid-line demarcation on forehead. (K.C.G.H.)
(*Bottom*) Zoster of the mandibular branch of the trigeminal nerve.

KAPOSI'S VARICELLIFORM ERUPTION

This virus disease is an uncommon but severe complication of children who have atopic eczema. It results from self-inoculation by scratching, due to the virus of either herpes simplex or vaccinia (Fig. 62). In the former type a history of exposure to fever blisters may or may not be obtained. With the vaccinia form a history of vaccination of the child or the sibling is commonly obtained. With either type, the child is acutely ill, has a high fever and has generalized umbilicated chickenpoxlike skin lesions. Supportive therapy consists of antibiotics systemically, intravenous infusions, and a nonalcoholic white shake lotion locally. Systemic corticosteroid therapy should not be given in the early stage of the disease but may be given later. Gamma globulin injections may be beneficial.

ZOSTER

Shingles is a common viral disease characterized by the appearance of several groups of vesicles distributed along a cutaneous nerve segment (Fig. 63). Zoster and chickenpox are thought to be caused by the same virus. Susceptible children who are exposed to cases of zoster often develop chickenpox. Less commonly, older individuals exposed to chickenpox may get zoster.

Primary Lesions. Multiple groups of vesicles or crusted lesions.

Secondary Lesions. Bacterial infection with pustules, rarely progressing to gangrenous ulcers and scarring.

Distribution. Unilateral eruption following a nerve distribution, frequently in the thoracic region, the face, the neck and less frequently the lumbosacral area and elsewhere. Eye involvement can be serious. Bilateral involvement of the body is rare but not fatal, contrary to the old wives' tale.

Course. New crops of vesicles can appear for 3 to 5 days. The vesicles then dry up and form crusts which take 3 weeks on the average to disappear. The general health is seldom affected except for low-grade fever and malaise. Recurrences are rare. The postherpetic pain can persist for months in aged patients.

Subjective Complaints. Pain of a neuritic type can precede the eruption and, if in the abdominal area, can lead to erroneous diagnoses and surgical procedures. The common simple pain of young persons with shingles is readily treated and soon disappears. On the other hand, the severe true postherpetic pain of older patients can be very serious. In order to evaluate critically the therapeutic response to the many agents said to relieve this severe pain, *a nerve distribution pain should not be labeled as the true postherpetic type unless it has been present for over 30 days.* If this strict criterion is adhered to, many newly proclaimed treatments for such pain will be found to be of limited value.

Etiology. Caused by a virus similar to the one that causes chickenpox. Trauma is thought to play a role in development of some cases of shingles. "Nervousness" plays little if any role.

Contagiousness. The interrelationship between shingles and chickenpox has been referred to above.

Laboratory Findings. Isolation and identification of the virus is not an office procedure.

Differential Diagnosis

OF THE NEURITIC-TYPE PAIN THAT PRECEDES THE SKIN LESIONS: *appendicitis, ureteral colic, sciatica, migraine, etc.*

OF THE ERUPTION: *herpes simplex* (see single group of vesicles, recurrence history, p. 121); *blistered burn from hot application for neuritic pain* (very commonly the patient really has shingles and erroneously attributes the blisters as due to the hot application for the preceding herpetic pain).

Treatment

1. Forty-year-old female with multiple grouped vesicles on right cheek and forehead, causing moderately severe pain.

A. Reassure the patient that shingles is not a serious disease and advise her not to believe what her well-meaning friends will tell her about the disease.

B. Supply the name of an ophthalmologist to consult to rule in or out eye complications.

C. Chlortetracycline (Aureomycin) 500 mg.
Alcoholic white shake lotion q.s. 60.0
Sig: Apply locally to skin b.i.d. (The Aureomycin is added to help prevent secondary infection.)

D. Empirin tablets #50
Sig: 1 tablet q.i.d. for pain.

E. Meprobamate tablets, 200 mg. #30
Sig: 1 tablet q.i.d. (For the anxious apprehensive patient.)

2. Seventy-year-old male patient with severe postherpetic pain of 5 weeks' duration.

A. Acthargel, 80 units. Inject subcutaneously on the first visit and repeat in 2 days if necessary.

B. Hydrocortisone tablets, 20 mg. #20
Sig: 1 tablet t.i.d. for 4 days then decrease dose slowly as symptoms subside.
C. Tuinal capsule, 50 mg. #10
Sig: 1 capsule h.s. for sleep.
D. For resistant cases, consult larger texts for additional therapy.

CHICKENPOX

This common viral disease of childhood is characterized by the development of tense vesicles first on the trunk and then spreading to a milder extent to the face and the extremities, appearance of new crops of vesicles for 3 to 5 days, and healing of the individual lesions in a week. The disease occurs 10 to 14 days after exposure to another child with chickenpox or to an adult with zoster. The clear vesicle becomes a pustule, then a crusted lesion before dropping off. Itching is more prominent during the healing stage.

Treatment

1. Usually nothing indicated, or
2. Menthol 0.25%
   Nonalcoholic white shake lotion q.s. 120.0
   Sig: Apply locally t.i.d. for itching.
3. Benadryl elixir 60.0
   Sig: 1 tsp. t.i.d. for moderately severe itching.

SMALLPOX

Smallpox is an uncommon viral disease characterized by the development, after an incubation period of 1 to 3 weeks, of prodromal symptoms of high fever, chills and various aches. After 3 to 4 days a rash develops with lowering of the fever. The individual lesions are most extensive on the face and the extremities; they come out as a single shower and progress from papule to vesicle and in 5 to 10 days to pustule. With the occurrence of the pustule the fever goes up again with a high white blood cell count. Hemorrhagic lesions usually indicate a severe form of the disease.

Alastrim is a mild form of smallpox resulting from a less virulent strain of the virus.

Varioloid is a mild form of smallpox which occurs in vaccinated individuals. However, this strain of virus is very virulent and when transmitted to a nonvaccinated person often causes a fulminating disease.

Severe systemic complications of smallpox include pneumonia, secondary bacterial skin infection and encephalitis.

Treatment. This consists of systemic antibiotics, parenteral infusions and locally applied white shake lotion containing an antibiotic.

Prophylactic treatment consists of vaccination. The best technic is by multiple puncture. *Never vaccinate a patient who has active atopic eczema; scratching of the vaccination can lead to development of Kaposi's varicelliform eruption.*

VACCINIA

Vaccinia is produced by the inoculation of the vaccinia virus into the skin of a person who has no immunity.

The *primary vaccination reaction* follows this timetable. The multiple puncture technic should be used. A red papule on a red base develops on the 4th day, becomes vesicular in 3 more days, pustular in 2 to 3 more days, and then gradually dries to form a crust which drops off within 3 to 4 weeks after the vaccination. A mild systemic reaction may occur during the pustular stage. The vaccination site should be kept dry and uncovered. Generalized vaccinia is rare but can occur from auto-inoculation by scratching in atopic eczema patients (see Kaposi's varicelliform eruption, p. 124). A biologic false-positive serologic test for syphilis develops in approximately 20% of vacci-

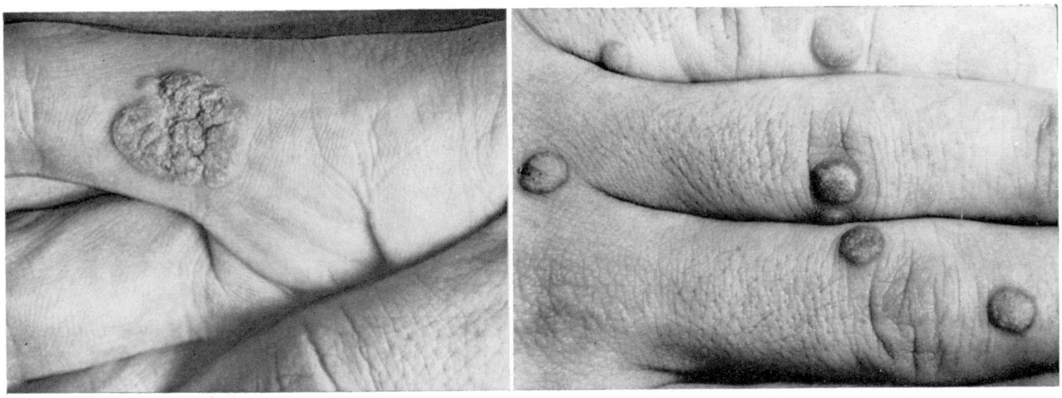

Fig. 64. Common warts on the hand.

nated persons. The test becomes negative within 2 to 4 months.

A *vaccinoid reaction* develops in a partially immune individual. A pustule with some surrounding redness occurs within 1 week.

An *immune reaction* consists of a papule that develops in 2 days which may or may not persist for 1 week.

An *absent reaction* indicates that the vaccine was inactivated by the procedure (alcohol used in cleaning the site, etc.), or that the vaccine was impotent.

A successful vaccination offers protection from smallpox within 3 weeks, and this immunity lasts for approximately 7 years.

COWPOX

Jenner used the cowpox virus to vaccinate humans against smallpox. For that reason, the vaccinia virus and the cowpox virus have been thought to be the same. Evidence now exists that proves these viruses to be different, presumably as a result of a change in the vaccinia virus through years of passage. The term "cowpox" is now reserved for the viral disease of cows that occurs in Europe. Man can get the disease from infected teats and udders. A solitary nodule appears, usually on the hand, which eventually suppurates and then heals in 4 to 8 weeks.

WARTS (VERRUCAE)
(Plate 22 B)

Warts or verrucae are very common small tumors of the skin. It is doubtful if any human escapes this viral infection. Warts have been played with for centuries, and cures have been attributed to burying a dead black cat in the graveyard at midnight and other such similar feats. The interesting fact is that these examples of psychotherapy do work. Physicians attempt the same type of therapy under more professional guise and are pleased but not surprised when such therapy is effective. Children, fortunately, are most amenable to this suggestion therapy. On the other hand, however, every physician is also familiar with the stubborn wart that has been literally blasted from its mooring in the skin but keeps recurring.

The various clinical types of warts relate to the appearance of the growth and to its location. The treatment varies somewhat for each type of wart and will be discussed separately for each type.

COMMON WART (FIG. 64)

The appearance is a papillary growth, slightly raised above the skin surface, varying from pinhead size to large clusters of pea-sized tumors. These warts are seen most commonly on the hands.

Rarely, they have to be differentiated from *seborrheic keratoses* (flatter, darker, velvety tumors of older adults, p. 221) and *pigmented verrucous nevi* (projections are not dry and rough to touch, longer duration, biopsy may be indicated, p. 227).

Treatment

1. Suggestion therapy can be attempted, particularly with children. One form of such therapy consists of the application by the doctor of a colored solution, such as podophyllum in alcohol, 25% solution. This has the added benefit of being a cell-destroying chemical.

2. Electrosurgery. Single warts in adults or older children are removed best by this method. The recurrence rate is minimal, and one treatment usually suffices. The technic is to cleanse the area, anesthetize the site with 1% procaine, destroy the tumor with any form of electrosurgery (see p. 39), snip off or curette out the dead tissue, and desiccate the base. Recurrences can be attributed to failure to remove the dead tissue and to destroy the lesion adequately to its full depth. No dressing should be applied. The site will heal in 5 to 14 days with only minimal bacterial infection and scar formation. Warts around the nails have a high recurrence rate, and cure usually requires removal of part of the overlying nail.

3. Salicylic acid 10%
   Flexible collodion q.s. 30.0
   Sig: Apply to warts cautiously every night for 5 nights out of 7. The dead tissue can be removed with scissors.

This type of treatment is applicable to the case with 20 or more warts on one hand. The purpose is to remove as many warts as possible in this manner over a period of several weeks. Any remaining warts can be removed by electrosurgery.

4. Bistrimate tablets #50
   Sig: 1 t.i.d., p.c. (Watch for gastric upset and check urine occasionally for albuminuria. Tell the patient that his stools will turn black.)

It is difficult to evaluate whether Bistrimate therapy orally is effective as a result of suggestion or as a result of the metallic bismuth. Nonetheless, in cases where many warts are present or recurrences have been common, occasionally this medication works.

Filiform Warts

These are warts with long fingerlike projections from the skin that most commonly appear on the eyelids, the face and the neck. They are to be differentiated from *cutaneous horns* (seen in elderly patients with senile keratosis or prickle cell epithelioma at the base; has a hard keratin horn, p. 213), and *pedunculated fibromas* (on the neck and the axillae of middle-aged men and women, p. 221).

Treatment

1. Snip off with scissors and apply acid. Without anesthesia, snip off the wart with a small scissors and apply trichloracetic acid solution (saturated) cautiously to the base. This is a fast and effective method, especially for children.

2. Electrosurgery. As above for common warts. An annoying variant of this type of wart is the case with multiple small *filiform warts of the beard area*. Electrosurgery without anesthesia is well tolerated and effective for these warts. However, in order to achieve a permanent cure, the patient should be seen again in 3 to 4 weeks to remove the young warts that are in the process of enlarging. The physician's job is to keep ahead of these warts and eliminate the reinfection that occurs from shaving.

Flat Warts

These small flat tumors are often barely visible but can occur in clusters of 10 to

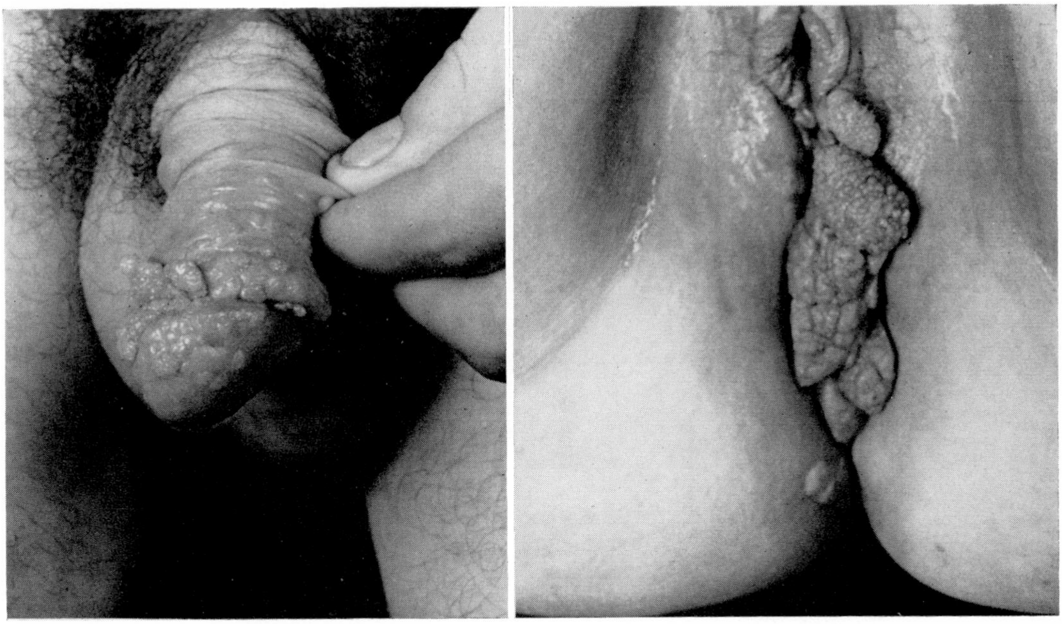

Fig. 65. Condyloma acuminata or moist warts.
(*Left*) Of the penis.
(*Right*) Of the vulva.

30 or more. They are commonly seen on the forehead and the dorsum of the hand and should be differentiated from small *seborrheic keratoses* or *nonpigmented nevi*.

Treatment

1. Suggestion therapy. This form of treatment is very effective for these warts in children. The following bland lotion has been used with excellent results:

Alcoholic white shake lotion q.s. 60.0

Sig: Apply to warts b.i.d.

2. Electrosurgery lightly. Some adult cases can exhaust your therapeutic modalities only to have the warts disappear with time.

Moist Warts (Condyloma Acuminata) (Fig. 65)

These are quite characteristic single or multiple, soft, nonhorny masses that appear in the anogenital areas and less commonly between the toes and the corners of the mouth. They are not always of a venereal nature.

Treatment

1. Podophyllum resin in alcohol (25% solution). Apply once to the warts cautiously. Second or third treatments are rarely necessary. To prevent excessive irritation, the site should be bathed within 6 hours after the application.

Plantar Warts (Fig. 66)

(This is the layman's "planter's warts" which I am sure they believe are related to "Planter's Peanuts.") As the name signifies, this wart occurs on the sole of the foot, is flat, extends deep into the thick skin and, on superficial trimming, reveals small pinpoint-sized bleeding points. Varying degrees of disability can be produced from the pressure type of pain. Single or multiple lesions can be present.

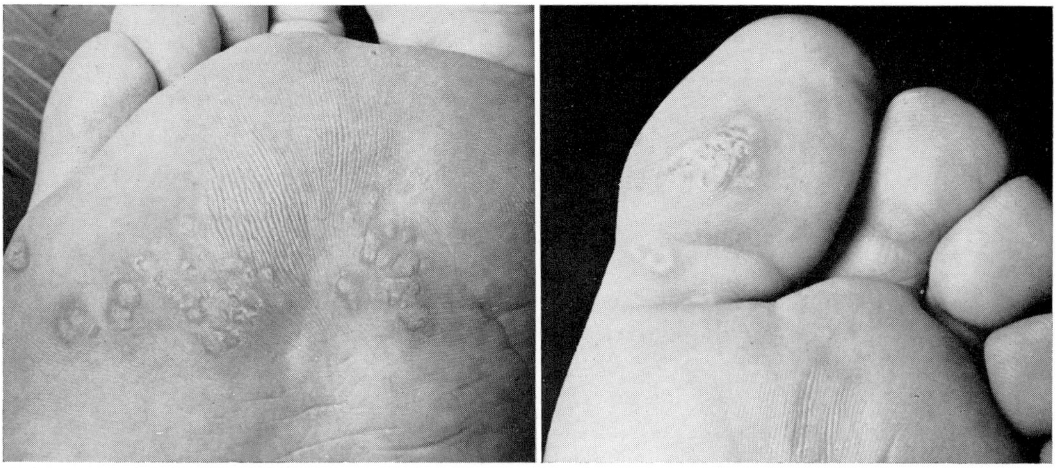

Fig. 66. Plantar warts.

(*Left*) Such a large number of warts should be treated with a peeling local agent and Bistrimate orally.
(*Right*) These warts can be removed by electrosurgery.

One of the most vexing problems in dermatology is the patient with half of the sole of a foot covered with these warts. Plantar warts are to be differentiated from a *callus* (no bleeding points visible on superficial trimming, and from *scar tissue from a previous treatment* (no bleeding points seen). *Never treat a plantar lesion as a wart until you have proved your diagnosis by trimming.*

Treatment

1. Electrosurgery. This is the simplest and most successful form of therapy for a single plantar wart. The procedure is the same as for common warts except that the downgrowth of the plantar wart is greater. The disadvantage of this type of treatment, as with any treatment except x-ray, is that healing takes from 3 to 4 weeks to be complete. Some bleeding is to be expected a few days after the surgery. Most patients do not complain of much pain during the healing stage.

2. Trichloracetic acid—tape technic. Useful for children and cases with multiple plantar warts. The procedure is as follows: pare down the wart with a sharp knife, apply trichloracetic acid solution (saturated) to the wart, then cover the area with plain tape. Leave the tape on for 5 days without getting it wet. The physician then removes the tape and curettes out the dead wart tissue. Usually, more wart will remain, and the procedure is repeated until the wart is destroyed. This course of treatment may take from 3 to 6 weeks. After the first 2 visits the site may become tender and secondarily infected. If the disability and the infection are severe, therapy should be stopped temporarily and hot soaks instituted.

3. X-ray therapy. This painless form of therapy can be used for single warts. Only a dermatologist or a radiologist should administer this treatment. Once x-ray therapy is given in the usual dose, which varies with the size of the wart, the dose never should be repeated to that site. The cure rate is fairly high.

MOLLUSCUM CONTAGIOSUM

This uncommon viral infection of the skin is characterized by the occurrence, usually in children, of one or multiple small skin tumors (Fig. 67).

Primary Lesion. An umbilicated, firm, waxy, skin-colored, raised papule varying in diameter from 2 mm. to 5 mm. and, rarely, larger.

Secondary Lesion. Inflamed from bacterial infection.

Distribution. Most commonly on trunk, face and arms but can occur anywhere.

Course. Onset of lesions is insidious, due to lack of symptoms. Trauma or infection of a lesion causes it to disappear. Recurrences are rare if lesions are removed adequately.

Contagiousness. Unusual.

Differential Diagnosis

Warts: no umbilication, not waxy (p. 127).

Keratoacanthoma: most commonly in older adults, larger lesion, biopsy characteristic (p. 220).

Basal Cell Epithelioma: in older adults, slow growing, biopsy characteristic (p. 214).

Treatment. A 6-year-old child has 10 small molluscum papules on his arms and upper trunk.

1. Curettement. Rapidly curette each lesion, apply pressure to stop bleeding, then apply bandage. A small amount of trichloracetic acid (saturated solution) on the broken pointed end of a swab stick helps to stop prolonged bleeding. Two or 3 visits may be necessary to treat recurrent lesions and new ones that have popped up.

2. Electrosurgery. Done lightly and rapidly, this is another effective method. It is not necessary to destroy the entire lesion as for a wart but only to induce some trauma and mild infection.

LYMPHOGRANULOMA VENEREUM

This uncommon venereal disease occurs mainly in Negroes and is characterized by a primary lesion on the genitals and secondary changes involving the

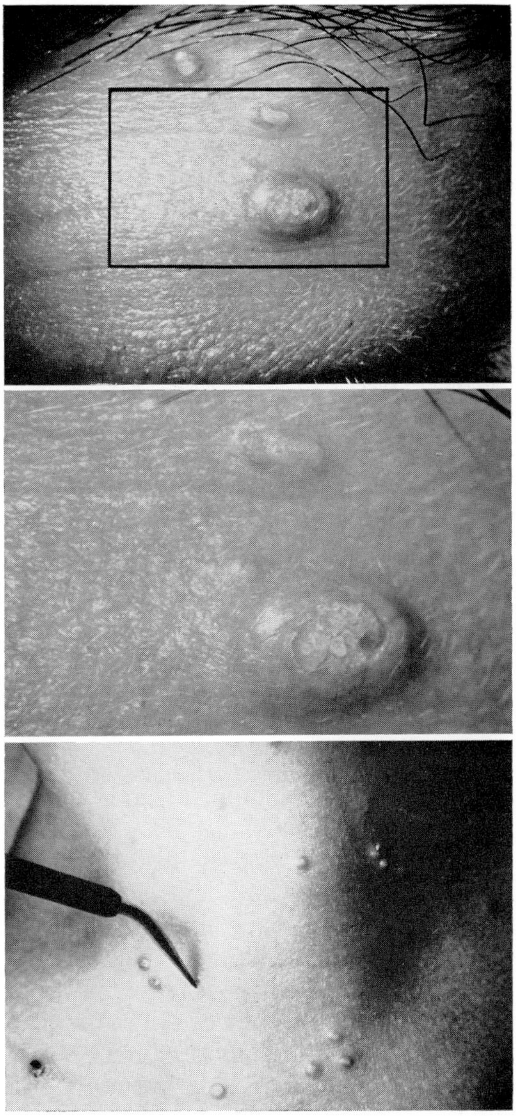

Fig. 67. Molluscum contagiosum.

(*Top*) Three molluscum contagiosum lesions on upper eyelid (Drs. Calkins, Lemoine and Hyde).

(*Center*) Close-up of area marked in top photograph (Drs. Calkins, Lemoine and Hyde).

(*Bottom*) Demonstrating the use of electrosurgery in treating multiple lesions on the neck and the shoulder.

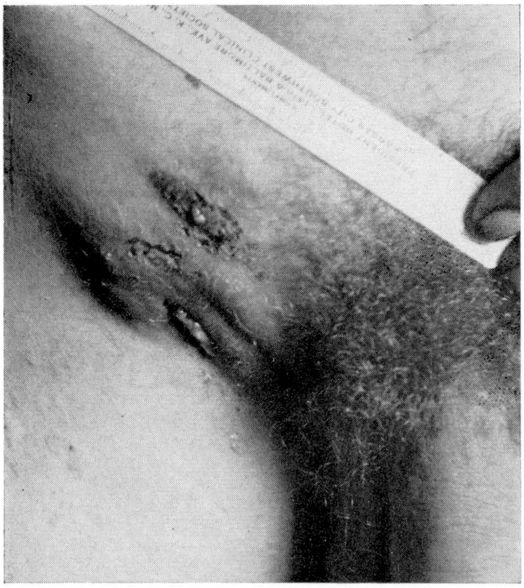

Fig. 68. Lymphogranuloma venereum, showing lymph node involvement.
(*Dr. T. B. Hall.*)

draining lymph channels and glands (Fig. 68).

The primary erosion or blister is rarely seen, especially on the female. Within 10 to 30 days after exposure the inguinal nodes, particularly in the male, enlarge unilaterally. This inguinal mass may rupture if treatment is delayed. In the female the lymph drainage most commonly is toward the pelvic and perirectal nodes, and their enlargement may be overlooked. Low-grade fever, malaise and generalized lymphadenopathy frequently occur during the adenitis stage. Scarlatinalike rashes and erythema nodosum lesions also may develop. The later manifestations of lymphogranuloma venereum occur as the result of scarring of the lymph channels and fibrosis of the nodes. These changes result in rectal stricture, swelling of the penis or the vulva, and ulceration.

Etiology. Lymphogranuloma venereum is caused by one of the chlamydozoaceae, *Miyagawanella lymphogranulomatis,* which is related to the rickettsiae. Previously, the organism was classified as a "large" virus.

Diagnostic Skin Test. The Frei intradermal test is positive in any patient who has had the disease for 3 weeks. The test is performed by injecting 0.1 cc. of the antigen (Lygranum, Squibb) and 0.1 cc. of the control material intradermally. The reaction is of the delayed tuberculin-type. To be positive the papule should exceed 6 mm. in diameter within 48 hours (the surrounding zone of erythema is not important), and the control site should not exceed 3 mm.

Treatment. Sulfonamides, chlortetracycline (Aureomycin), and oxytetracycline (Terramycin) are effective in the early stages when continued for several weeks.

MEASLES

A very common childhood disease. The characteristic points are as follows. The incubation period averages 14 days before the appearance of the rash. The prodromal stage appears around the 9th day after exposure and consists of fever, conjunctivitis, running nose, Koplik spots and even a faint red rash. The Koplik spots measure from 1 to 3 mm. in diameter, are bluish white on a red base and occur bilaterally on the mucous membrane around the parotid duct and on the lower lip. With increasing fever and cough the "morbilliform" rash appears, first behind the ears and on the forehead, then spreads over face, neck, trunk and extremities. The fever begins to fall as the rash comes out. The rash is a faint reddish, patchy eruption, occasionally papular. Scaling occurs in the end stage. Complications consist of secondary bacterial infection and encephalitis.

Differential Diagnosis

German Measles: postauricular nodes,

milder fever and rash, no Koplik spots (see below).

Scarlet Fever: circumoral pallor, rash brighter red and confluent (p. 106).

Drug Eruption: history of new drugs, usually no fever (p. 55).

Infectious Mononucleosis: rash similar, see characteristic blood picture, high titer of heterophile antibodies.

Treatment

Prophylactic. Gamma globulin can be administered to prevent the infection by giving large doses within 6 days after exposure. Modification of the disease, which is usually most desired, can be produced by giving a smaller dose with a longer time interval after exposure.

Active. Supportive therapy for the cough, bed rest, and protection from bright light are measures for the active disease. The antibiotics have eliminated most of the bacterial complications. Corticosteroids are of value for the rare but serious complication of encephalitis.

GERMAN MEASLES

While this is a benign disease of children, it is serious if it develops in a pregnant woman during the first trimester, since it causes anomalies in a low percentage of newborns.

The incubation period is around 18 days and, as with measles, there may be a short prodromal stage of fever and malaise. The rash also resembles measles since it occurs first on the face and then spreads. However, the redness is less intense, and the rash disappears within 2 to 3 days. Enlargement of the cervical and the postauricular nodes is a characteristic finding. Serious complications are rare.

Differential Diagnosis

Measles: see Koplik spots, the fever and the rash are more severe, no postauricular nodes (p. 132).

Scarlet Fever: has high fever, perioral pallor, rash may be similar (p. 106).

Drug Eruption: get new drug history, usually no fever (p. 55).

Treatment. Usually unnecessary. Gamma globulin given to a pregnant woman in the first trimester might prevent malformations in the unborn child.

ROSEOLA

This is a common exanthem of children of 6 to 18 months of age. The incubation period is 10 days, but a contact history is rarely helpful. Characteristically, there is a high fever up to 105° for 4 to 5 days. With the appearance of the rash the fever and the malaise subside. The rash is mainly on the trunk as a faint red macular eruption. It fades in a few days. There are no severe complications.

Differential Diagnosis. Measles, German measles, scarlet fever, infectious mononucleosis and drug eruption.

Treatment. Not necessary except to reduce the high fever.

ERYTHEMA INFECTIOSUM

Also known as fifth disease, this exanthem occurs in epidemics and is thought to be caused by a virus.

It affects children primarily, but in a large epidemic many cases are seen in adults. In the Kansas City epidemic of the Spring of 1957 over 1,000 cases occurred, and this description is based on personal observation of that epidemic.

The incubation period varies from 1 to 7 weeks. In children the prodromal stage lasts from 2 to 4 days and is manifested by low-grade fever and occasionally joint pains. When the red macular rash develops it begins on the arms and the face and then spreads to the body. The rash in children is measleslike on the body, but on the face it looks as though the cheeks had been slapped. On the arms and the legs the rash is more red and confluent on the extensor surfaces. A low-grade fever persists for a few days after the onset of the rash, which lasts for approximately 1 week.

In adults the rash on the face—the "slap"—is less conspicuous, joint complaints are more common, and itching is present.

Etiology. A virus etiology has not been proved.

Differential Diagnosis

Drug Eruption (p. 55)

Measles (coryza, eruption begins on face and behind ears, p. 132)

Other Measleslike Eruptions

Treatment. Not necessary.

Dermatologic Mycology*

CHAPTER 15

FUNGI can be present as part of the normal flora of the skin or as abnormal inhabitants. We are concerned with the abnormal inhabitants or pathogenic fungi.

Pathogenic fungi have a predilection for certain body areas; most commonly it is the skin, but the lungs, the brain and other organs can be infected. Pathogenic fungi can invade the skin *superficially* and *deeply* and are thus divided into these two groups.

SUPERFICIAL FUNGUS INFECTIONS

The superficial fungi live on the dead horny layer of the skin and elaborate an enzyme that enables them to digest keratin, causing the superficial skin to scale and disintegrate, the nails to crumble, and the hairs to break off. The deeper reactions of vesicles, erythema and infiltration are presumably due to the fungi liberating an exotoxin. Fungi are also capable of eliciting an allergic or "id" reaction.

It will be necessary to define a few mycologic terms before proceeding further. When a skin scraping, a hair or a culture growth is examined with the microscope in a wet preparation (see p. 9 and Fig. 6) the two structural elements of the fungi will be seen: the spores and the hyphae.

Spores are the reproducing bodies of the fungi. Sexual and asexual forms occur. Spores are rarely seen in skin scrapings.

Hyphae are threadlike, branching, filaments that grow out from the fungus spore. The hyphae are the identifying filaments seen in skin scrapings in potassium hydroxide (KOH) solution.

Mycelia are matted clumps of hyphae that grow on culture plates.

Culture media vary greatly in context, but modifications of Sabouraud's dextrose agar are used to grow the superficial fungi (Fig. 7). Sabouraud's agar and cornmeal agar are both used for the deep fungi. Hyphae and spores grow on the media, and identification of the species of fungi is established by the gross appearance of the mycelia, the color of the substrate, and the microscopic appearance of the spores and the hyphae when a sample of the growth is placed on a slide.

CLASSIFICATION

The latest classification divides the superficial fungi into three genera: *Microsporum, Epidermophyton* and *Trichophyton.* Only two of these species invade the hair: *Microsporum* and *Trichophyton.* As seen in a KOH preparation *Microsporum* causes an ectothrix infection of the hair shaft, whereas *Trichophyton* causes either an ectothrix or an endothrix infection. The ectothrix fungi cause the formation of an external spore sheath around the hair, whereas the endothrix fungi do not. The filaments or mycelia penetrate the hair in both types of infection.

* An excellent book on this subject has been written by Conant, N. F., Smith, D. T., Baker, R. D., Callaway, J. L., and Martin, D. S.: Manual of Clinical Mycology, ed. 2, Philadelphia, Saunders, 1954.

TABLE 1—RELATIONSHIP OF FUNGI TO BODY AREAS

	Feet and Hands	Nails	Groin	Smooth Skin	Scalp	Beard
Microsporum						
1. *M. audouini*	0	0	0	Mod. common	Common	0
2. *M. canis*	0	0	0	Common	Mod. common	Rare
3. *M. gypseum*	0	0	0	Rare	Rare	0
Epidermophyton						
E. floccosum	Mod. common	Rare	Common	Mod. common	0	0
Trichophyton						
1. Endothrix species						
a. *T. schoenleini*	0	Rare	0	Rare	(Favus) rare	0
b. *T. violaceum*	0	Rare	0	0	Rare	Rare
c. *T. tonsurans*	0	Rare	0	Rare	Mod. common	0
2. Ectothrix species						
a. *T. mentagrophytes*	Common	Mod. common	Common	Rare	Rare	Mod. common
b. *T. rubrum*	Common	Common	Mod. common	Rare	0	Rare
c. *T. verrucosum*	0	0	0	Rare	Rare	Rare

Table 1 correlates the species of fungi with the clinical diseases. The organism causing tinea versicolor is not included in this table because it does not liberate a keratolytic enzyme.

Clinically, the treatment of a fungus infection varies according to the site that is involved. Therefore, the fungus diseases are classified as to the location of the dermatitis. These clinical types are as follows:

Tinea of the feet and the hands (Tinea pedis and manus)

Tinea of the nails (Onychomycosis)

Tinea of the groin (Tinea cruris)

Tinea of the smooth skin (Tinea corporis)

Tinea of the scalp (Tinea capitis)

Tinea of the beard (Tinea barbae)

Dermatophytid

Tinea versicolor (see p. 90)

Tinea of the external ear (see External Otitis, p. 63)

TINEA OF THE FEET AND THE HANDS (Plate 23)

Tinea of the feet is a very common skin infection, whereas tinea of the hands is uncommon. The clinical appearance and treatment of both conditions is the same (Figs. 69 and 70).

Primary Lesions. Acute: blisters on the soles and the palms or between the toes and the fingers. Chronic: lesions are dry and scaly.

Secondary Lesions. Bacterial infection of the blisters very common; also maceration and fissures.

Course. Recurrent acute infections can lead to chronic infection. If the nails become infected, a cure is highly improbable, since this focus is very difficult to irradicate.

The species of fungus determines the response to therapy. Most vesicular, acute fungus infections are due to *Trichophyton*

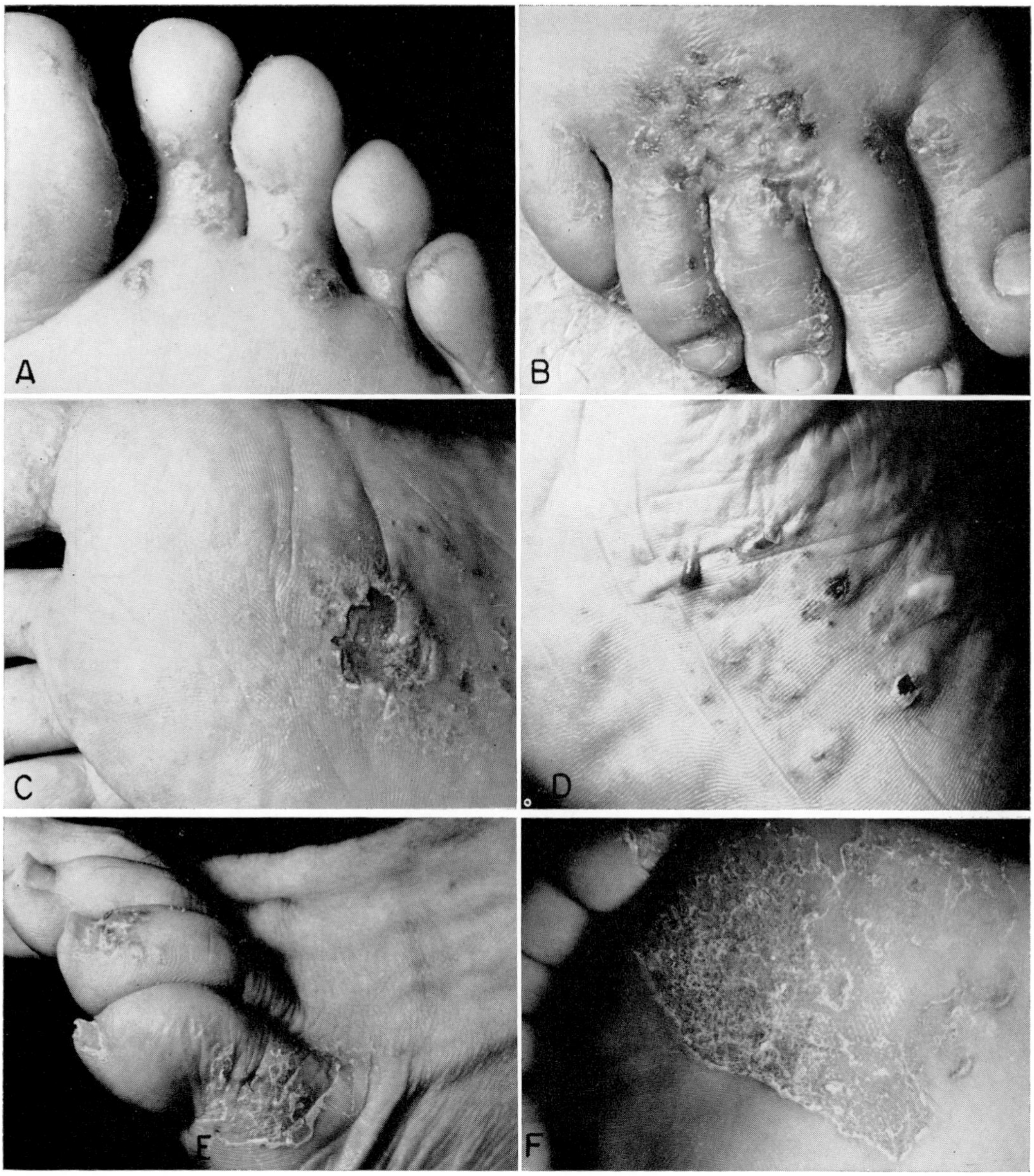

Fig. 69. Tinea of the foot.

The top 4 photographs demonstrate acute infection, and the bottom 2 show chronic tinea infection.

mentagrophytes and respond readily to correct treatment. The chronic scaly type of infection is usually due to *T. rubrum* and is exceedingly difficult, if not impossible, to cure.

Contagiousness. Experiments have shown that there is a susceptibility factor necessary for infection. Children and adult females are only slightly susceptible and seldom become infected, even when exposed.

Laboratory Findings. KOH prepara-

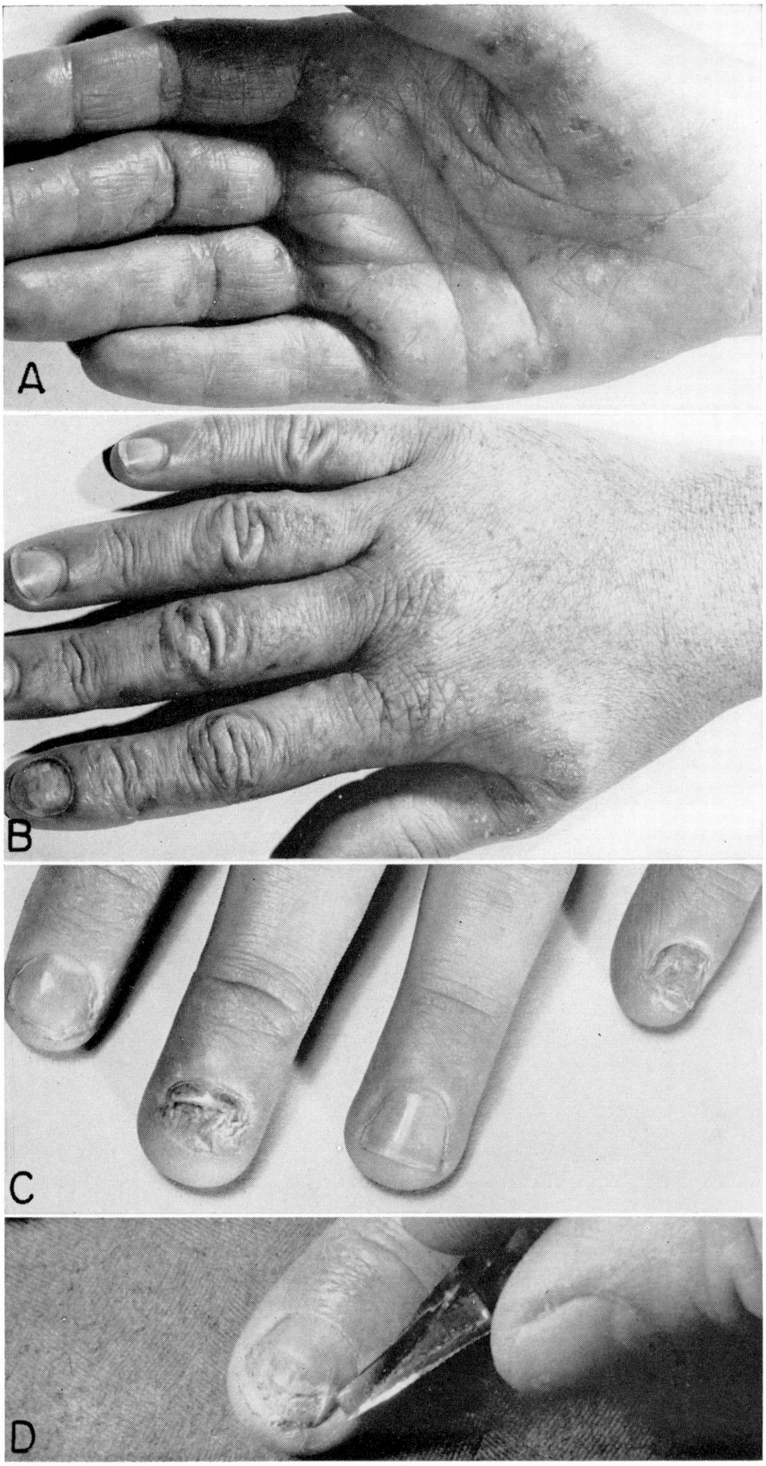

Fig. 70. Tinea of the hand and the nails.

(A) *T. rubrum* infection of palm of hand. Note blisters at the sharp border of the infection. See Figure 71 B for buttocks of same patient. (K.U.M.C.)

(B) Dorsum of hand in Figure A. Note involvement of nail of index finger. (K.U.M.C.)

(C) *T. rubrum* infection of fingernails.

(D) Demonstration of use of piece of glass for débridement of infected nail.

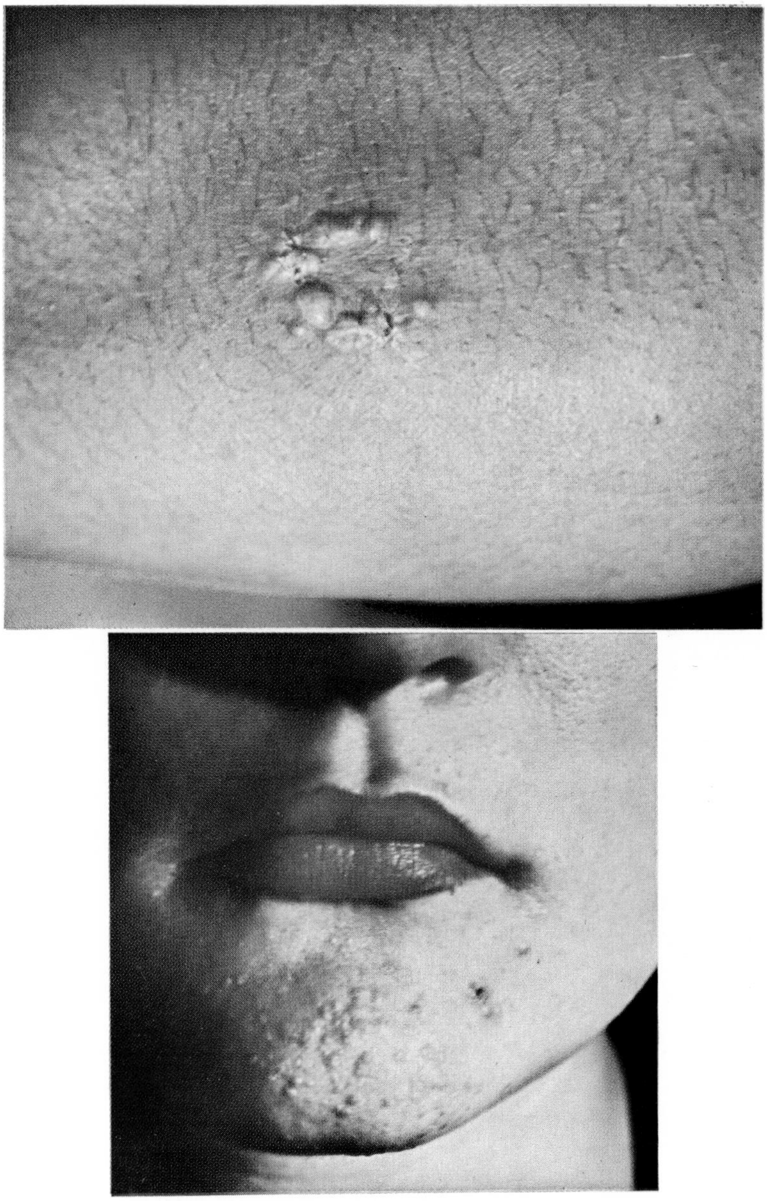

Plate 22. Dermatologic virology.

A. Herpes simplex on the forearm. (K.U.M.C.)

B. Flat warts on the chin. (K.U.M.C.)

(E. R. Squibb & Sons)

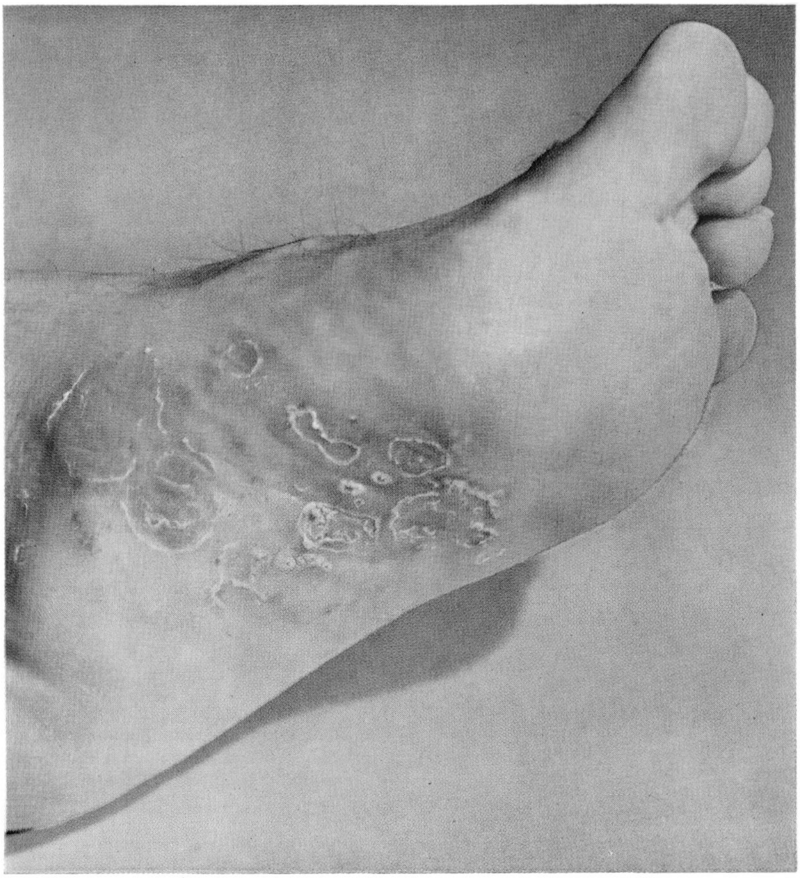

Plate 23. Tinea of the foot.

This dry scaly form of fungus infection is usually due to *T. rubrum*.

(Smith, Kline & French Laboratories)

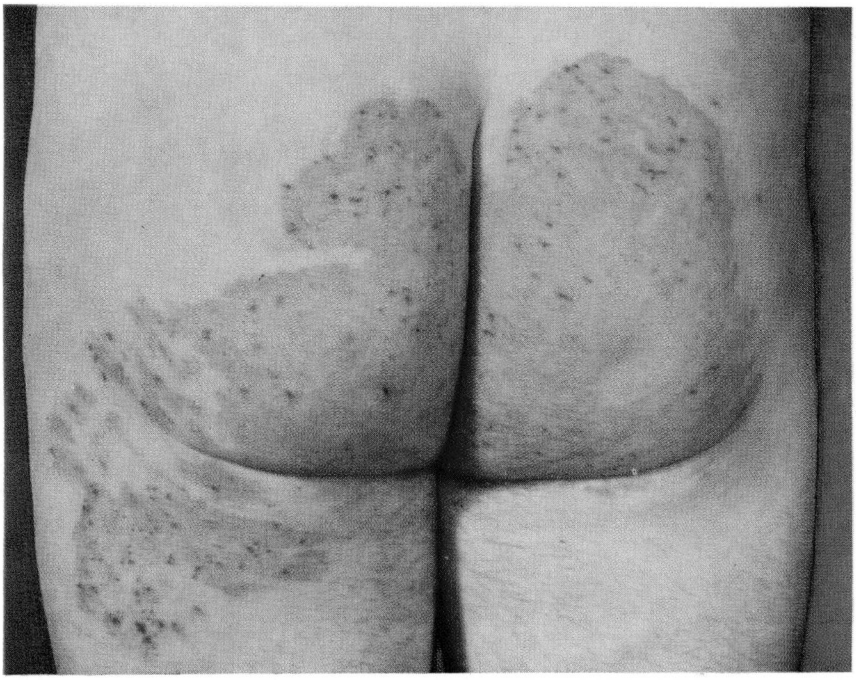

Plate 24. Tinea of the smooth skin.

This infection on the buttocks had spread from the crural region.

(Smith, Kline & French Laboratories)

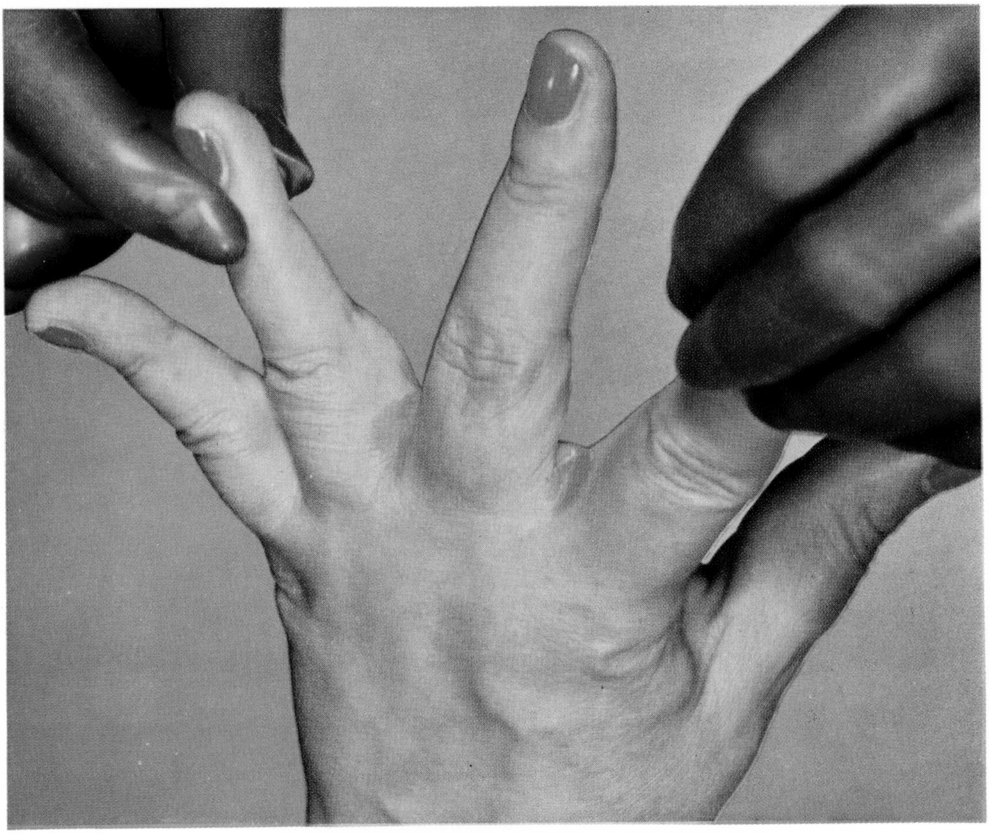

Plate 25. Monilial intertrigo of the webs of the fingers.

(Smith, Kline & French Laboratories)

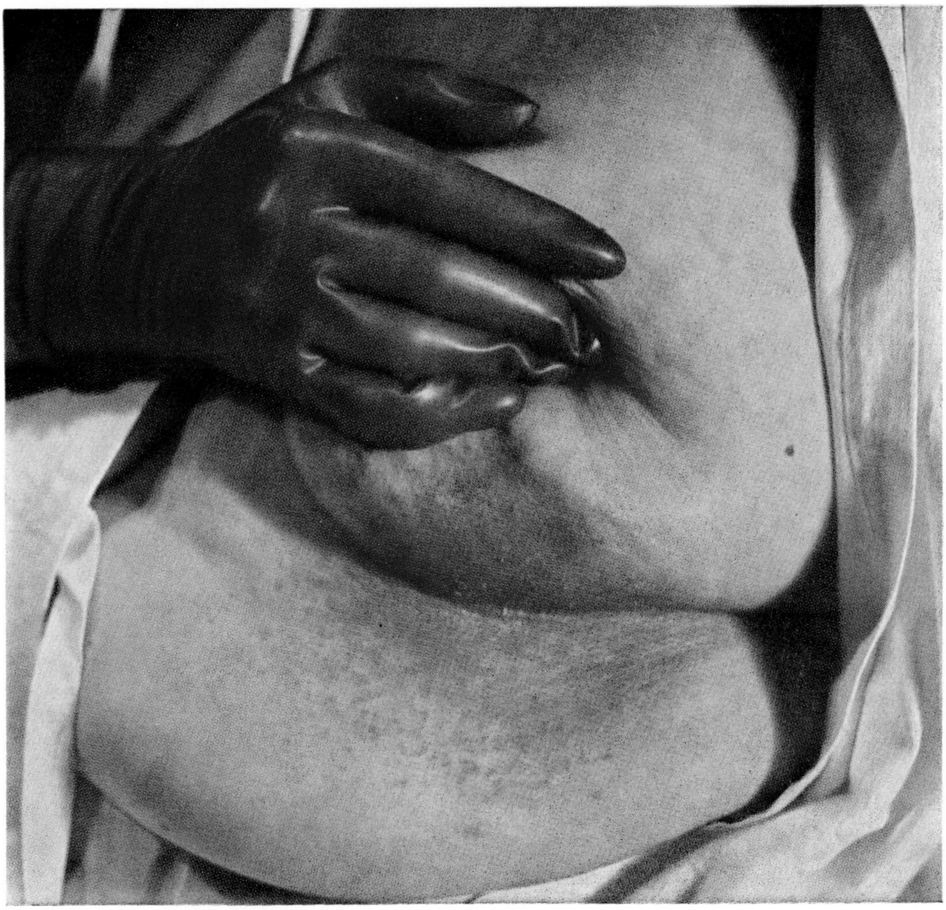

Plate 26. Monilial intertrigo under the breast.

(*Smith, Kline & French Laboratories*)

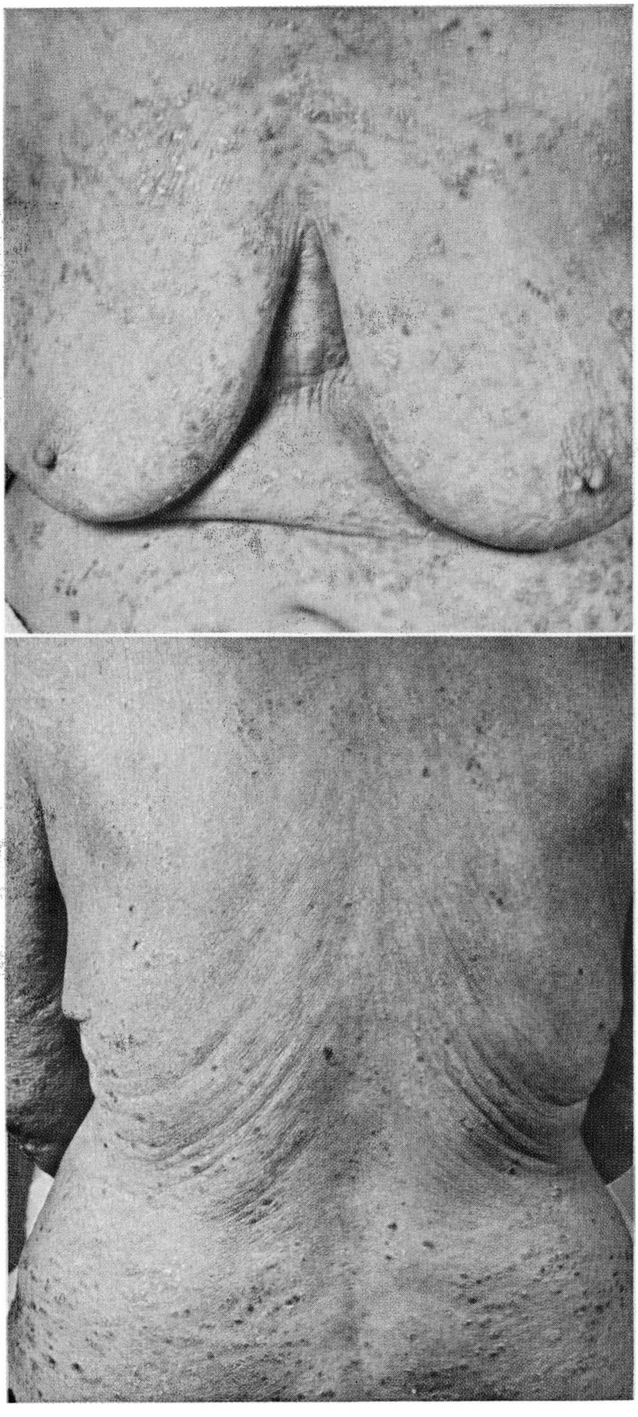

Plate 27. Exfoliative dermatitis due to psoriasis.

The primary scaly lesions of psoriasis can be seen on the back and the chest. (K.U.M.C.)
(*Texas Pharmacal*)

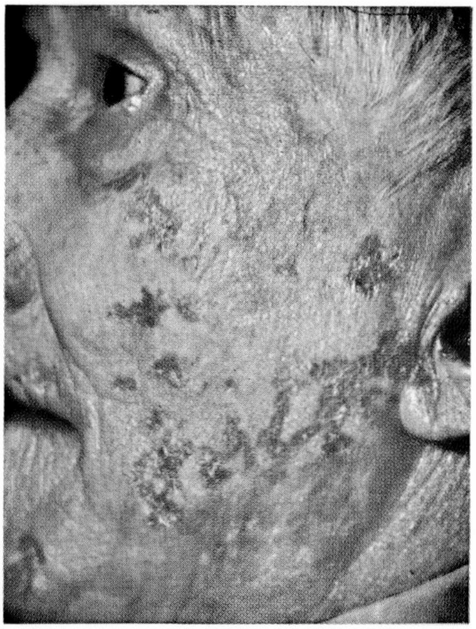

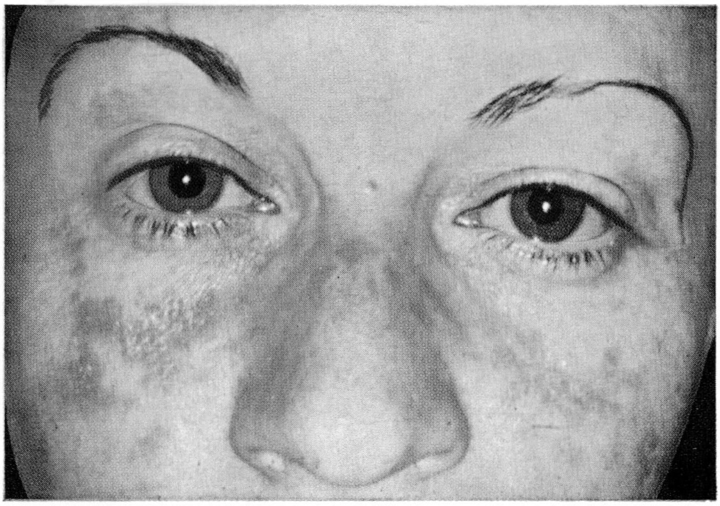

Plate 28. Lupus erythematosus.

A. Chronic discoid lupus erythematosus on the cheek of an elderly male. (K.C.G.H.)

B. Acute disseminated lupus erythematosus showing classic "butterfly" eruption. (Dr. Sloan Wilson)

(Smith, Kline & French Laboratories)

tions of scrapings and cultures on Sabouraud's media serve to demonstrate the presence of fungi and the specific type. A KOH preparation is a very simple office procedure and should be resorted to when the diagnosis is uncertain or the response to therapy is slow (see p. 9).

Differential Diagnosis

Contact dermatitis due to shoes, socks, gloves, foot powder (usually on dorsum of feet or hands, history of new shoes or new foot powder, fungi not found, p. 42).

Psoriasis of soles and palms (rarely vesicular or pustular, thickened, well-circumscribed lesions, psoriasis elsewhere on body, fungi not found, p. 83).

Pustular bacterid: pustular lesions only, chronic, resistant to local therapy, fungi not found.

Dyshidrosis of palms: feet clear, recurrent, seasonal incidence, fungi not found.

Treatment

1. AN ACUTE VESICULAR, PUSTULAR FUNGUS INFECTION of 2 weeks' duration on the soles of the feet and between the toes in a 16-year-old boy. This clinical picture is usually due to the organism *T. mentagrophytes*.

A. Minimize the fear of the infectiousness of athlete's feet but emphasize normal cleanliness, including the wearing of slippers over bare feet, wiping the feet last after a bath (not the groin last), and changing socks daily (white socks are not necessary).

B. Débridement. The doctor or the patient should snip off the tops of the blisters with small scissors. This enables the pus to drain out and allows the medication to reach the organisms. The edges of any blister should be kept trimmed, since the fungi spread under these edges. Follow this débridement by a foot soak.

C. Boric acid crystals
Sig: 1 tablespoon of boric acid crystals to 1 quart of warm water. Soak feet for 10 minutes twice a day. Dry skin carefully afterward.

D. Sulfur, ppt. 5%
Neosporin or other antibiotic ointment q.s. 15.0
Sig: Apply b.i.d. locally to feet after soaking. (The sulfur is antifungal, and the Neosporin is antibacterial for the secondary bacterial infection.)

E. Rest at home for 2 to 4 days may be advisable.

F. Place small pieces of cotton sheeting or cotton between the toes when wearing shoes.

SUBSEQUENT TREATMENT 5 days later. The secondary infection and blisters have decreased.

A. The soaks may be continued for another 3 days or stopped if no marked redness or infection is present.

B. Substitute the following salve for the first milder one:
Sulfur, ppt. 5%
Benzoic and salicylic acid oint. (U.S.P.) 7.5
Desenex ointment 7.5
Sig: Apply small amount b.i.d. locally to feet. (Other antifungal ointments can be substituted for Desenex, such as Timofax, Asterol, Enzactin and Salundek.)

C. Boric acid 2%
Sulfur, ppt. 4%
Timofax powder q.s. 45.0
Sig: Supply in powder can. Apply small amount to feet over the salve and to the shoes in the morning. (Other powder bases can be substituted for Timofax such as Asterol, Desenex, Sopronal, Vioform, etc.)

2. A CHRONIC, SCALY, THICKENED FUNGUS INFECTION of 4-years' duration that has in the past week developed a few small tense blisters on the sole of the feet.

This type of clinical picture probably is due to the organism *T. rubrum*. This form of infection can occur on the palms.

A. Tell the patient that you can clear up the acute flare-up (the blisters) but that it will be very difficult and time-consuming on his part to cure the chronic infection. If the toenails are found to be infected, the prognosis for cure is even poorer. (See "Tinea of the Nails," below.)

B. Débride and trim the blisters with manicure scissors.

C. Sulfur, ppt. 5%
Benzoic and salicylic acid oint. (U.S.P.) 15.0
Sig: Apply locally to soles b.i.d.

D. Soaks in the following solution will soften the scales and aid in the penetration of the salve:

Sodium Thiosulfate (Hypo) 240.0
Sig: 2 tablespoons to 1 quart of warm water. Soak feet for 10 minutes once a day.

SUBSEQUENT VISIT OF RESISTANT CASE

A. 0.5% Anthralin ointment (Abbott) 15.0
Sig: Apply to soles of feet h.s. Caution: Wash hands thoroughly afterward and do not touch eyes —an irritant.

B. Griseofulvin therapy. See note concerning this at end of present section.

TINEA OF THE NAILS

Tinea of the toenails is very common but tinea of the fingernails is uncommon. Tinea of the toenails is almost inevitable in patients who have recurrent attacks of tinea of the feet. Once developed, the infected nail serves as a resistant focus for future skin infection.

Primary Lesions. Begin as distal or lateral detachment of nail with subsequent thickening and deformity.

Secondary Lesions. Bacterial infection can result from the pressure of shoes on the deformed nail and surrounding skin.

Distribution. The infection usually begins in the 5th toenail and may remain there or spread to involve the other nails.

Course. Tinea of the toenails can rarely be cured. Aside from the deformity and an occasional mild flare-up of acute tinea, treatment is not necessary. Progression is slow, and spontaneous cures are rare. Tinea of the fingernails can be cured, but the treatment usually takes months.

Etiology. Usually due to *T. rubrum* and, less importantly, to *T. mentagrophytes*.

Laboratory Findings. These organisms can be found in a KOH preparation of a scraping and occasionally can be grown on culture media. The material should be gathered from the debris under the nail plate.

Differential Diagnosis

Nail injury: get history of such, although tinea infection often starts in an injured nail, absence of fungi.

Psoriasis of Fingernails: see pitting, red areas under nail with resulting detachment, psoriasis elsewhere usually, no fungi found (p. 195).

Psoriasis of Toenails: impossible to differentiate from tinea, since most psoriatic nails have some secondary fungal invasion.

Moniliasis of Fingernails: common in housewives, paronychial involvement common, monilia found (p. 150).

Treatment. A tinea infection of 6-months' duration in 3 fingernails of a young salesman. There is a mild amount of scaling of the skin around these nails.

1. Warn the patient that cure of the infection will require months of treatment.

2. Débridement. This is the most important factor. Twice a week the dead, thickened, crumbly debris must be removed. This can be accomplished by picking away with a broken piece of glass (Fig. 70 D), a sharp knife, a razor blade, or a motor-driven drill (see p. 236).

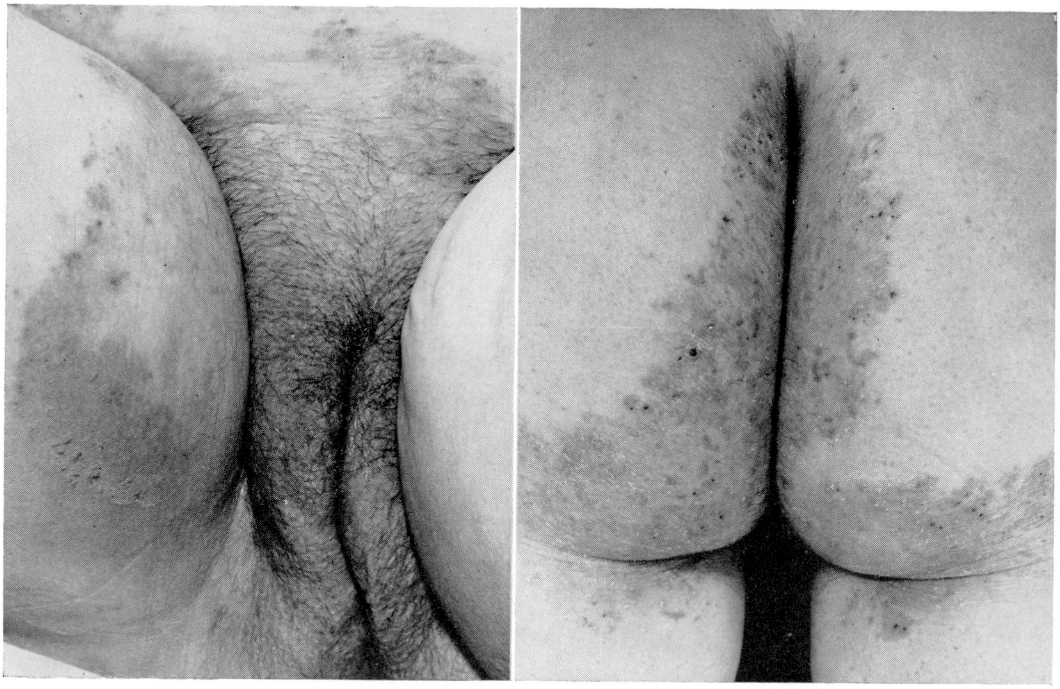

Fig. 71. Tinea of the groin area and the buttocks.

(A, *left*) Fungus infection of the thigh and the pubic area in a female.

(B, *right*) Fungus infection that has spread from the crural area to the buttocks. See Figure 70 A and B for hand of same patient. (K.U.M.C.)

3. A. Onychophytex 30.0
   or
   B. Chrysarobin 2%
   Chloroform 10%
   Asterol Tincture q.s. 15.0
   Sig: Apply to involved fingernails in A.M. Caution: Keep fingers away from the eyes.

4. Double Strength Whitfield's Ointment (benzoic acid 12% and salicylic acid 6%), q.s. 15.0
   Sig: Apply to nails h.s.

5. Surgical evulsion of the fingernail is curative in some cases if reinfection can be eliminated. Care should be taken to scrape away all the infected debris, particularly from the lateral grooves. This salve can be used following surgery:
   Sulfur, ppt. 4%
   Enzactin ointment, q.s. 15.0
   Sig: Apply b.i.d. locally.

6. Griseofulvin therapy. See note concerning this at the end of present section.

Tinea of the Groin
(Plate 24)

This is a common, itching, annoying fungus infection of the groin appearing usually in males and often concurrently with tinea of the feet (Fig. 71). Home remedies often result in a contact dermatitis that adds fuel to the fire.

Primary Lesions. Bilateral fan-shaped, red, scaly patches with a sharp, slightly raised border. Small vesicles may be seen in the active border.

Secondary Lesions. Oozing, crusting, edema and secondary bacterial infection.

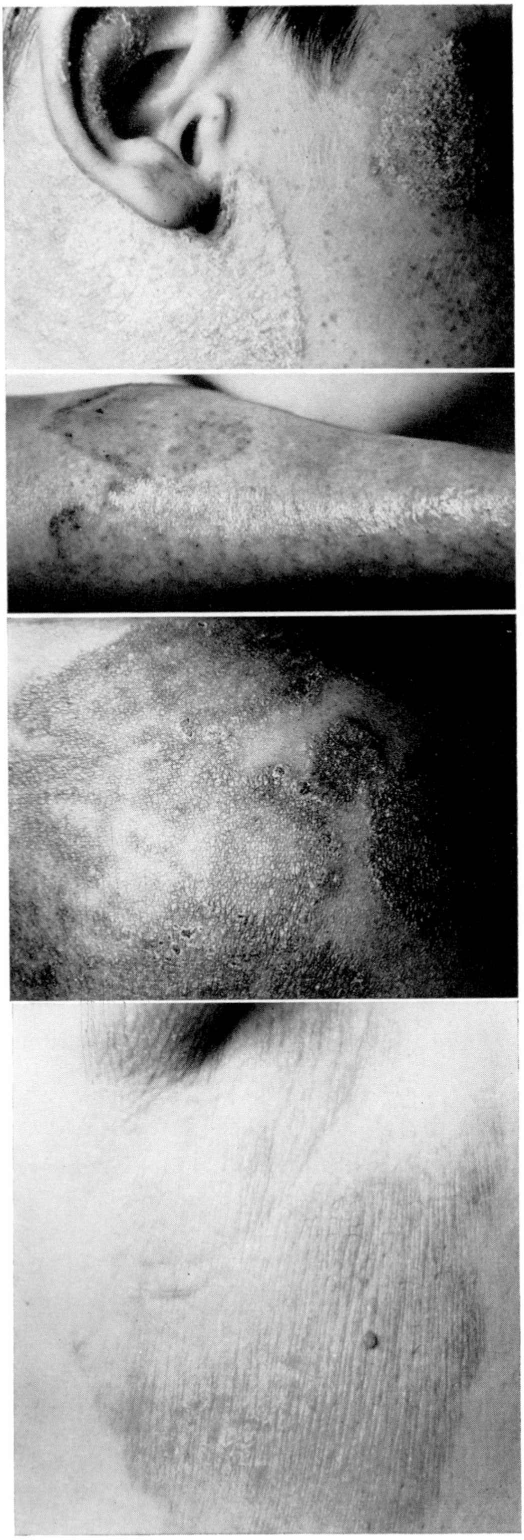

Fig. 72. Tinea of the smooth skin. (Top to bottom.)

A. Tinea of the face in a farm boy.
B. Tinea of the leg due to *T. rubrum*. (K.U.M.C.)
C. Tinea of the shoulder in a Negro woman.
D. Erythrasma of axilla.

In chronic cases lichenification may be marked.

Distribution. Crural fold and extending to involve scrotum, penis, thighs, perianal area and buttocks.

Course. The type of fungus influences the course, but most acute cases respond rapidly to treatment. Other factors that affect the course and recurrences are obesity, hot weather, sweating, and chafing garments.

Etiology. Commonly due to the fungi of tinea of the feet, *T. rubrum* and *T. mentagrophytes,* and also the fungus *E. floccosum*.

Infectiousness. Minimal, even between husband and wife.

Laboratory Findings. The organism is found in KOH preparations of scrapings and can be grown on culture. Take material from the active border (see p. 9).

Differential Diagnosis

Contact Dermatitis: often coexistent but can be separate entity, new contactant history, no fungi found, no active border (p. 42).

Prickly Heat: pustular, papular, no active border, no fungi, may also be present with tinea (p. 206).

Neurodermatitis: unilateral usually, may have resulted from old chronic tinea, no fungi (p. 62).

Psoriasis: usually unilateral, may or may not have raised border, psoriasis elsewhere, no fungi (p. 83).

Moniliasis: no sharp border, see fine scales, oozing, redness, commoner in obese females, monilia found (p. 150).

Erythrasma (Fig. 72): no redness, only fine scaling with no border, also commonly in axilla, due to a petite fungus that cannot be cultured, *Nocardia minutissimum*.

Treatment. Oozing, red dermatitis with sharp border in crural area of young man.

1. Since the infection usually comes from chronic tinea of the feet, to prevent recurrences advise the patient to dry the feet last and not the groin area last when taking a bath.
2. Boric acid wet packs
   Sig: 1 tablespoon of boric acid crystals to 1 quart of warm water. Wet the sheeting or thin toweling and apply to area for 15 minutes twice a day.
3. Sulfur, ppt. 5%
   Nonalcoholic white shake lotion, q.s. 90.0
   Sig: Apply locally b.i.d.

SUBSEQUENT VISIT, oozing gone.

Apply in the office:

Chrysarobin	3%
Chloroform q.s.	15.0

This is very effective for resistant, dry, scaly patches. It stings after application. Caution patient to avoid touching area with fingers and then rubbing eyes.

TINEA OF THE SMOOTH SKIN

The familiar ringworm of the skin is most common in children because of their intimacy with animals and other children (Fig. 72). The lay public believes that most skin conditions are "ringworm," and many physicians erroneously agree with them.

Primary Lesions. Round, oval, or semicircular scaly patches with slightly raised border that commonly is vesicular. Rarely, deep ulcerated granulomatous lesions are due to superficial fungi.

Secondary Lesions. Bacterial infection, particularly at the advancing border, is common in association with certain fungi, such as *M. canis* and *T. mentagrophytes*.

Course. Infection is short-lived if treated correctly. Recurrence seldom unless treatment is inadequate.

Etiology. Most commonly due to *M. canis* from kittens and puppies; to *M. audouini* from other children who usually also have scalp infection; and less commonly due to *E. floccosum* and *T. mentagrophytes* from groin and foot infections.

Infectiousness. Incidence is high.

Laboratory Findings. Same as for previously discussed fungus diseases.

Differential Diagnosis

Pityriasis Rosea: history of herald patch, sudden shower of oval lesions, fungi not found (p. 87).

Impetigo: vesicular, crusted, most commonly on face, no fungi found (p. 96).

Contact Dermatitis: no sharp border or central healing; may be coexistant with ringworm due to overtreatment (p. 42).

Treatment. A child has several 2 to 4-cm. sized scaly lesions on his arms of 1 week's duration. He has a new kitten which he holds and plays with.

1. Examine the scalp, preferably with a Wood's light, to rule out scalp infection.
2. Advise the mother regarding moderate isolation procedures in relation to the family and others.
3. Sulfur, ppt. 5%
   Desenex ointment q.s. 15.0
   Sig: Apply b.i.d. locally. (Other antifungal bases can be used such as Asterol, Timofax, Salundek, Enzactin, etc.)

SUBSEQUENT VISIT OF RESISTANT CASE

1. Sulfur, ppt. 5%
   Benzoic and salicyclic acid oint. (U.S.P.) 15.0
   Sig: Apply b.i.d. locally. Warn about possible irritation.

Tinea of the Scalp

Tinea of the scalp is the commonest cause of patchy hair loss in children (Fig. 73). Endemic cases are with us always, but epidemics, usually due to the human type, are the real therapeutic problem.

Tinea capitis infections can be divided into two clinical types: *noninflammatory* and *inflammatory*. The treatment, the cause and the course varies for these two types.

Noninflammatory Type

Primary Lesions. Grayish, scaly, round patches with broken-off hairs, causing balding areas. The size of the areas varies.

Secondary Lesions. Bacterial infection and "id" reactions are rare. A noninflammatory patch can become inflamed spontaneously or as the result of strong treatment. Scarring almost never occurs.

Distribution. Commonest in posterior scalp region. Body ringworm from the scalp lesions is common, particularly on the neck and the shoulders. *Perform Wood's light examination of scalp on any child with ringworm of the smooth skin.*

Course. The incubation period in and on the hair is short, but clinical evidence of the infection cannot be expected under 3 weeks after inoculation. Parents often do not notice the infection for another 3 weeks to several months, particularly in girls. Spontaneous cures are rare in 2 to 6 months but after that time occur with greater frequency. Some cases last for years if untreated. Recurrence of the infection after the cure of a previous episode is rare but not impossible, since adequate immunity does not develop.

Age Group. Infection of the noninflammatory type is commonest between the ages of 3 and 8 and is rare after the age of puberty. This adult resistance to infection is attributed in part to the higher content of fungistatic fatty acids in the sebum after puberty. This research laboratory finding had great therapeutic significance, and the direct outgrowth was the development of Desenex, Timofax, Salundek and other fatty acid ointments and powders.

Etiology. The noninflammatory type of scalp ringworm is caused most commonly by *M. audouini,* occasionally by *M. canis* and rarely by *T. tonsurans*. *M. audouini* and *T. tonsurans* are anthropophilic fungi (human-to-human passage only), whereas *M. canis* is a zoophilic fungus (animals are the original source, mainly kittens and puppies).

Contagiousness. High incidence in children. The case can be a part of a large urban epidemic.

Laboratory Findings. Microscopic examination of the infected hairs in 20% potassium hydroxide solution shows an ectothrix arrangement of the spores when due to the *Microsporum* species, and endothrix spores when due to *T. tonsurans*. Culture is necessary for species identification but is not practical in most offices. Treatment by x-ray epilation of the scalp should not be done without cultural identification of the species. The cultural characteristics of the various fungi can be found in many larger dermatologic or mycologic texts and will not be presented here.

Wood's light examination of the scalp is an important diagnostic test. The Wood's light is a specially filtered ultraviolet light. The hairs infected with *M. audouini* and *M. canis* fluoresce with a bright yellowish-green color. Over 90% of the tinea capitis in the United States and Canada is due to these fungi, so very few cases will be missed by this light. The bright fluorescence of fungus-infected hairs is not to be confused with the white or dull yellow color emited by lint particles or sulfur-laden scales. An inexpensive but excellent Wood's light is described on page 236.

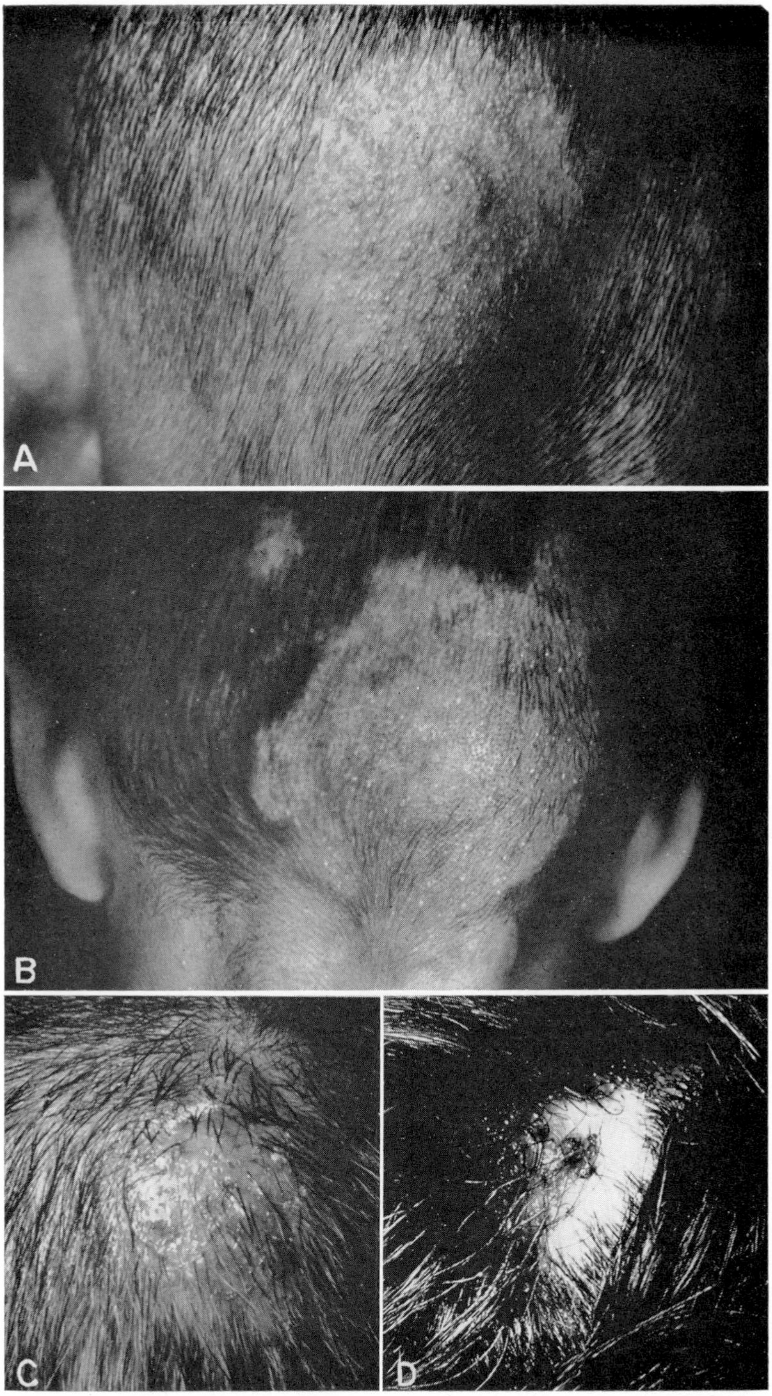

Fig. 73. Tinea of the scalp.

A. Due to *M. audouini*. Note absence of visible inflammation.

B. Due to *T. tonsurans*. Wood's light examination revealed no fluorescence.

C. Due to *T. mentagrophytes*. Note inflammation.

D. Favus, due to *T. schoenleini,* of 11-years' duration.

Differential Diagnosis

	Wood's Light	Scales	Redness	Hair Loss	Remarks
Tinea capitis	+	Dry or crusted	Uncommon	Yes	Back of scalp, child
Alopecia areata (p. 188)	—	None	No	Yes	Exclamation point hairs at edges
Seborrheic derm. (p. 73)	—	Greasy	Yes	No	Diffuse scaling
Psoriasis (p. 83)	—	Thick and dry	Yes	No	Look at elbows, knees and nails
Trichotillomania (p. 190)	—	None	No	Yes	Psychoneurotic child
Pyoderma (p. 96) (with or without lice)	—	Crusted	Yes	Occasional	Poor hygiene

Prophylactic Treatment

1. Infected individuals may attend school, provided that (a) the child wears a cotton stockinette cap at all times (no swapping allowed), and (b) a note must be presented from the physician every 3 weeks, stating that the child is under a doctor's care. Infected children should be restricted from theaters, church and other public places. Consult your own Health Department for specific rulings.

2. Inspection of all susceptible school children with a Wood's light by school nurse every 4 weeks during an epidemic.

3. Wash hair after every haircut at a barber shop.

4. Provide parent-and-teacher education on methods of spread of disease, particularly during an epidemic.

5. Suggest provision for individual storage of clothing, particularly caps, in school and home.

Active Treatment. (See note on griseofulvin oral therapy at the end of this section. If griseofulvin is administered, many of the instructions that follow are fortunately not necessary, such as shaving the hair, nightly shampoos, application of salve, x-ray epilation of scalp hairs, etc. However, in view of the preliminary nature of the reports on griseofulvin therapy to date, it was felt advisable to retain the following therapy suggestions.)

1. Parent and child instructions:

A. The entire scalp hair should be shaved or cut off. This can be emotionally traumatic, particularly for girls. It could be deferred if the infection is minimal or if the child or parent objects too strenuously.

B. Shampoo the hair every night.

C. Apply the salve as directed.

D. Make white cotton stockinette cap and wash it daily.

E. Separate child's towels, bedding, etc., from noninfected children.

F. Remove salve from the scalp before the visit to the doctor.

2. Salundek ointment, q.s. 30.0
Sig: Apply to infected areas b.i.d. (Other antifungal ointments such as Desenex, Timofax, Enzactin, etc., can be substituted for Salundek.)

Subsequent Visit of Resistant Case

1. Sulfur, ppt. 5%
Benzoic and salicyclic acid oint. (U.S.P.) 15.0
Sig: Apply to infected areas b.i.d. (Watch for irritation, although some irritation is good because it can result in cure.)

2. X-ray epilation (Kienbock-Adamson technic). If there is no evidence of improvement in 6 to 8 weeks of active local therapy, it is wise to send the child to a

qualified dermatologist or radiologist for epilation of the hairs by x-rays. This is accomplished in one visit, using a 5-point method with superficial type x-rays. About 3 weeks after the epilating exposure the hairs fall out and begin to return in another 3 weeks. This middle 3-week interim is the important one for ensuring that the cure will be complete.

Inflammatory Type

Primary Lesions. Pustular, scaly round patches with broken-off hairs, causing bald areas.

Secondary Lesions. Bacterial-like infection is common. When the secondary reaction is marked the area becomes swollen and tender. This inflammation is called a *kerion*. Minimal scarring sometimes remains.

Distribution. Any scalp area. Concurrent body ringworm infection is common.

Course. Duration much shorter than the noninflammatory type of infection. Spontaneous cures will result after 2 to 4 months in majority of cases, even if untreated.

Etiology. The inflammatory type of scalp ringworm is most commonly caused by *M. canis,* occasionally by *M. audouini,* rarely by *M. gypseum, T. mentagrophytes* and *T. verrucosum*. Except for *M. audouini* the species are zoophilic, that is, passed from infected animals or soil.

Contagiousness. High incidence in children and farmers. Endemic except for cases due to *M. audouini*.

Laboratory Findings. Microscopic examination of the infected hairs in 20% potassium hydroxide solution shows an ectothrix arrangement of the spores. The hairs infected with *M. canis* and *M. audouini* fluoresce with a bright yellowish-green color under the Wood's light.

Differential Diagnosis (See chart on p. 146)

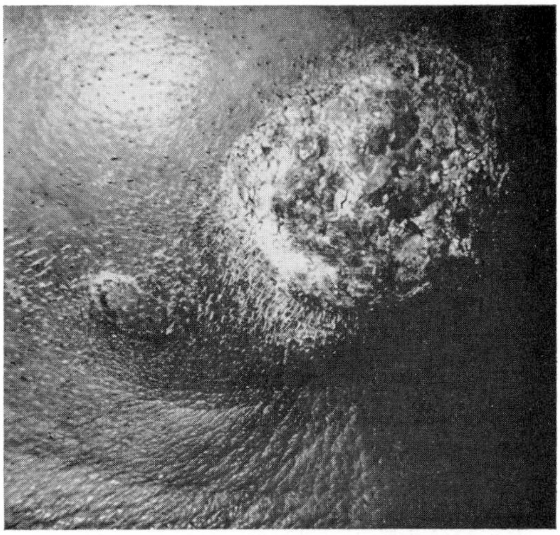

Fig. 74. Tinea of the beard (chin).

Prophylactic Treatment

1. Same as for noninflammatory cases but less stringent.

Active Treatment. (See note on griseofulvin therapy at the end of this section.)

1. Parent-and-child instructions:
   A. Boys should have their scalp hair shaved or cut off. Girls can have the hair trimmed only in the infected patch.
   B. Further instructions the same as for the noninflammatory type.
2. Sulfur, ppt. 5%
   Sterosan ointment, q.s. 15.0
   Sig: Apply locally b.i.d.
3. If kerion is severe:
   A. Boric acid wet packs
      Sig: 1 tablespoon of boric acid to 1 quart of warm water. Apply soaked cloths for 15 minutes twice a day.
   B. Sulfonamide tablets such as
      Kynex 0.5 Gm.
      Sig: 2 tablets stat, then 1 a day. (Dose depends on the weight of the child.)
4. X-ray epilation is rarely necessary.

Tinea of the Beard

Fungus infection is a rare cause of dermatitis in the beard area. Farmers occasionally contract it from infected cattle (Fig. 74). The course of such an infection is long. Any presumed bacterial infection of the beard that does not respond readily to proper treatment should be examined for fungi.

Primary Lesions. Follicular pustular lesions, or sharp bordered ringworm-type lesions, or deep boggy inflammatory masses.

Secondary Lesions. Bacterial infection is common. Scarring is unusual.

Etiology (see table, p. 136)

Differential Diagnosis

Bacterial Folliculitis: acute onset, rapid spread, no definite border, responds rather rapidly to local therapy, no fungi found on examination of hairs or culture (p. 98).

Treatment. Farmer with a quarter-sized boggy inflammatory, pustular mass on chin of 3-weeks' duration.

1. Have veterinarian inspect cattle if farmer is not aware of source of infection.
2. Boric acid wet packs
   Sig: 1 tablespoon of boric acid to 1 quart of hot water. Apply wet cloths to area for 15 minutes twice a day.
3. Sulfur, ppt. 5%
   Asterol ointment, q.s. 15.0
   Sig: Apply locally b.i.d.

Resistant Case

1. Sulfur, ppt. 5%
   Benzoic and salicylic acid oint. (U.S.P.) q.s. 15.0
   Sig: Apply locally b.i.d.
2. X-ray therapy by dermatologist or radiologist. From 4 to 6 superficial treatments of 75 to 100 r each appear to be effective in some cases. An epilating dose never should be given.
3. Griseofulvin therapy. See note at the end of this section.

Dermatophytid

During an acute episode of any fungus infection, an id eruption can develop over the body. This is a manifestation of an allergic reaction to the fungus infection. The commonest id reaction occurs on the hands during an acute tinea infection on the feet. To assume a diagnosis of an id reaction the following criteria should be followed: (1) the primary focus should be acutely infected with fungi, not chronically infected; (2) the id lesions must not contain fungi; and (3) the id eruption should disappear or wane following adequate treatment of the acute focus.

Primary Lesions. Vesicular eruption of the hands (primary on the feet); papulofollicular eruption on body (primary commonly is scalp kerion); pityriasis rosealike id eruptions and others are seen less commonly.

Secondary Lesions. Excoriation and infection when itching is severe, which is unusual.

Treatment

1. Treat the primary focus of infection.
2. For a vesicular id reaction on the hands:
   A. Boric acid soaks
   Sig: 1 tablespoon of boric acid to 1 quart of cool water. Soak hands for 15 minutes twice a day.
3. For an id reaction on the body that is moderately pruritic:
   A. Linit starch bath
   Sig: ½ of small box of Linit starch to 6 to 8 inches of cool water in a tub, once daily.
   B. Alcoholic white shake lotion 120.0
   Sig: Apply locally b.i.d. Menthol 0.25% or phenol 0.5%, or camphor 2% could be added to this lotion.
4. For a severely itching generalized id eruption:
   A. Hydrocortisone or related corticosteroid tablets #20
   Sig: 1 tablet q.i.d. for 2 days then 1 t.i.d. for 4 days (or longer if necessary).

GRISEOFULVIN (FULVICIN, GRIFULVIN) THERAPY. As this book goes to press, the author and other dermatologists in this country and overseas are in the process of evaluating the effectiveness of a penicillin-related antibiotic, griseofulvin, administered orally for the treatment of superficial fungus infections. Many superficial fungus infections are readily cured by appropriate local therapy, but there is an impressive group of fungus diseases that respond poorly, if at all, to such therapy. As the result of less than a year's clinical trial of griseofulvin, it appears that this chemical is a long-sought-for oral medicine for such stubborn fungus infections as tinea of the scalp due to *M. audouini,* tinea of the nails, tinea of the groin due to *T. rubrum,* etc. Aside from mild headaches and a rare urticarial eruption, there appears to date to be no serious side-effects due to this therapy. It would be advisable to consult the latest medical journals for further information regarding toxicity as more is learned about this drug.

Based on preliminary data, the following therapy schedules can be listed.

Tinea of the scalp in children. Griseofulvin, 250 mg. b.i.d. or 500 mg. once a day for 6 weeks, appears to be adequate. The use of this agent should not preclude the use of fungus cultures and Wood's light examinations. The child should not be dismissed from the physician's care until fluorescence, if present, has disappeared. For those rarer cases of scalp ringworm where no fluorescence is present, a negative culture is necessary before a cure can be pronounced.

Tinea of feet, hands, groin, body and beard. For adults, griseofulvin, 250 mg. q.i.d. or 500 mg. b.i.d. for 4 to 6 weeks, appears to be adequate. Some resistant cases may require larger doses. The basis for a cure should be the absence of fungi on scrapings or cultures.

Tinea of the nails. Due to the fact that the nails grow slowly, the adult dosage (1 Gm. per day) should be continued for 3 to 6 months for this disease.

In summary, it appears that an effective oral agent for treating resistant superficial fungus infections has been found. A considerable amount of additional research will be forthcoming, and, undoubtedly, improvements will be made upon this original antibiotic. It is not premature to stress at this time that the cure of many of the resistant fungus infections will still require the knowledge necessary to make a correct diagnosis, the application of suitable local medications and other supportive therapy, and the intelligent use of laboratory procedures. Griseofulvin, and the griseofulvinlike agents to come, will not be panaceas.

DEEP FUNGUS INFECTIONS

Those fungi that invade the skin deeply and go into living tissue are also capable of involving other organs. Only the skin manifestations of these deeply invading fungi will be the concern of this book.

The following diseases are included in this group of deep fungus infections. Other rarer deep mycotic diseases will be found in the Dictionary-Index.

Moniliasis
Sporotrichosis
Actinomycosis
North American blastomycosis

MONILIASIS
(Plates 25 and 26)

Moniliasis is a fungus infection caused by *Candida albicans* which produces lesions in the mouth, the vagina, the skin, the nails, the lungs, the gastro-intestinal tract, or occasionally, a septicemia. The latter condition apparently has been seen in increasing frequency since the advent of the oral antibiotics. Since *C. albicans* exists commonly as a harmless skin inhabitant, the laboratory finding of this organism is not adequate proof of its pathogenicity

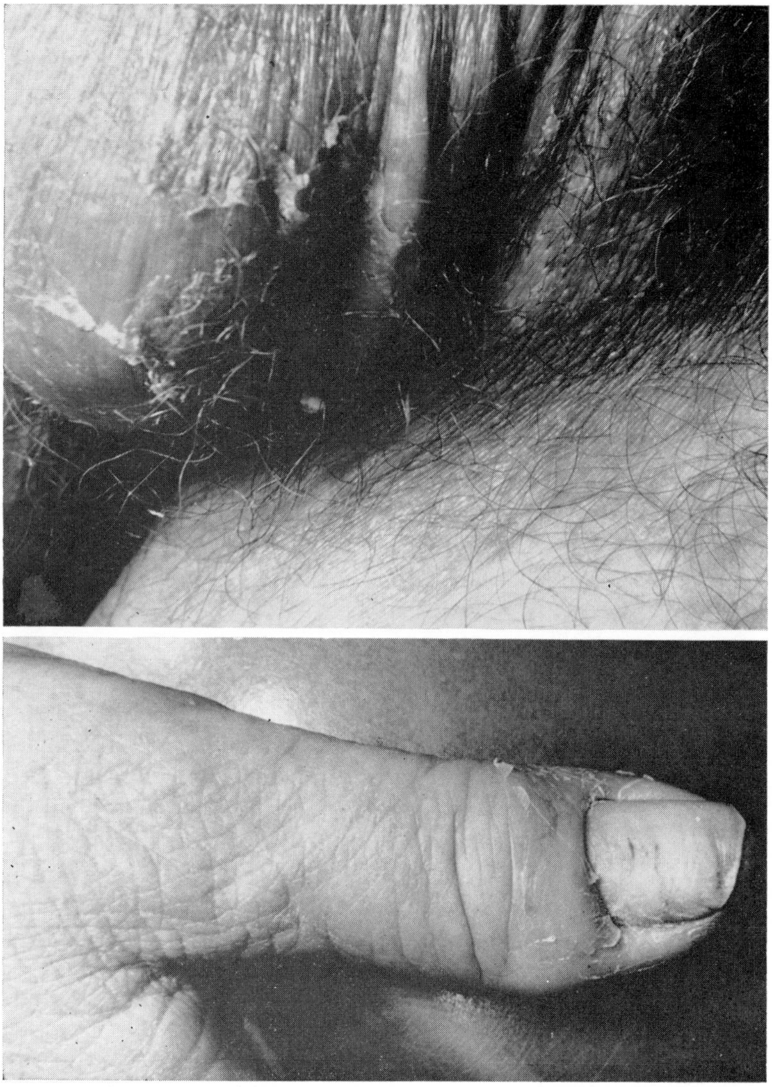

Fig. 75. Moniliasis.

(A, *top*) Monilial intertrigo of scrotum and adjacent thigh. Note the characteristic thin scale on the scrotum.

(B, *bottom*) Chronic monilial paronychia of the thumb.

and etiologic role. Monilia commonly seed pre-existing disease conditions. This book will be concerned with the *cutaneous* and the *mucocutaneous* monilial diseases. The following classification will be helpful.

1. Cutaneous moniliasis

A. Localized diseases

a. Monilial paronychia (Fig. 75 B). A common monilial infection which is characterized by development of painful, red swellings of the skin around the nail plate. In chronic infections the nail becomes secondarily thickened and hardened. Monilial paronychia is commonly seen in housewives and those individuals whose occupations predispose to frequent immersions of the hands in water. This nail involvement is to be differentiated from *superficial tinea of the nails* (the monilial infection does not cause the nail to lose its luster or to become crumbly, and debris does not accumulate beneath the nail), and from *bacterial paronychia* (this is more acute in onset and throbs with pain).

b. Monilial intertrigo (Fig. 75 A). A moderately common condition characterized by well-defined, red, eroded patches, with scaly, pustular or pustulo-vesicular diffuse borders. The commonest sites are axillae, inframammary areas, umbilicus, genital area, anal area, and webs of toes and fingers. Obesity and diabetes predispose to the development of this intertriginous type. It is to be differentiated from *superficial tinea infections,* which are not as red and eroded, and from *seborrheic dermatitis.*

B. Generalized cutaneous moniliasis. This rare infection involves the smooth skin, mucocutaneous orifices and intertriginous areas. It follows in the wake of general debility and is very resistant to treatment.

2. Mucous membrane moniliasis

A. Oral moniliasis (thrush and perlèche). Thrush is characterized by creamy white flakes on a red, inflamed mucous membrane. The tongue may be smooth and atrophic, or the papillae may be hypertrophic as in the condition labeled "hairy tongue." Perlèche is seen as cracks or fissures at the corners of the mouth, usually associated with monilial disease elsewhere and a dietary deficiency. A nonmonilial clinically similar condition is commonly seen in elderly people with ill-fitting dentures where the corners of the mouth override. Oral moniliasis is also to be differentiated from *allergic conditions,* such as those due to tooth paste or mouthwash.

B. Monilial vulvovaginitis. The clinical picture is an oozing, red, sharply bordered skin infection surrounding an inflamed vagina that contains a buttermilklike discharge. This type of monilial infection is frequently seen in pregnant women and diabetics. It is to be differentiated from an *allergic condition,* or from *trichomonal vaginitis.*

Laboratory findings for all of above monilial diseases: Skin or mucous membrane scrapings placed in 20% potassium hydroxide solution and examined with the high-power microscope lens will reveal small, oval, budding, thin-walled yeastlike cells with occasional mycelia. Culture on Sabouraud's media will produce creamy dull-white colonies in 4 to 5 days. Further cultural studies on cornmeal agar are necessary to identify the species as *Candida albicans.*

Treatment

Monilial paronchia of 2 fingers in a 37-year-old male bartender.

1. Advise patient concerning avoiding exposure of his hands to soap and water by wearing cotton gloves under rubber gloves, hiring a dishwasher, etc.
2. Chrysarobin 2%
   Chloroform 10%
   Asterol Tincture q.s. 15.0
   Sig: Apply b.i.d. with cotton-tipped applicator to nails and surrounding skin. Caution: avoid rubbing eyes with fingers. (Continue this treatment for several weeks.)

Monilial intertrigo of inframammary and crural region in an elderly obese female.

1. Advise patient to wear pieces of cotton sheeting under breasts. Frequent bathing with thorough drying is helpful.
2. Gentian violet 1%
   Distilled water, q.s. 30.0
   Sig: Apply locally b.i.d. followed by this powder:
3. Mycostatin powder 15.0
   Sig: Apply powder b.i.d. locally.

Monilial vulvovaginitis in a 6-month pregnant woman.

1. Mycostatin vaginal tablets, 100,000 U. #20
   Sig: Insert one tablet b.i.d. in vagina.
2. Sulfur, ppt. 4%
   Calamine lotion, q.s. 90.0
   Sig: Apply b.i.d. locally to skin.

Sporotrichosis

Sporotrichosis is a granulomatous fungus infection of the skin and the subcutaneous tissues. Characteristically, a primary chancre precedes more extensive

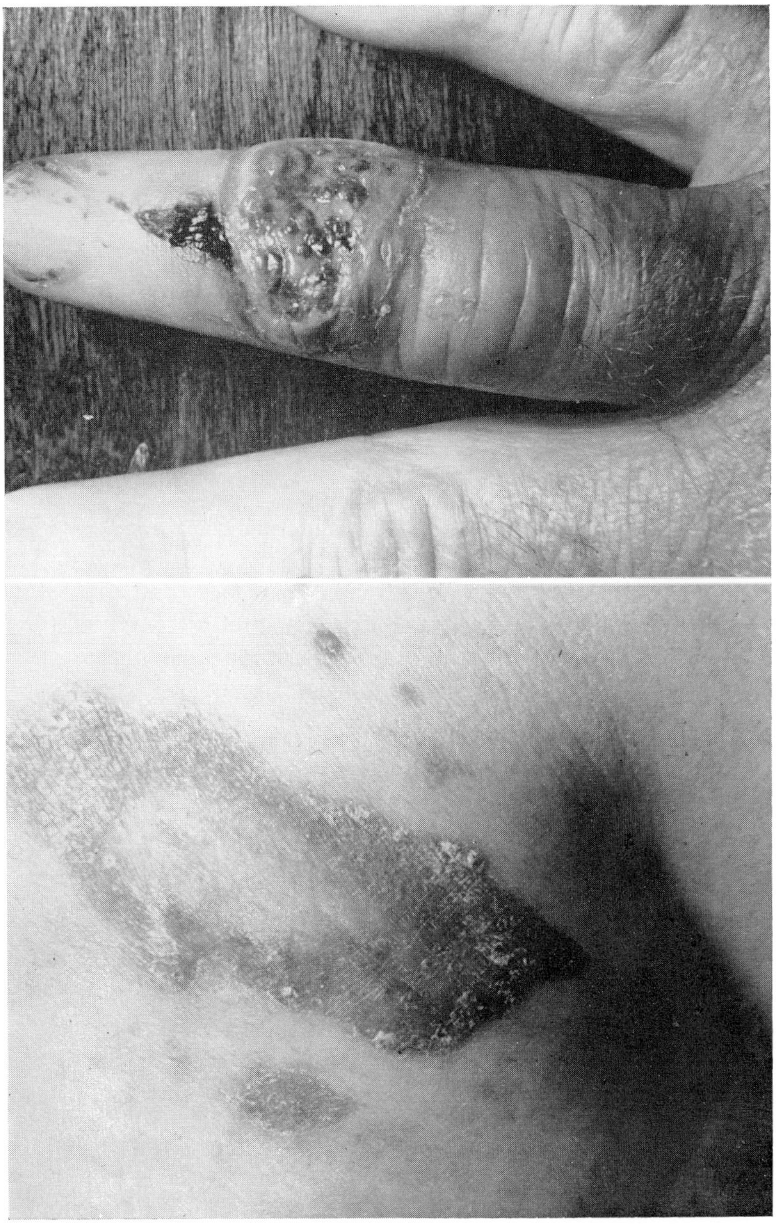

Fig. 76. Deep fungus infections.

(A, *top*) Sporotrichotic chancre of the finger.

(B, *bottom*) North American blastomycosis lesion on the posterior aspect of the shoulder.

skin involvement (Fig. 76 A). Invasion of the internal viscera is rare.

Primary Lesion. A sporotrichotic chancre develops at the site of skin inoculation, which is commonly the hand, less commonly the face or the feet. The chancre begins as a painless, movable, subcutaneous nodule that eventually softens and breaks down to form an ulcer.

Secondary Lesions. Within a few weeks subcutaneous nodules arise along the course of the draining lymphatics and form a chain of tumors that eventuate into ulcers. This is the classic clinical picture, of which there are variations.

Course. The development of the skin lesions is slow and rarely affects the general health.

Etiology. *Sporotrichum Schenckii,* a fungus that grows on wood and in the soil. It involves open wounds and is an occupational hazard of farmers, laborers and miners.

Laboratory Findings. Cultures of the purulent material from unopened lesions readily grow on Sabouraud's media.

Differential Diagnosis. Consider any of the skin granulomas such as pyodermas, syphilis, tuberculosis, sarcoidosis and leprosy. An ioderma or bromoderma can cause a similar clinical picture.

Treatment

1. Saturated solution of potassium iodide 60.0 cc.

   Sig: On the first day, 10 drops t.i.d., p.c. added to milk or water. Second day, 15 drops t.i.d.; third day, 20 drops t.i.d. and increase until 30 to 40 drops t.i.d. are given. Watch for gastric irritation and ioderma. Continue this very specific treatment for 1 month after apparent cure.

Actinomycosis

Actinomycosis is a deep fungus disease that characteristically causes the formation of a granulomatous draining sinus. The commonest location of the draining sinus is in the jaw region, but thoracic and abdominal sinuses do occur.

Primary Lesion. Red, firm, nontender tumor in jaw area that slowly extends locally to form a "lumpy jaw."

Secondary Lesions. Discharging sinuses that become infected with bacteria and, if untreated, may eventuate into osteomyelitis.

Course. General health is usually unaffected unless extension occurs into bone or deeper neck tissues. Recurrence is unusual if treatment is continued long enough.

Etiology. *Actinomyces bovis,* which is an anaerobic fungus that lives as a normal inhabitant of the mouth, particularly in individuals who have poor dental hygiene. Injury to the jaw or a tooth extraction usually precedes the development of the infection. Infected cattle are nct the source of human infection. The disease occurs twice as frequently in males.

Laboratory Findings. Pinpoint-sized "sulfur" granules, which are colonies of the fungi, can be seen grossly and microscopically in the draining pus. A gram stain of the pus will show masses of interlacing gram-positive fibers with or without club-shaped processes at the tips of these fibers. The organism can be cultured anaerobically on special media.

Differential Diagnosis. Consider pyodermas, tuberculosis and neoplasm.

Treatment

1. Penicillin, 2,400,000 units intramuscularly daily until definite improvement is noted. Then oral penicillin in the same dosage should be continued for 3 weeks after the infection apparently has been cured.
2. Incision and drainage of the lumps and the sinuses.
3. Institute good oral hygiene.
4. In resistant cases, broad-spectrum antibiotics can be used alone or in combination with the penicillin.

North American Blastomycosis

Two cutaneous forms of this disease are seen: primary cutaneous blastomycosis and secondary localized cutaneous blastomycosis.

Primary cutaneous blastomycosis occurs in laboratory workers and physicians following accidental innoculation. A primary chancre develops at the site of the inoculation, and the regional nodes enlarge. In a short time the primary lesion and nodes heal spontaneously, and the cure is complete.

The following discussion will be confined to the *secondary cutaneous form.*

Systemic blastomycosis is rarer than the cutaneous forms.

Primary Lesion (secondary localized cutaneous form): Begins as a papule that ulcerates and slowly spreads peripherally with a warty, pustular, raised border. The face, the hands and the feet are involved most commonly (Fig. 76 B).

Secondary Lesion. Central healing of the ulcer occurs gradually with resultant thick scar.

Course. Takes months to develop large lesion. Therapy is moderately effective on a long-term basis. Relapses are common.

Etiology. The fungus *Blastomyces dermatitidis* is thought to invade the lungs primarily and the skin secondarily as a metastatic lesion. High native immunity prevents the development of more than one skin lesion. This immunity is low in the rare systemic form of blastomycosis where multiple lesions occur in the skin, the bones and other organs. This fungus disease affects adult males most frequently.

Laboratory Findings. Collect the material for a 20% potassium hydroxide solution mount from the pustules at the border of the lesion. Round budding organisms can be found in this manner or in a culture mount. A chest roentgenogram is indicated in every case.

Differential Diagnosis. Consider any of the granuloma producing diseases such as tuberculosis, syphilis, iodide or bromide drug eruption, pyoderma and neoplasm.

Treatment

1. Surgical excision and plastic repair of early lesions is quite effective.
2. 2-Hydroxystilbamidine suppresses the chronic lesion more effectively than any other drug. It is administered by intravenous infusion daily in varying schedules which are described in larger texts or reviews.

Dermatologic Parasitology

CHAPTER 16

THIS IS a very extensive subject and includes the dermatoses due to 3 main groups of organisms: protozoa, helminths and arthropods.

The *protozoal dermatoses* are exemplified by the various forms of trypanosomiasis and leishmaniasis.

Helminthic dermatoses include those due to roundworms (ground itch, creeping eruption, filariasis and other rare tropical diseases), and those due to flatworms (schistosomiasis, swimmer's itch and others).

Arthropod dermatoses are divided into those caused by 2 classes of organisms: the arachnids (spiders, scorpions, ticks and mites) and the insects (lice, bugs, flies, moths, beetles, bees and fleas).

In this chapter we shall discuss scabies caused by a mite and pediculosis caused by lice. In Chapter 25, "Geographic Dermatoses," the following will be presented: flea bites, chigger bites, creeping eruption and swimmer's itch.

SCABIES

This parasitic infestation is more prevalent in a populace ravaged by war, famine, or disease, when personal hygiene becomes unimportant. In normal times scabies is rarely seen except in school children or in poorer people under crowded conditions. *Scabies should be ruled out in any generalized excoriated eruption.* (See Figs. 77 and 78.)

Primary Lesions. A minute burrow caused by the female of the mite *Sarcoptes scabiei*. The burrow measures approximately 2 mm. in length and can be hidden by the secondary eruption. Small vesicles may overlie the burrows.

Secondary Lesions. Excoriations of the burrows may be the only visible pathology. In severe, chronic cases bacterial infection may be extensive and take the form of impetigo, cellulitis and furunculosis.

Distribution. Most commonly, the excoriations are seen on the lower abdomen and the back with extension to the pubic and the axillary areas, the legs, the arms and the webs of the fingers. In this day of only mild cases of scabies the eruption is not commonly seen in the webs of the fingers.

Subjective Complaints. Itching is intense, particularly at night when the patient is warm in bed and the mite more active. However, many skin diseases itch worse at night, presumably due to a lower itch threshold when relaxation occurs.

Course. The mite can persist for months and years ("seven-year itch") in untreated, unclean individuals.

Contagiousness. Other members of the family may or may not have the disease, depending on the cleanliness and the severity of the infestation.

Laboratory Findings. The female scabies mite and ova may be seen in curetted burrows examined under the low-power magnification of the microscope. Potassium hydroxide (20% solution) can be used to clear the tissue as

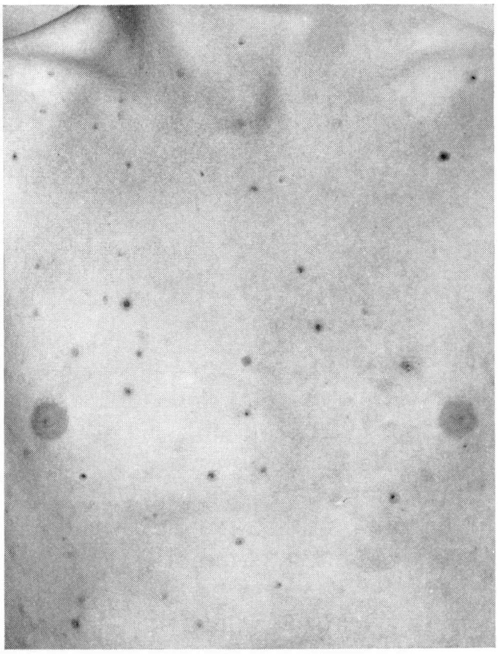

Fig. 77. Scabies lesions on a boy's chest. (K.C.G.H.)

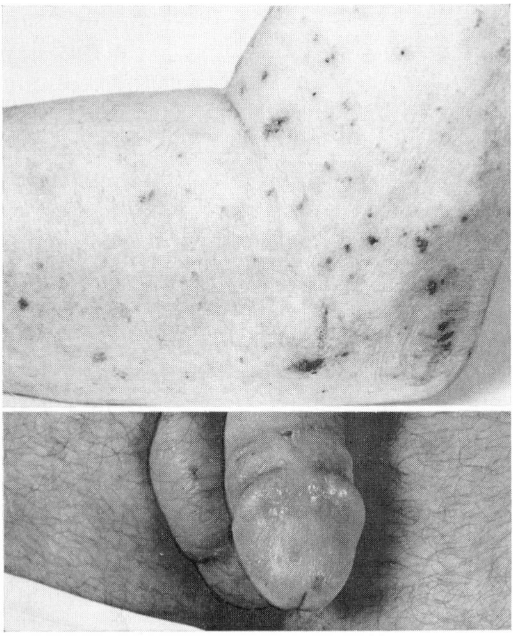

Fig. 78. Scabies.

(*Top*) On arm. Note excoriations. (K.U.M.C.)

(*Bottom*) On penis.

with fungus smears. Skill is necessary to uncover the mite by curetting.

Differential Diagnosis

Pyoderma: examine the patient carefully to rule out concurrent parasitic infestation, positive history of high carbohydrate diet, only mild itching (p. 96).

Pediculosis Pubis: see lice and eggs on and around hairs, distribution different (p. 157).

Winter Itch: see no burrows, seasonal incidence, elderly patient usually, worse on legs and back (p. 60).

Dermatitis Herpetiformis: see vesicles, urticaria, excoriated papules, eosinophilia, no burrows (p. 163).

Neurotic Excoriations: nervous individual, patient admits picking at lesions, no burrows.

Treatment

1. Inspect or question concerning other members of family to rule out infestation in them.
2. Instruct patient to bathe thoroughly, scrubbing the involved areas with a brush.
3. Topicide (Benzyl benzoate D.D.T. lotion, U.S.P. 180.0

   Sig: Apply to the entire body from the neck down at night.
4. Do not bathe for 24 hours. Old clothes may be reworn.
5. After 24 hours bathe carefully and change to clean clothes and bedding.
6. Washing, dry cleaning or ironing of clothes or bedding is sufficient to destroy the mite. Sterilization is unnecessary.
7. Itching may persist for a few days in spite of the destruction of the mite. For this apply:

A. Sulfur, ppt.	4%
Camphor	1%
Alcoholic white shake lotion, q.s.	120.0
or	
B. Eurax cream, q.s.	60.0

This cream has scabiecidal power and antipruritic action combined.

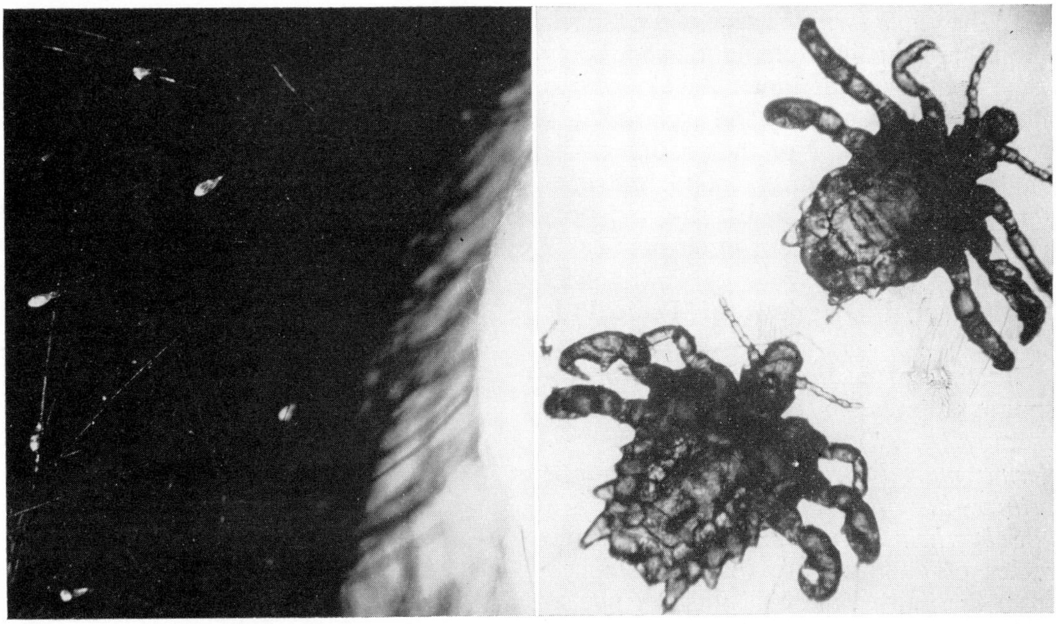

Fig. 79. Pediculosis.

(*Left*) Nits on scalp hair behind ear. (Dr. Lawrence Hyde) (*Right*) Head louse or *Pediculus humanus capitis* as seen with 7.5X lens of microscope. (Dr. James Boley)

8. If itching persists for 1 to 2 weeks, re-examine patient carefully for burrows and retreat if necessary.

PEDICULOSIS

Lice infestation affects people of all ages but usually those in the lower-income strata because of lack of cleanliness and infrequent changes of clothing. Three clinical entities are produced, (1) infestation of the hair by the head louse, *Pediculus humanus capitis* (Fig. 79), (2) infestation of the body louse, *P. humanus corporis* and (3) infestation of the pubic area by the pubic louse, *Phthirus pubis*. Since lice bite the skin and live on the blood, it is impossible for them to live without human contact. The readily visible oval eggs or nits are attached to hairs or to clothing fibers by the female. After the eggs hatch the newly born lice mature within 30 days. Then the female can live for another 30 days, depositing a few eggs daily.

Primary Lesions. The bite is not unusual and is seldom seen because of the secondary changes produced by the resulting intense itching. In the *scalp and pubic form* the nits are found on the hairs, but the lice are found only occasionally. In the *body form* the nits and the lice can be found after careful searching in the seams of the clothing.

Secondary Lesions. In the *scalp form* the skin is red and excoriated, with such severe secondary bacterial infection in some cases that the hairs become matted together in a crusty, foul-smelling "cap." Regional lymphadenopathy is common. A morbilliform rash on the body, an "id" reaction, is seen in long-standing cases.

In the *body form,* linear excoriations and secondary infection seen mainly on the shoulders, the belt-line and the buttocks mask the primary bites.

In the *pubic form* the secondary excoriations are again dominant, producing some matting of the hairs. This louse can also infest body, axillary and eyelash hairs. An unusual eruption on the abdomen, the thighs and the arms, called *maculae cerulae* because of the bluish-gray, pea-sized macules, can occur in chronic cases of pubic pediculosis.

Differential Diagnosis of Pediculosis Capitis

Bacterial Infection of the Scalp: responds rapidly to correct antibacterial therapy (p. 96). *All cases of scalp pyoderma must be examined closely for a primary lice infestation.*

Seborrheic Dermatitis or *Dandruff:* the scales of dandruff are readily detached from the hair, while oval nits are not so easily removed (p. 73).

Hair Casts: resemble nits but can be pulled off more easily; no eggs seen on microscopic examination.

Differential Diagnosis of Pediculosis Corporis

Scabies: may see small burrows, distribution of lesions different, no lice in clothes (p. 155).

Senile or Winter Itch: history helpful, see dry skin, aggravated by bathing, will not find lice in clothes (pp. 60 and 61, respectively).

Differential Diagnosis of Pediculosis Pubis

Scabies: will not see nits, see burrows in pubic area and elsewhere (p. 155).

Pyoderma Secondary to Contact Dermatitis from condoms, contraceptive jellies, new underwear, douches (history important, acute onset, on nits, p. 96).

Seborrheic Dermatitis when in eyebrows and eyelashes (no nits found, p. 73).

Treatment

1. *Pediculosis capitis*
   A. Topocide liquid 60.0
   or Kwell lotion 60.0
   Sig: Shampoo and comb hair thoroughly, then when dry apply medicine. Shampoo again in 3 days and repeat application.
   B. For secondary scalp infection:
   a. Trim hair as much as is possible and agreeable with the patient.
   b. Shampoo hair twice a day with Dial Shampoo.
   c. Neosporin or other antibiotic ointment 15.0
   Sig: Apply to scalp b.i.d.
   C. Change and clean bedding and headwear after 24 hours of treatment. Storage of headwear for 30 days will destroy the lice and the nits.
2. *Pediculosis corporis*
   A. Phenol 0.5%
   Calamine lotion, q.s. 120.0
   Sig: Apply locally b.i.d. for itching. (The lice and the nits are in the clothing.)
   B. Have the clothing laundered or dry cleaned. If this is impossible, dusting with 10% DDT or 10% lindane powder will kill the parasites. Care should be taken to prevent reinfestation. Storage of clothing for 30 days will kill both nits and lice.
3. *Pediculosis pubis:* Same as for scalp form.

Bullous Dermatoses

CHAPTER 17

TO MEDICAL STUDENTS and practitioners alike, the bullous skin diseases are the most dramatic. One of these diseases, pemphigus, is undoubtedly greatly responsible for the aura that surrounds the exhibition and the discussion of an unfortunate patient with a bullous disease. Happy would the instructor be who could behold such student interest when a case of acne or hand dermatitis is being presented.

Three bullous diseases will be discussed in this chapter: *pemphigus, erythema multiforme bullosum* and *dermatitis herpetiformis*. However, other bullous skin diseases do occur, and in this introduction they will be differentiated from these three.

Bullous Impetigo. The name of *pemphigus neonatorum* has been attached to this pyodermic skin infection because of the resemblance of the large bullae in this disease to pemphigus. This term should be abandoned. Bullous impetigo is to be differentiated from the other bullous diseases by occurring in infants and children, rapid development of the individual bullae, presence of impetigo lesions in siblings, and rapid response to local antibiotic therapy (p. 96).

Contact Dermatitis Due to Poison Ivy or Similar Plants. Bullae and vesicles are seen in linear configuration; history of pulling weeds or burning brush is usually obtained; past history of poison ivy or related dermatitis is common; duration of disease is only 7 to 14 days (p. 42).

Drug eruption, particularly from sulfonamides and iodides. Elicit drug history; eruption usually clears on discontinuing drugs; bullae appear rapidly (p. 55).

Epidermolysis Bullosa. This rare chronic hereditary skin disease is manifested by the formation of bullae, usually on the hands and the feet, following mild trauma. The *simple form* can begin in infancy or adulthood with the formation of tense, slightly itching bullae at the sites of pressure, which heal quickly without scarring. Forced marches during war can initiate this disease in patients who have the heredity factor. Such cases are usually treated erroneously as athlete's feet. The disease is worse in the summer or may be present only at this time. The *dystrophic form* begins in infancy like the simple form, but as time elapses the bullae become hemorrhagic, heal slowly, leave scars which can amputate digits, and death can result from secondary infection. Mucous membrane lesions are more common in the dystrophic form than in the simple form. Treatment is supportive.

Familial Benign Chronic Pemphigus (Hailey-Hailey Disease). This is a rare hereditary bullous eruption most common on the neck and in the axillae. It can be distinguished from pemphigus by its chronicity and benign nature, and by its histologic picture. Some consider this disease to be a bullous variety of keratosis follicularis (Darier's disease).

Impetigo Herpetiformis. One of the rarest of skin diseases, this is characterized by groups of pustules mainly seen in the

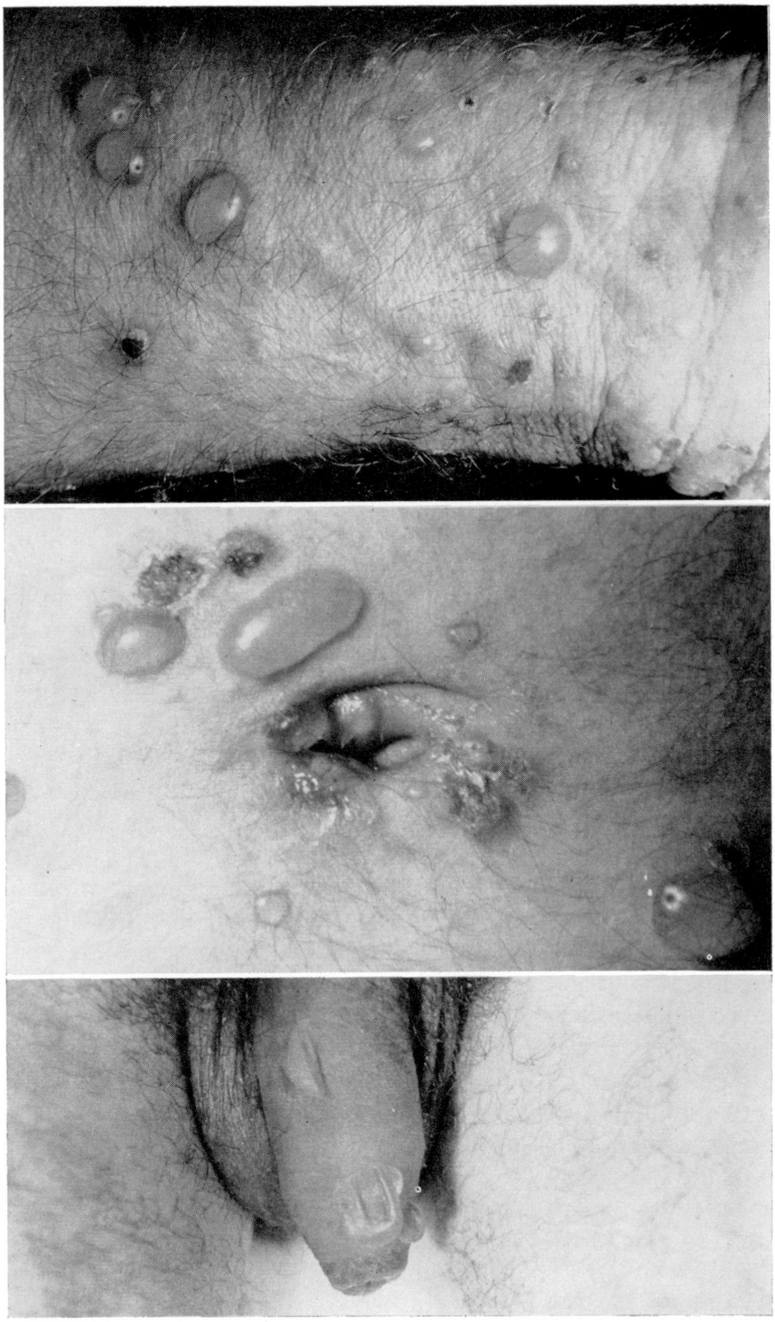

Fig. 80. Pemphigus and erythema multiforme bullosum.

(*Top*) Pemphigus vulgaris bullae on wrist.

(*Center*) Pemphigus vulgaris bullae and crusted lesions around umbilicus. Same patient as above.

(*Bottom*) Erythema multiforme bullosum on penis.

axillae and the groin, high fever, prostration, severe malaise and generally a fatal outcome. It occurs most commonly in pregnant or postpartum women. It can be distinguished from pemphigus vegetans or dermatitis herpetiformis by the fact that these diseases do not produce such general, acute, toxic manifestations.

In spite of high student and general practitioner interest in the bullous skin conditions, the diagnosis and the management of the 3 main diseases, particularly pemphigus and dermatitis herpetiformis, should be the problem of the dermatologist. Indeed, it is one of the greatest problems in the field of dermatology. The problem of therapy is difficult enough, but the differential diagnosis between these 3 diseases is often not proved until an individual case has been followed for months or years. It will be the purpose of the author in this chapter to present the salient features of these diseases, with therapy skimmed over lightly.

PEMPHIGUS VULGARIS
(Plate 1 F)

Even though this disease is rare, most doctors see several cases of pemphigus early in their career. Pemphigus cases have to be hospitalized at one time or another during the course of the disease and, as a result, the hospital personnel and staff are exposed to this most miserable, odiferous, debilitating skin disease. Prior to the advent of corticosteroid therapy the disease was eventually fatal (Fig. 80).

Primary Lesions. The early lesions of pemphigus are small vesicles or bullae on apparently normal skin. Redness of the base of the bullae is unusual. Without treatment the bullae enlarge and spread, and new ones balloon up on different areas of the skin or the mucous membranes. Rupturing of the bullae leaves large eroded areas.

Secondary Lesions. Bacterial infection with crusting is marked and accounts in part for the characteristic mousy odor. Lesions that heal spontaneously or under therapy do not leave scars.

Course. When untreated, pemphigus can be readily fatal or assume a slow lingering course with debility, painful mouth and body erosions, systemic bacterial infection and toxemia. Spontaneous temporary remissions do occur without therapy.

Three variations of common pemphigus exist. *Pemphigus foliaceus* appears as a scaly, moist, generalized exfoliative dermatitis. The characteristic mousy odor of pemphigus is dominant in this variant, which is also remarkable for its chronicity. The response to steroid therapy is less favorable in the foliaceus form than in the other types.

Pemphigus vegetans is characterized by the development of large granulomatous masses in the intertriginous areas of the axillae and the groin. Secondary bacterial infection, while present in all cases of pemphigus, is most marked in this form. Pemphigus vegetans is to be differentiated from a granulomatous ioderma or bromoderma (p. 58) and from impetigo herpetiformis (p. 159).

Pemphigus erythematosus clinically resembles a mixture of pemphigus, seborrheic dermatitis and lupus erythematosus. The distribution of the red, greasy, crusted and eroded lesions is on the butterfly area of the face, the sternal area, the scalp and occasionally in the mouth. The course is more chronic than for pemphigus vulgaris, and remissions are common.

Etiology. Unknown.

Laboratory Findings. The histopathology of early cases is quite characteristic and serves to differentiate most cases of pemphigus from dermatitis herpetiformis and the other bullous diseases.

Differential Diagnosis. See Introduction to this chapter; also *dermatitis herpetiformis* and *erythema multiforme bullosum*.

Treatment of Pemphigus

1. If possible, a dermatologist or an internist should be called in to share the responsibility of the care.

2. Hospitalization is necessary for the patient with large areas of bullae and erosions. Early cases of pemphigus can be managed in the office.

3. Triamcinolone, 4 mg., or related corticosteroids #30

Sig: One tablet q.i.d. for 4 days;

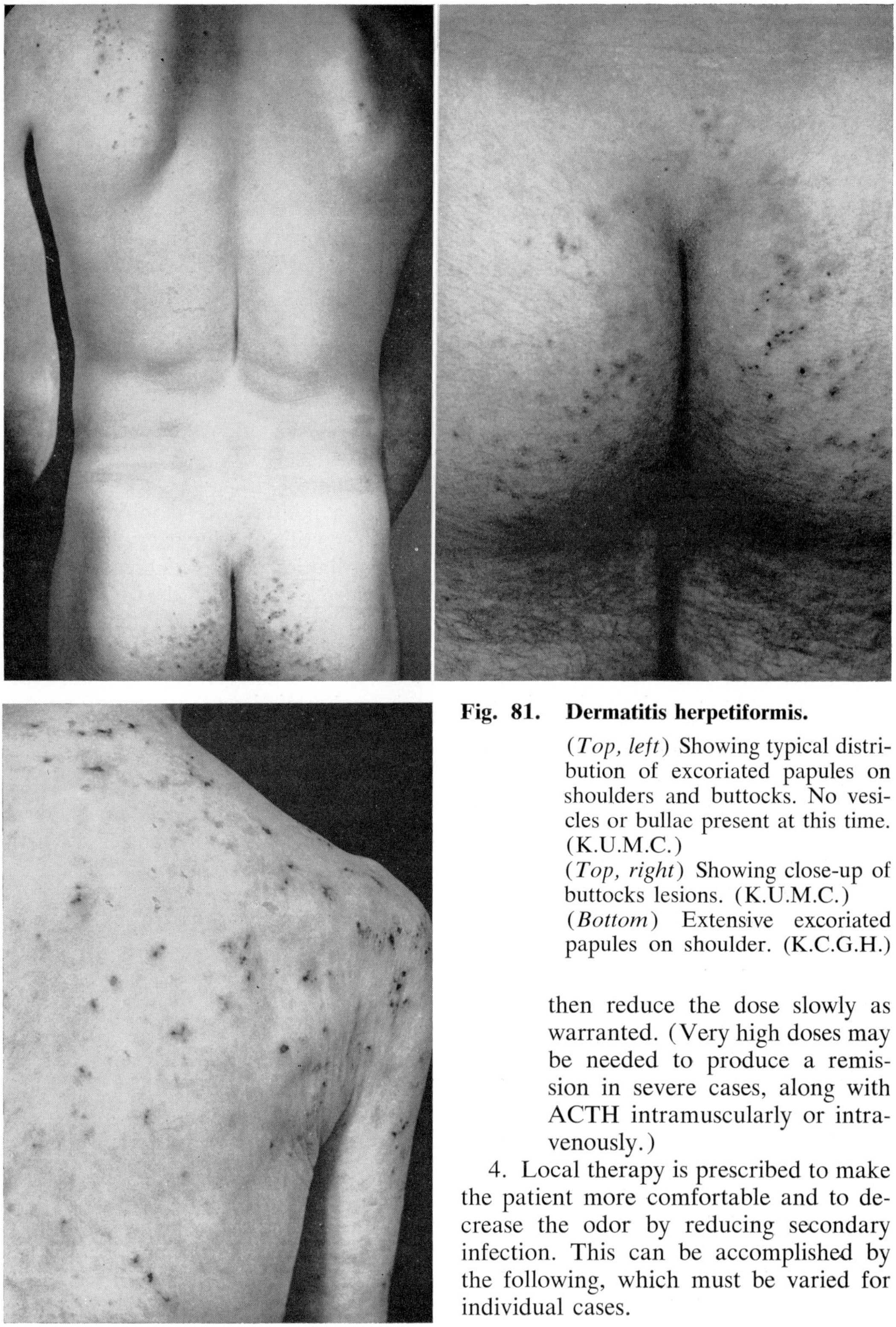

Fig. 81. Dermatitis herpetiformis.

(*Top, left*) Showing typical distribution of excoriated papules on shoulders and buttocks. No vesicles or bullae present at this time. (K.U.M.C.)
(*Top, right*) Showing close-up of buttocks lesions. (K.U.M.C.)
(*Bottom*) Extensive excoriated papules on shoulder. (K.C.G.H.)

then reduce the dose slowly as warranted. (Very high doses may be needed to produce a remission in severe cases, along with ACTH intramuscularly or intravenously.)

4. Local therapy is prescribed to make the patient more comfortable and to decrease the odor by reducing secondary infection. This can be accomplished by the following, which must be varied for individual cases.

A. Potassium permanganate crystals 60.0
Sig: Place 2 teaspoons of the crystals to the bathtub with approximately 10 inches of lukewarm water. (To prevent crystals from burning the skin they should be dissolved completely in a glass of water before adding to the tub. The solution should be made fresh daily. The tub stains can be removed by applying acetic acid or "hypo" solution.)

B. Talc 120.0
Sig: Dispense in powder can. Apply to bed sheeting and to erosions twice a day. (Called a "powder bed.")

C. Sulfur, ppt. 3%
Neo-Polycin or other antibiotic ointment, q.s. 30.0
Sig: Apply to small infected areas b.i.d.

6. Supportive therapy should be used when necessary. This includes vitamins, iron, blood transfusions and oral antibiotics.

7. Nursing care of the highest caliber is a prerequisite for the severe case of pemphigus with generalized erosions and bullae. The nursing personnel should be told that this disease is not contagious or infectious.

DERMATITIS HERPETIFORMIS

Dermatitis herpetiformis is a rare, chronic, markedly pruritic, papular, vesicular and bullous skin disease of unknown etiology (Fig. 81). The patient describes the itching of a new blister as a burning itch which disappears when the blister top is scratched off. The severe scratching results in the formation of excoriations and papular hives which may be the only visible pathology of the disease. Individual lesions heal, leaving an area of hyperpigmentation which is very characteristic. The typical distribution of the blisters or excoriations is on the scalp, the sacral area, the scapular area, the forearms and the thighs. In severe cases, the resulting bullae may be indistinguishable from pemphigus. The duration of dermatitis herpetiformis varies from months to as long as 40 years, with periods of remission scattered in between. Laboratory tests should include a biopsy which is quite characteristic, and a blood count which shows an eosinophilia.

Herpes gestationis is dermatitis herpetiformis that occurs in relation to pregnancy. It usually develops during the 2nd or the 3rd trimester, and commonly disappears after birth, only to return with subsequent pregnancies. This variation of dermatitis herpetiformis may be related to an Rh incompatibility.

Differential Diagnosis of Dermatitis Herpetiformis

Pemphigus: see large, flaccid bullae, mouth involvement more commonly in pemphigus, debilitating course, biopsy quite characteristic, eosinophilia uncommon (p. 161).

Erythema Multiforme Bullosum: bullae usually arise on a red irislike base; burning itch is absent; residual pigmentation is minor; course is shorter (p. 164).

Neurotic Excoriations: if this diagnosis is being considered, it is very important to rule out dermatitis herpetiformis, and usually this can be done by finding no scalp lesions, no blisters at any time, no eosinophilia.

Scabies: see no vesicles or bullae; see burrows, lesions in other members of family (p. 155).

Treatment. A dermatologist should be consulted to establish the diagnosis and to outline therapy. This would consist of local and oral measures to control itching, and a course of one of the following quite effective drugs: sulfapyridine (0.5 Gm. q.i.d.) or Diasone (0.33 Gm. q.i.d.).

These initial doses should be decreased in relation to the patient's response. These drugs can be toxic, and the patient must be under the close surveillance of the physician. Corticosteroids are often used for a short period to give relief in acute flare-ups.

ERYTHEMA MULTIFORME BULLOSUM

This entity presents a distinct clinical picture and course from erythema multiforme (p. 69). Many drugs can cause an "erythema multiforme bullosumlike" picture, but then this manifestation should be labeled a "drug eruption." True erythema multiforme bullosum has no known cause (Fig. 80 C). Clinically, it differs from erythema multiforme by the development of large vesicles and bullae usually overlying red irislike macules. The lesions most commonly appear on the arms, the legs and the face but can occur elsewhere, including, on occasion, the mouth. Erythema multiforme bullosum can last from days to months. Slight malaise and fever may precede a new shower of bullae, but for the most part the patient's general health is unaffected. Itching may be mild or severe enough to interfere with sleep. When the characteristic iris lesions are absent, it is difficult to differentiate this bullous eruption from early pemphigus, dermatitis herpetiformis and bullous hives.

Treatment. These patients should be referred to a dermatologist or an internist to substantiate the diagnosis and initiate therapy. Corticosteroids orally and by injection are the single most effective drugs in use today. For widespread cases that must be hospitalized, the local care is similar to that for pemphigus.

Exfoliative Dermatitis

CHAPTER 18

AS THE term implies, exfoliative dermatitis is a generalized scaling eruption of the skin. The causes are many. This diagnosis never should be made without additional qualifying etiologic terms.

This is a rather rare skin condition, but many general physicians, residents and interns see these cases because they are frequently hospitalized. The purpose of hospitalization is twofold: (1) to perform a diagnostic workup, since the cause in many cases is difficult to ascertain, and (2) to administer intensive therapy under close supervision.

Classification of the cases of exfoliative dermatitis is facilitated by dividing them into primary and secondary forms.

PRIMARY EXFOLIATIVE DERMATITIS

These cases develop in apparently healthy individuals from no ascertainable cause.

Skin Lesions. Clinically, it is impossible to differentiate this primary form from the one where the etiology is known or suspected. Various degrees of scaling and redness are seen, ranging from fine generalized granular scales with mild erythema, to scaling in large plaques with marked erythema and lichenification. Generalized adenopathy is usually present. The nails become thick and lusterless, and the hair falls out in varying degrees.

Subjective Complaint. Itching in most cases is intense.

Course. The prognosis for early cure of the disease is poor. The mortality rate is high in older patients, due to generalized debility and secondary infection.

Etiology. Various authors have studied the relationship of lymphomas to cases of exfoliative dermatitis. Some believe the incidence to be low, but others state that from 35% to 50% of these exfoliative cases, particularly those in patients over the age of 40, are the result of lymphomas. However, years may pass before the lymphoma becomes obvious.

Laboratory Findings. There are no diagnostic changes, but the usual case has an elevated white blood cell count with eosinophilia. Biopsy of the skin is not diagnostic in the primary type. Biopsy of an enlarged lymph node, in either the primary or the secondary form, will reveal *lipomelanotic reticulosis.*

Treatment. A male aged 50 has had a generalized, pruritic, scaly, erythematous eruption for 3 months.

1. A general medical workup is indicated, either in the office or in the hospital. A focus of infection in the teeth, the tonsils, the gallbladder or the genitourinary tract should be ruled out.

2. A high protein diet should be prescribed, because these patients have a high basal metabolic rate and catabolize protein.

3. Bathing instructions are variable. Some patients prefer a daily cool bath in a colloid solution for relief of itching (1 box of Linit Starch or 1 cup of Aveeno

to 10 inches of water), but for most cases generalized bathing dries the skin and intensifies the itching.

4. Provide extra blankets for the bed. These patients lose a lot of heat through their red skin and consequently feel chilly.

5. Locally, an ointment is most desired, but some prefer an oily liquid. Formulas for both follow:

A. White petrolatum 240.0
Sig: Apply locally b.i.d. (As time progresses more antipruritic effect can be gained by adding menthol 0.25%, or camphor 2%, or phenol 0.5%, or coal tar solution 1% to 5%. Watch for sensitivity to these chemicals, with intensification of itching and erythema.)

B. Zinc oxide 40%
Olive oil q.s. 240.0
Sig: Apply locally with hands or a paint brush b.i.d. (Antipruritic chemicals can also be added to this.)

6. Oral antihistamine, for example:
Temaril, 2.5 mg. #20
Sig: 1 tablet q.i.d. for itching.

Subsequent Care

1. Systemic steroids. For resistant cases the corticosteroids have consistently provided more relief than any other single form of therapy. Any of the preparations can be used, for example:

Triamcinolone (Kenacort or Aristocort), 4 mg. #30
Sig: 1 tablet q.i.d. for 5 days; then 1 tablet b.i.d. or as indicated.

2. Systemic antibiotics may or may not be indicated.

SECONDARY EXFOLIATIVE DERMATITIS
(Plate 27)

The majority of patients with secondary exfoliative dermatitis have had a previous skin disease which became generalized because of overtreatment or unknown reasons. There always remain a few cases of exfoliative dermatitis where the cause is unknown but suspected.

Skin Lesions. The clinical picture of this secondary form is undistinguishable from the primary form unless some of the original dermatitis is present. It is important to look for such diagnostic evidence at the edge of an advancing early exfoliative dermatitis or on mildly involved areas.

Course. The prognosis in the secondary form is better than for the primary form, particularly if the original cause is definitely known and more specific therapy can be administered.

Etiology and Treatment. A list follows of the commoner causes of secondary exfoliative dermatitis. The treatment of these cases would be a combination of those listed above for the primary form of exfoliative dermatitis plus a cautious institution of stronger therapy directed toward the original causative skin condition. This therapy should be reviewed in the section devoted to the specific disease.

Contact dermatitis (p. 42)
Drug eruption (p. 55)
Psoriasis (p. 83)
Atopic eczema (p. 51)
Pyoderma with "id" reaction (p. 96)
Fungous disease with "id" reaction (p. 148)
Seborrheic dermatitis (p. 73)
Lymphoma (p. 231)

Pigmentary Dermatoses

CHAPTER 19

THERE are two variants of pigmentation of the skin: hyperpigmentation and hypopigmentation. The predominant skin pigment to be discussed in this chapter is melanin, but other pigments can be present in the skin. A complete classification is listed under "Pigmentary Disorders" in the Dictionary-Index.

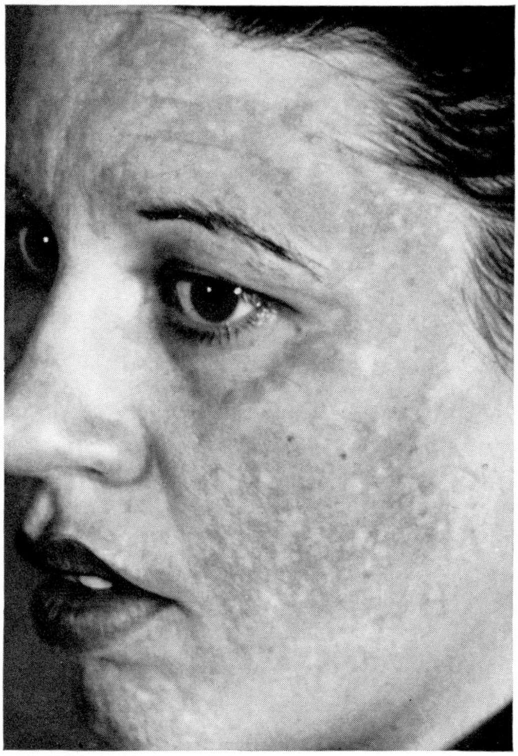

Fig. 82. Chloasma.

This hyperpigmentation became prominent during pregnancy. (K.C.G.H.)

The common clinical example of abnormal hyperpigmentation is chloasma, but secondary melanoderma can result from many causes. The commonest form of hypopigmentation is vitiligo, but secondary leukoderma does occur.

CHLOASMA

Clinical Lesions. An irregular hyperpigmentation of the skin that varies in shades of brown (Fig. 82).

Distribution. Usually on the sides of the face, the forehead and the sides of the neck.

Course. Slowly progressive, but remissions do occur. More obvious in the summer.

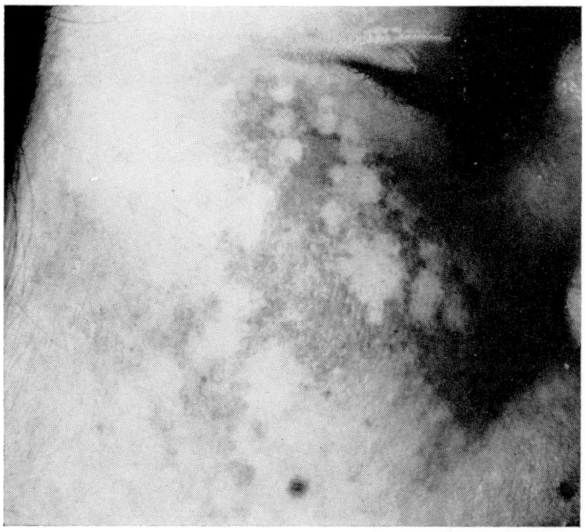

Fig. 83. Secondary hyperpigmentation.

An example of berlock dermatitis on the face due to a photosensitivity reaction from a cosmetic.

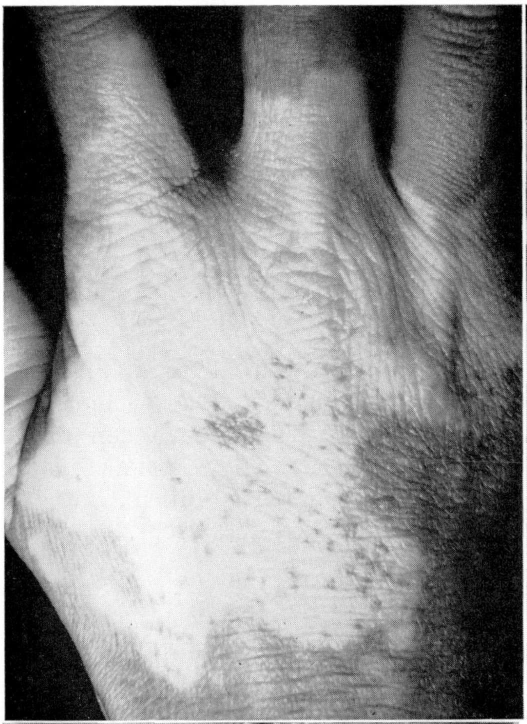

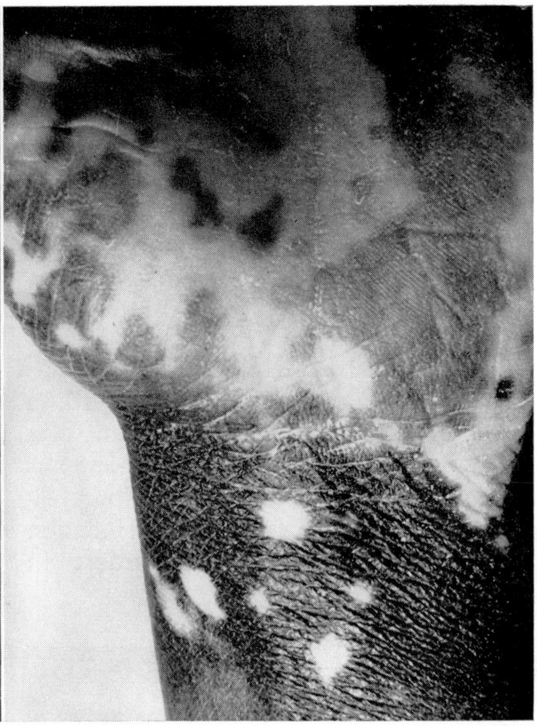

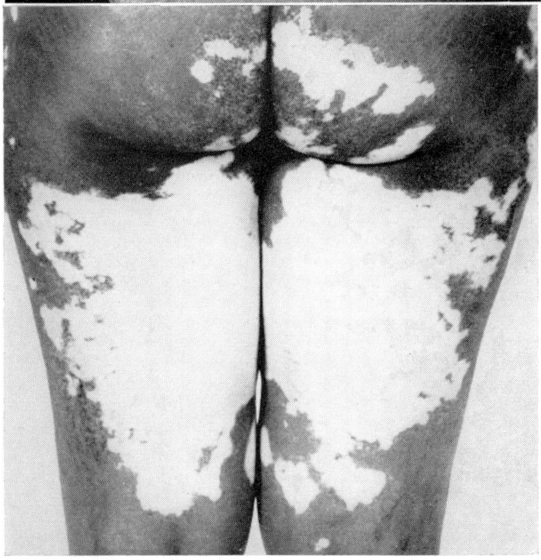

Fig. 84. Vitiligo.

(*Top, left*) On dorsum of hand of a white patient. Central brown dots show result of 2½ months of 8-MOP therapy.
(*Top, right*) On wrist and palm of Negro patient.
(*Bottom*) On posterior aspect of thighs of a Negro patient.

Etiology. Unknown, but some cases appear during pregnancy (called "mask of pregnancy") or with chronic illness. A lay term for chloasma is "liver spots," but there is no association with liver pathology. The melanocyte-stimulating hormone of the pituitary may be excessive and effect the tyrosine-tyrosinase enzyme system.

Differential Diagnosis. Rule out the causes of *secondary melanoderma* (see Dictionary-Index under "Pigmentary Disease"). (See Fig. 83.)

Treatment

1. Do not promise great therapeutic results to the patient. Most cases associated with pregnancy fade or disappear completely following delivery.
2. Benoquin ointment (Elder) 30.0
   Sig: Apply locally b.i.d. Stop if irritation develops.

The active chemical in this ointment, monobenzyl ether of hydroquinone, was discovered following an investigation of the cause of an occupational leukoderma which occurred in Negroes exposed to rubber-ageing compounds in the rubber industry.

Allergic contact reactions to this drug occur in an appreciable number of cases. If this happens, the 5% Benoquin lotion can be substituted, or a salve containing 5% ammoniated mercury in white petrolatum. A few patients cannot be helped.

VITILIGO

Clinical Lesions. Irregular areas of depigmented skin occasionally seen with a hyperpigmented border (Fig. 84).

Distribution. Most commonly on the face, dorsum of hands and feet, but can occur on all body areas.

Course. Slowly progressive, but remissions and changes are frequent. More obvious during the summer because of the tanning of adjacent normal skin.

Etiology. Unknown. Heredity is a factor in some cases.

Differential Diagnosis. Rule out causes of secondary hypopigmentation (see Dictionary-Index under "Pigmentary Disease"). (See Fig. 85.)

Treatment. An attractive young woman with large depigmented patches on her face and dorsum of hands asks if something can be done for her "white spots." Her sister has a few lesions.

1. Cosmetics. The use of the following covering or staining preparations is recommended: pancake type cosmetics, such as Covermark by Lydia O'Leary; walnut juice stain (Depelle); or potassium permanganate solution in appropriate dilution. Many patients with vitiligo become quite proficient in the application of these agents. If the patient desires a more specific treatment, the following can be suggested with certain reservations:

2. Psoralen derivatives. For many years Egyptians along the Nile River chewed certain plants to cause the disappearance of the white spots of vitiligo. Extraction of the chemicals from these plants revealed the psoralen derivatives to be the active agents, and one of these, 8-methoxy-

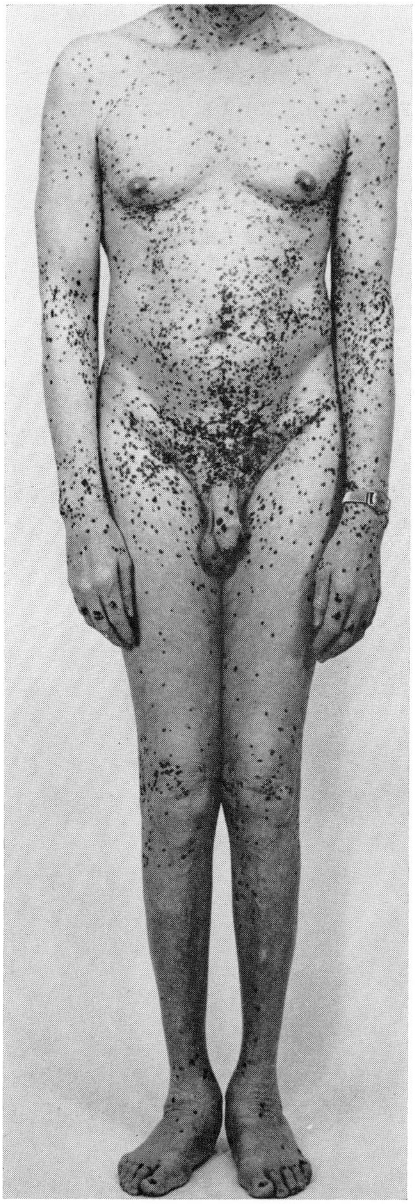

Fig. 85. Secondary hypopigmentation.

A marked example of loss of pigment that occurred in a Negro male following healing of an exfoliative dermatitis. Corticosteroids were used in the therapy.

psoralen, was found to be the most effective. This chemical has now been manufactured in this country under the names of Oxsoralen (Elder), Methoxa-Dome (Dome), and Meloxine (Upjohn) in 10-mg. capsules. A liquid form is also available for local application, but this form of treatment is not recommended. Therapy for a patient with vitiligo consists in taking 20 mg. of 8-methoxypsoralen a day, followed after 2 hours by exposure of the affected areas to ultraviolet light from the sun or from a home sun-lamp. The exposure should be cautious at first, usually 1 to 5 minutes, depending on the quality and the quantity of the light source, and increased slowly by 1 to 5 minute increments up to 30 minutes. Beginning repigmentation is noted in 50 to 70% of patients after 6 to 12 weeks of treatment. The disadvantages of this therapy are the time-consuming element and the cost of medication. As a result, only a few patients complete therapy. After repigmentation occurs, usually not 100% complete, the pigmentation can be maintained by 2 to 3 months of therapy annually, utilizing the summer sun, which is more effective than artificial ultraviolet. The side-effects include a blistering reaction from overzealous ultraviolet exposure and, rarely, liver function impairment. To discover and minimize the latter, cephalin flocculation or bromsulphalein tests should be run at biweekly intervals for the first 4 to 6 weeks.

A short 2-week course of this therapy is advocated for the purpose of acquiring an increased suntan. The value of such a course has not been proved. Liver function tests are not necessary during this short treatment.

Collagen Diseases

CHAPTER 20

THE DISEASES commonly included in this group are lupus erythematosus, scleroderma and dermatomyositis. The skin manifestations are usually a dominant feature of these diseases, but in some cases, particularly acute L. E., skin lesions may be absent. Rheumatoid arthritis and periarteritis nodosa are often included in the collagen disease group but only occasionally are accompanied by skin lesions, usually of the erythema multiformelike group (p. 69).

The onset of the collagen diseases is insidious, and the prognosis as to life is serious. It is not unusual to attach the label of "collagen disease" to a patient who has only minimal subjective and objective findings (malaise, weakness, vague joint and muscle pains, biologic false positive serology and high sedimentation rate) with the realization by the physician that months and years will have to elapse before a more exacting diagnosis of one of the above diseases can be made.

	Chronic Discoid L. E.	Acute Disseminated L. E.
Primary lesions	Red, scaly, thickened, well-circumscribed patches with enlarged follicles and elevated border	Red, mildly scaly, diffuse, puffy lesions. Purpura also seen
Secondary lesions	Atrophy, scarring and pigmentary changes	No scarring. Mild hyperpigmentation
Distribution	Face, mainly in "butterfly" area, but also on scalp, ears, arms and chest. May not be symmetrical	Face in "butterfly" area, arms, fingers and legs. Usually symmetrical
Course	Very chronic with gradual progression; slow healing under therapy; no effect on life	Acute onset with fever, rash, malaise and joint pains. Most cases respond rather rapidly to steroid and supportive therapy, but the prognosis for life is poor
Season	Aggravated by intense sun exposure or radiation therapy	Same
Sex incidence	Almost twice as common in females	Same
Systemic pathology	None obvious	Nephritis, arthritis, epilepsy, pancarditis, hepatitis, etc.
Laboratory findings	Biopsy characteristic in classic case. L. E. cell test negative, as are other laboratory tests	Biopsy less useful. L. E. cell test positive. Leukopenia, anemia, albuminuria, increased sedimentation rate, and biologic false-positive serologic test for syphilis

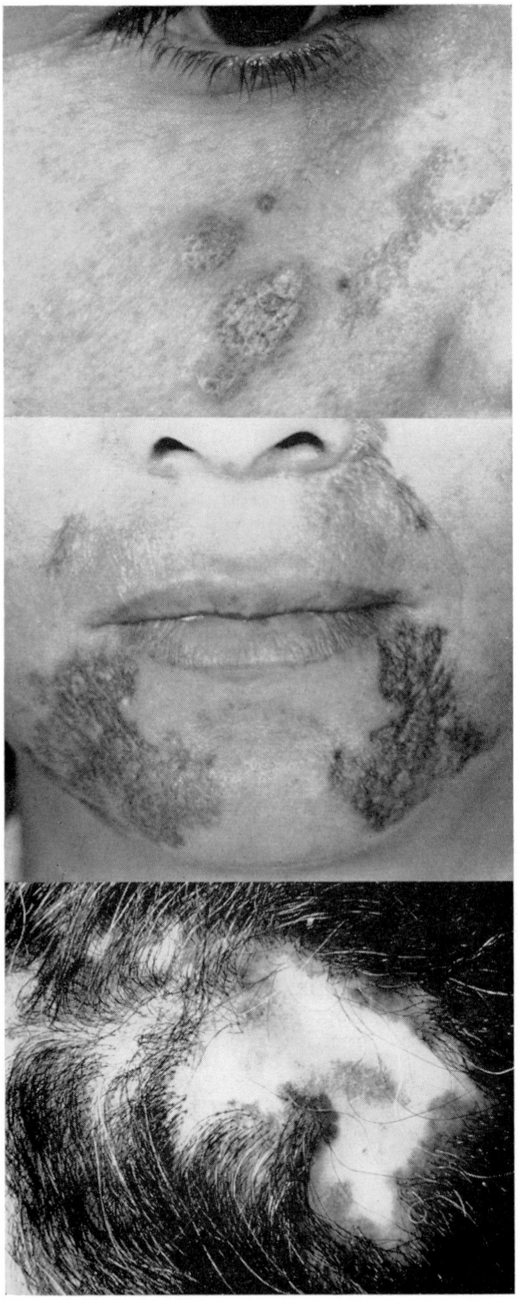

Fig. 86. Chronic discoid lupus erythematosus.

(*Top*) Typical active red, scaly patches on cheek.
(*Center*) Marked hyperpigmentation and scarring following healing.
(*Bottom*) Permanent hair loss and atrophic hypopigmentation following healing in Negro's scalp.

LUPUS ERYTHEMATOSUS (Plate 28)

Acute disseminated L. E. and chronic discoid L. E. are clinically dissimilar but basically related diseases. The two diseases differ in regard to characteristic skin lesions, subjective complaints, other organ involvement, L. E. cell test findings, response to treatment, and eventual prognosis. However, rare cases of clinically classic chronic discord L. E. show laboratory evidence of the pathology seen with the acute form of L. E. and can terminate as the disseminated disease. Certain early borderline cases are difficult to categorize, but eventually the majority of these subacute forms develop into the acute disseminated disease. The variations of the acute and the chronic forms of L. E. are shown in the chart on page 171.

CHRONIC DISCOID LUPUS ERYTHEMATOSUS (Fig. 86)

Differential Diagnosis

Acute Disseminated L. E. (see chart, p. 171)

Actinic Dermatitis: many cases are grossly and histologically similar to acute or chronic L. E. but get history of presence only in summer; see faster response to antimalarial drugs and locally applied sun-screening agents.

Seborrheic Dermatitis: lesions greasy, red, scaly, associated with scalp dandruff; see in eyebrows and scalp without hair loss; rapid response to antiseborrheic local therapy (p. 73).

Any Cutaneous Granulomas: such as sarcoidosis (p. 110), secondary and tertiary syphilis (p. 113) and lupus vulgaris (p. 109).

Cases with scarring alopecia are to be differentiated from *alopecia cicatrisata* (p. 191), *old tinea capitis of endothrix type* (p. 144), *lichen planus* (p. 92) and *folliculitis decalvens* (p. 191).

Treatment. Young female patient

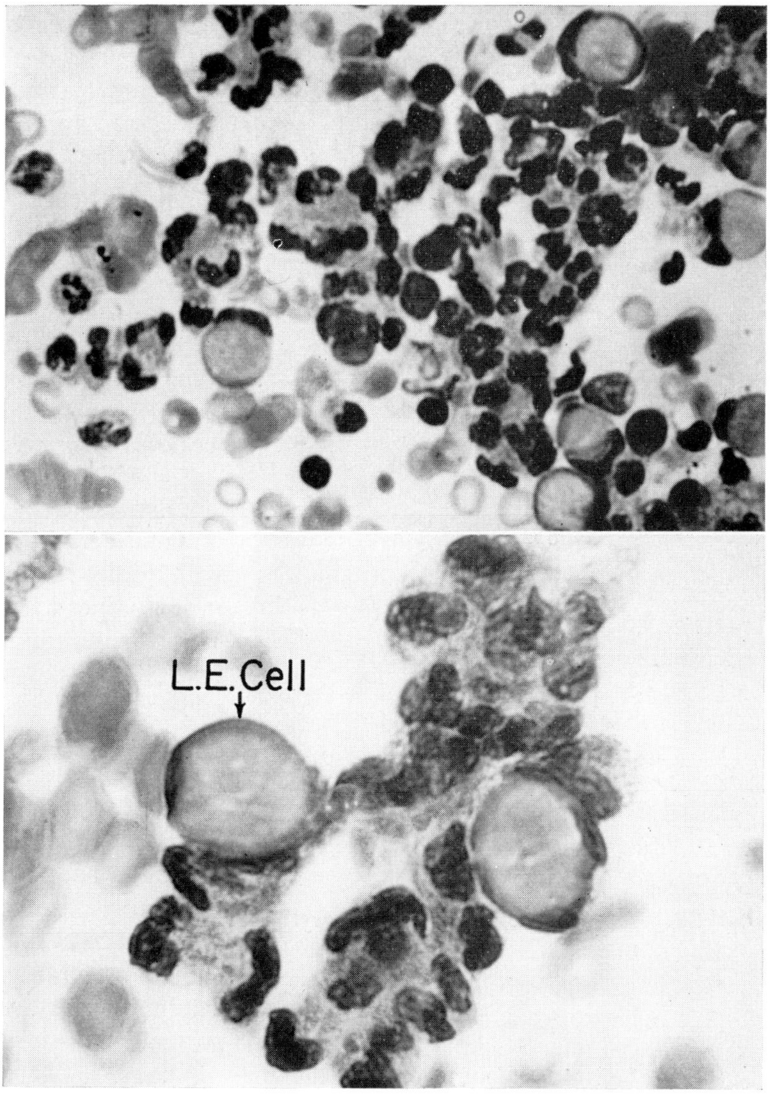

Fig. 87. L. E. cells under low power (top) and high power (bottom) lens of microscope.

(Dr. Sloan Wilson)

with 2 red, scaly, dime-sized lesions on right cheek of 3-months' duration.

1. Laboratory workup should include a complete blood count, urinalysis, serology, L. E. cell test (Fig. 87), sedimentation rate and, uncommonly, a biopsy. The tests should be normal, but the biopsy rather characteristic of chronic discoid L. E. The assistance of a dermatologist to corroborate the diagnosis might be indicated.

2. Aralen (chloroquine), 250 mg. #30

Sig: 1 tablet t.i.d. for 1 week, then 1 b.i.d. for 2 or 3 weeks, and then adjust dose according to response. (For resistant cases can use Atabrine, 100 mg. t.i.d., or Plaquenil, 200 mg. b.i.d. Watch for side-effects with Aralen (blurred vision, gastric upset, leukopenia) and with Atabrine (yellow sclera and skin, skin eruption similar to lichen planus, and agranulocytosis).

3. Skolex cream 30.0

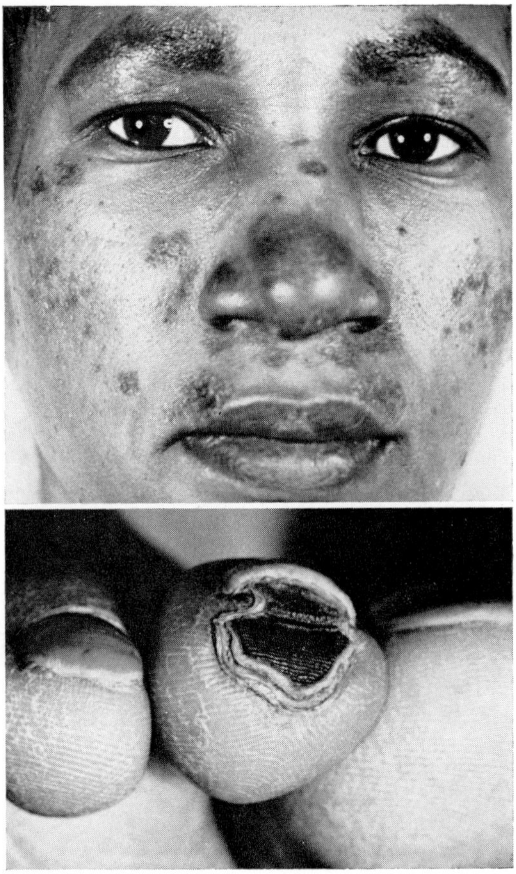

Fig. 88. Acute disseminated lupus erythematosus.

(*Top*) Scaly, dark red lesions in Negro woman with positive L. E. cell test. (K.U.M.C.)
(*Bottom*) Gangrene of toe due to Raynaud's phenomenon in fatal case. (Dr. Robert Jordan)

or

Afil cream 30.0
Sig: Apply to face as sun screen for protection. (Effect of cream lasts for 4 to 6 hours.)

ACUTE DISSEMINATED LUPUS ERYTHEMATOSUS (Fig. 88)

Differential Diagnosis

Chronic discoid L. E. (see preceding chart)

Actinic Dermatitis: skin lesions may be very similar in appearance, usually only in summer; find no altered laboratory studies; more rapid response to antimalarial drugs.

Seborrheic Dermatitis: associated with scalp dandruff; responds to local antiseborrhea therapy (p. 73).

Contact Dermatitis: due to cosmetics, paint sprays, vegetation, hand creams, etc.; acute onset with no systemic symptoms; history helpful (p. 42).

Dermatomyositis: muscle soreness and weakness, negative L. E. cell test (p. 176).

Drug Eruption Due to Apresoline: can simulate acute L. E.; take history.

Treatment. Young female patient with diffuse red, puffy eruption on cheeks, nose, forehead and at base of fingernails of 1-week's duration. Complains of malaise, fever, joint pains, headache and ankle edema which has become progressively worse in the past 3 weeks.

1. The patient should be hospitalized and, following careful diagnostic workup, should be treated with corticosteroids and any other supportive therapy as indicated for the organs involved. Sulfonamide therapy is contraindicated. Such patients should preferably be in the hands of an internist, with assistance from the other specialties as needed.

SCLERODERMA

As with lupus erythematosus, there are two forms of scleroderma that are clinically unrelated except for some common histopathologic changes in the skin. *Localized scleroderma (morphea)* is a benign disease. *Diffuse scleroderma* is a serious disease.

Localized Scleroderma

Morphea is an uncommon skin disease of unknown etiology with no systemic involvement.

Primary Lesions. Single or multiple, violaceous colored, firm, inelastic macules and plaques that enlarge slowly. The progressing border retains the violaceous hue, while the center becomes whitish and slightly depressed beneath the skin surface. Bizarre lesions occur, such as long linear bands on extremities, saber-cut type lesions in scalp, or lesions involving one side of the face or the body, causing hemiatrophy.

Secondary Lesions. Mild or severe scarring after healing is inevitable. Scalp lesions result in permanent hair loss. Ulceration is rare.

Distribution. Trunk, extremities and head most frequently involved.

Course. Disability is confined to the area involved. Lesions tend to involute slowly and spontaneously. Relapses are rare.

Differential Diagnosis. Guttate macular form from *lichen sclerosis et atrophicus* (histopathology rather characteristic); plaque type from *traumatic scars* (history important, no violaceous border).

Treatment. Nothing specific, but bismuth can be used in oral form (Bistrimate), or intramuscular form (Bismuth Cevitamate); also gentle local massage. Time is the healer.

Diffuse Scleroderma

This uncommon systemic disease of unknown etiology is characterized by a long course of progressive disability due primarily to lack of mobility of the areas and the organs that are affected. The skin becomes hidebound, the esophagus and the gastro-intestinal tract semirigid, the lungs and the heart fibrosed, the bones resorbed, and the overlying tissue calcified (Fig. 89).

Primary Lesions. There is usually a long prodromal stage of swelling of the skin with progressive limitation of movement. The early stage may or may not be associated with Raynaud's phenomenon, which is worse in the winter.

Secondary Lesions. As months and years pass the limitation of movement be-

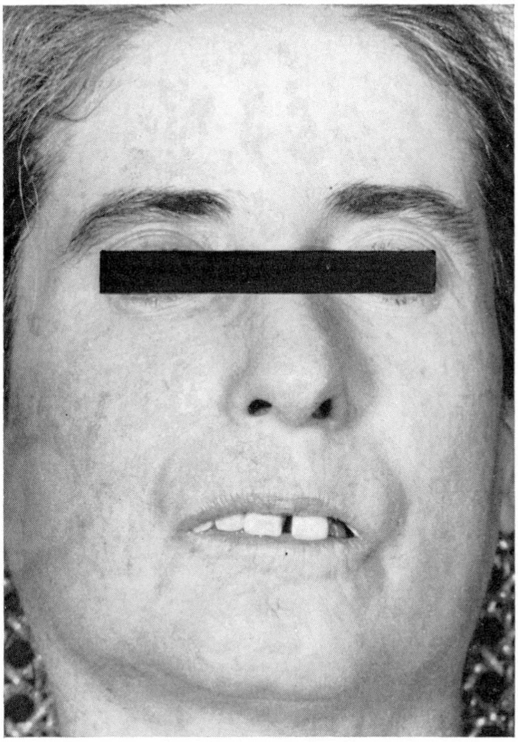

Fig. 89. Diffuse scleroderma.
Note apparent immobility of the skin and lack of facial lines.

comes marked, particularly of the hands, the feet and the face. The skin becomes atrophic, hidebound, develops sensory, vasomotor and pigmentary changes and, finally, ulcerations.

Distribution. The skin of the hands, the feet and the face is involved early, and in some rare cases the changes are confined only to the extremities ("acrosclerosis"). In the majority of patients, however, the entire skin becomes involved along with the internal organs.

Course. The prognosis is grave, and most cases die of the disease after years of disability. However, spontaneous or therapy-induced remissions can occur.

Sex Incidence. More common in females.

Laboratory Findings. Histologic examination of the skin shows generalized atrophy and hyalinization. The atrophic skeletal muscles lack the inflammatory component seen in dermatomyositis. The sedimentation rate is elevated early in the course of the disease. Other abnormal findings are related to the organs involved.

Differential Diagnosis

Dermatomyositis: find muscle tenderness, weakness, few skin changes, muscle biopsy rather characteristic (see below).

Early Rheumatoid Arthritis: swelling of joints and overlying skin, x-ray pictures helpful in determining diagnosis, as is time itself.

Treatment. No specific therapy is known. Protection of the skin from trauma, cold and infection is important. Physiotherapy may prevent contractures. Sympathectomy produces temporary benefits in some patients. Chelating agents are reported helpful for patients with extensive calcification. Bismuth orally or intramuscularly is an old form of treatment of doubtful value. Corticosteroids are not very beneficial.

DERMATOMYOSITIS

This is the rarest of the 3 collagen diseases. It is characterized by an acute or insidious onset of muscle pain, weakness, fever, arthralgia and in some cases a puffy erythematous eruption usually confined to the face and the eyelids. Progression of the disease results in muscle atrophy and contractures, skin telangiectasia and atrophy, and generalized organ involvement with death in 50% of cases. Dermatomyositis has a relationship to adenocarcinoma that is unexplained.

Laboratory Findings. These include increased sedimentation rate, rather characteristic muscle changes on biopsy study, albuminuria, anemia, negative L. E. cell test, and negative serologic test for syphilis. Degeneration of the muscles is accompanied by creatinuria.

Differential Diagnosis: *Acute lupus erythematosus, diffuse scleroderma, photosensitivity reactions, erysipelas, polyneuritis, myasthenia gravis* and others.

Treatment. Removal of an associated adenocarcinoma (present in 20% of cases of dermatomyositis) may result in a remission. Corticosteroid therapy, often in high doses as for acute L. E., may cause a remission.

The Skin and Internal Disease

CHAPTER 21

IT IS not possible to separate the skin and its diseases from the internal organs and their diseases. The physician who fails to recognize this union will end up treating a disease and not a patient. Even the common contact dermatitis from the poison ivy plant affects various people differently, and the person as a whole must be taken into consideration when treating the disease. This is the art of medicine, the learning of which comes slowly.

This union of the skin organ and the internal organs becomes most apparent when studying certain diseases that have both skin and internal components. Some internal diseases have skin manifestations, and a few skin diseases have internal manifestations. This close interrelationship can be extremely interesting and complex, but since these conditions do not form a common part of everyday office practice they will be presented here in summary form. For further reading it is suggested that the two books by Dr. Kurt Wiener should be consulted: *Skin Manifestations of Internal Disorders* and *Systemic Associations and Treatment of Skin Diseases.**

DERMATOSES DUE TO INTERNAL DISEASE

The skin manifestations of internal diseases may be specific or nonspecific. The specific skin changes contain the same pathologic process as the internal disease. An example is the lymphoblastomatous infiltrate in the skin of a patient with a lymphoblastoma.

More often, however, the skin changes are nonspecific. They do not contain the primary disease process. Therefore, these nonspecific skin changes are not diagnostic of the internal disease but when considered with other changes may be helpful in establishing the diagnosis.

The most important and common internal conditions and their related dermatoses are listed as follows:

Puberty State. In males at puberty the beard, the pubic and other body hair begins to grow in characteristic patterns which differ from the hair growth in females. Both sexes at this time notice increased activity of the apocrine glands with axillary perspiration and "B.O.," and increased development of the sebaceous glands with the formation of varying degrees of seborrhea and the comedones, the papules and the pustules of acne. Certain skin diseases disappear around the onset of puberty, such as the infantile form of atopic eczema, tinea of the scalp, and urticaria pigmentosa.

Pregnancy State. Certain physiologic skin changes occur, such as increased perspiration; hyperpigmentation of the abdominal mid-line, nipples, vulva, face (chloasma), and generally in some brunettes, with nevi and freckles also becoming more prominent; hypertrichosis which may be unnoticed until the excess hair begins to shed after delivery; and

* Published by C. V. Mosby Company, St. Louis, Mo.

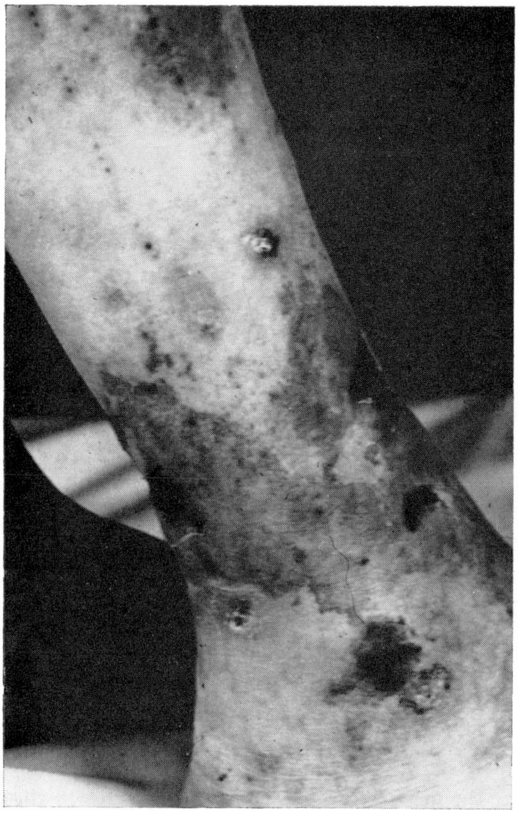

Fig. 90. Periarteritis nodosa with purpura and ischemic ulcers of the leg.

striae of breasts, abdomen and thighs. The skin diseases of pregnancy are dermatitis herpetiformis (herpes gestationis), impetigo herpetiformis, vulvar pruritus, often due to monilial infection, palmar erythema, spider hemangiomas and pedunculated fibromas. The following dermatoses are usually better or disappear during pregnancy: psoriasis, acne (can be worse), alopecia areata and possibly diffuse scleroderma.

Menopause State. Common physiologic changes in the skin of women during menopause include hot flashes, increased perspiration, increased hair growth on the face, and varying degrees of scalp hair loss. Other skin conditions associated with the menopause are chloasma, pedunculated fibromas, localized neurodermatitis, vulvar pruritus, keratoderma climactericum and rosacea.

Geriatric State. The diffuse atrophy of the skin that occurs in the aged individual is partially responsible for the dryness which results in senile pruritus and winter itch. Other changes include excessive wrinkling and hyperpigmentation of the skin. Specific dermatoses noted with increased frequency are seborrheic and senile keratoses, epitheliomas, senile purpura, pedunculated fibromas and papillary senile hemangiomas.

Rheumatic Fever. See nonspecific changes of increased sweating which results in prickly heat, also petechiae, urticaria, erythema nodosum, erythema multiforme, and rheumatic nodules.

Periarteritis Nodosa (Fig. 90). See periarteritic nodules which are specific, and nonspecific purpura, erythema and gangrene.

Thromboangiitis Obliterans (Buerger's Disease). See superficial migrating thrombophlebitis, pallor or cyanosis, gangrene and ulceration.

Fröhlich's Syndrome. Due to hypopituitarism in the male. Find feminine type smooth skin and scant hair growth, particularly in pubic and axillary regions, well-developed scalp hair, obesity and small thin fingernails.

Acromegaly. Due to hyperpituitarism and excess growth stimulating hormone. See skin changes due to overgrowth of the skeletal system, skin becomes coarse, lines deepened, increased sweating and oiliness, acne, increase in number of nevi, hyperpigmentation and hypertrichosis.

Cushing's Syndrome. Due to basophile adenoma of the pituitary gland. See purplish atrophic striae, hyperpigmentation, hypertrichosis in females and preadolescent males, and increased incidence of pyodermas.

Hyperthyroidism. The skin is moist, warm, has an evanescent erythema, hyper-

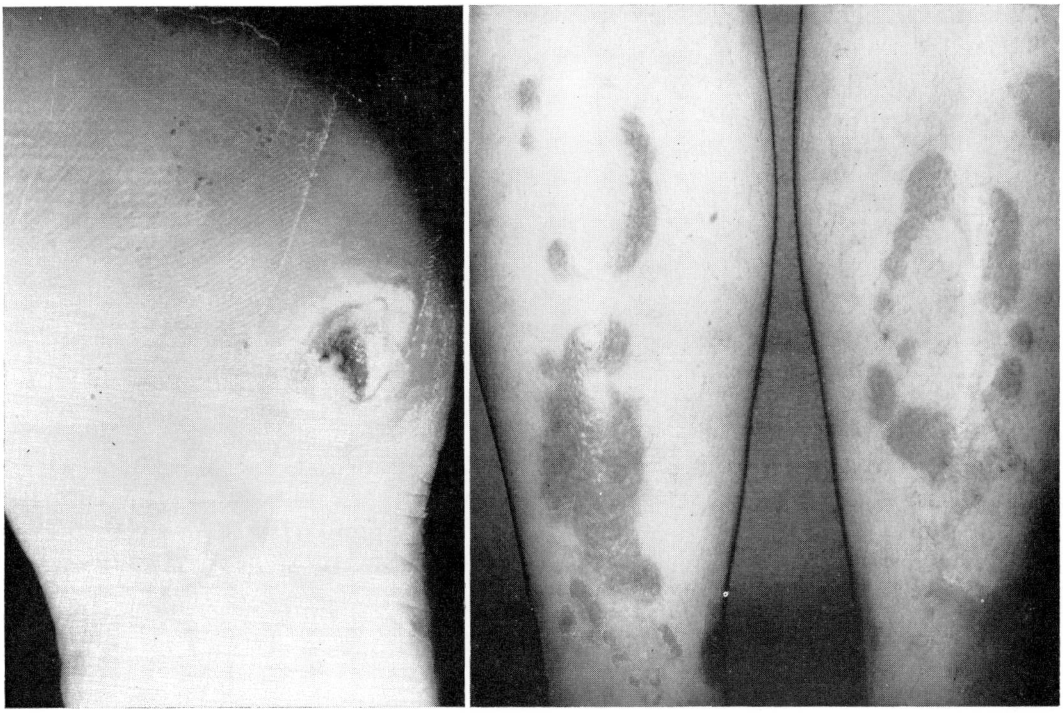

Fig. 91. Skin manifestations of diabetes mellitus.

(*Left*) Mal perforans of sole of foot of 3-years' duration.
(*Right*) Necrobiosis lipoidica diabeticorum on anterior tibial area of legs. (Dr. David Morgan)

pigmentation (hypopigmentation rarely), seborrhea, acne, toxic alopecia and nail atrophy. Localized myxedema of the pretibial area of the legs can develop and appears to be related to exophthalmos.

Hypothyroidism. The skin in generalized myxedema is cool, dry, scaly, thickened and hyperpigmented. Also see toxic alopecia with hair that is dull, dry and coarse, and increased incidence of pyodermas.

Addison's Disease. The most important dermatosis is hyperpigmentation which is first seen on areas of friction, pressure and irritation. Sweating is increased, and the axillary and pubic hair is shed.

Diabetes Mellitus (Fig. 91). Due to the increased amount of carbohydrate in the skin in patients with diabetes, skin infections occur with much higher frequency than in nondiabetic individuals. These infections include boils, carbuncles, ulcers, gangrene, moniliasis, tinea of the feet and the groin with or without secondary bacterial infection, and infectious eczematoid dermatitis. Other dermatoses seen are pruritus, xanthoma diabeticorum and necrobiosis lipoidica diabeticorum.

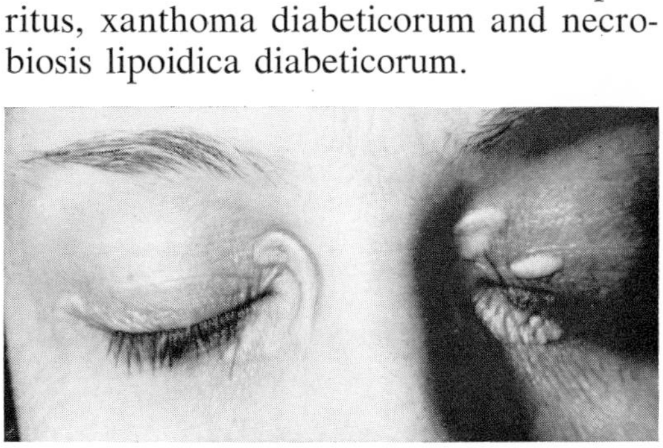

Fig. 92. Xanthelasma in woman with high blood cholesterol.

Lipidoses. This complex group of metabolic diseases causes varying skin lesions, depending somewhat on the basic metabolic fault. Thannhauser's classification* will be used to summarize these skin manifestations.

1. *Hypercholesteremic xanthomatoses* have lesions of xanthelasma of eyelids (Fig. 92), and papular, nodular and plaquelike xanthomas on the extensor surfaces of the extremities as seen in xanthoma tuberosum and also secondary to liver disease or hypothyroidism.

2. *Hyperlipemia* of the idiopathic type or secondary to diabetes mellitus, chronic pancreatitis or nephrosis is characterized by the sudden development of eruptive xanthomatoses consisting of single or multiple yellowish papules, nodules or plaques most commonly seen on the flexor surfaces of the extremities and on the trunk, the face and the scalp. Pruritus may be severe.

3. *Normocholesteremic xanthomatoses* include xanthoma disseminatum, Schüller-Christian syndrome, Letterer-Siwe disease and eosinophilic granuloma. Xanthelasma and flexural xanthomas occur. Vesicular lesions can be seen in cases of Schüller-Christian syndrome, and a seborrheic dermatitislike picture in Letterer-Siwe disease.

4. *Extracellular lipid accumulations* occur in lipoid proteinosis, extracellular cholesterosis and necrobiosis lipoidica diabeticorum. Skin lesions of the latter occur mostly in women on the anterior tibial area of the leg and are characterized by sharply circumscribed, yellowish plaques with a bluish border. Diabetes is present in the majority of cases.

5. *Disturbances of phospholipid metabolism* include Niemann-Pick disease and Gaucher's disease. Both develop a yellowish discoloration of the skin.

Vitamin Deficiencies. Dermatoses due to lack of vitamins are rare in the United States. However, a common question asked by many patients is, "Doctor, don't you think my trouble is due to lack of vitamins?" The answer in 99% of the cases is "No!"

VITAMIN A. Phrynoderma is the name for generalized dry hyperkeratoses of the skin due to chronic and significant lack of vitamin A. Clinically, the skin resembles the surface of a nutmeg grater. Eye changes are often present, including night blindness and dryness of the eyeball.

Large doses of vitamin A (25,000 to 50,000 units t.i.d.) are used in the treatment of patients with Darier's disease, pityriasis rubra pilaris, comedone acne and xerosis (dry skin). The value of this therapy has not been proved.

Hypervitaminosis A, due to excessively high and persistent intake of vitamin A in drug or food form, causes hair loss, dry skin, irritability, weight loss, and enlargement of the liver and the spleen.

VITAMIN B GROUP. Clinically, a patient with a true vitamin B deficiency is deficient in all of the vitamins of this group. Thus the classic diseases of this group, beriberi and pellagra, have overlapping clinical signs and symptoms.

VITAMIN B_1 (THIAMINE). This deficiency is clinically manifested by beriberi. The cutaneous lesions consist of edema and redness of the soles of the feet.

VITAMIN B_2 (RIBOFLAVIN). A deficiency of this vitamin has been linked with red fissures at the corners of the mouth and glossitis. This can occur in marked vitamin B_2 deficiency, but most cases with these clinical lesions are due to contact dermatitis or malocclusion of the lips from faulty dentures.

NICOTINIC ACID. This deficiency leads to pellagra, but other vitamins of the B group are contributory. The skin lesions are a prominent part of pellagra and include redness of the exposed areas of hands, face, neck and feet, which can go

* Thannhauser, S. J.: Lipidoses, ed. 2, New York, Oxford University Press, 1950.

on to a fissured, scaling, infected dermatitis. Local trauma may spread the disease to other areas of the body. The disease is worse in the summer and heals with hyperpigmentation and mild scarring. Gastro-intestinal and neurologic complications are serious.

The B group vitamins are administered with benefit to patients who have rosacea. Vitamin B_{12} in doses of 1,000 micrograms subcutaneously is somewhat effective for cases of severe seborrheic dermatitis.

VITAMIN C (ASCORBIC ACID). Scurvy is now a rare disease, and the skin lesions are not specific. They include a follicular papular eruption, petechia and purpura.

VITAMIN D. No skin lesions have been attributed to lack of this vitamin. Vitamin D and vitamin D_2 (calciferol) have been used in the treatment of lupus vulgaris.

VITAMIN K. Hypoprothrombinemia with purpura from various causes responds to vitamin K therapy.

Internal Cancer. Skin lesions may develop from internal malignancies either by metastatic spread or by the occurrence of nonspecific eruptions. The most interesting of the nonspecific dermatoses is the rare entity, *acanthosis nigricans*. The presence of the velvety, papillary, pigmented hypertrophies of this disease in the axillae, the groin and other moist areas of an adult will indicate an internal cancer, usually of the abdominal viscera, in over 50% of cases. A benign form of acanthosis nigrans exists in children and becomes most manifest at the age of puberty. This benign form is not associated with cancer.

Neuroses and Psychoses. A common belief among many members of the medical profession is that the majority of skin diseases are due to "nerves" or are a neurotic manifestation. This old idea is undoubtedly based on the familiar sight of the scratching skin patient; he just looks "nervous"; and it makes one nervous and itchy merely by looking at him. It is hard to know which came first for most patients, the itching or the nervousness. In my practice I tend to de-emphasize the nervous element but not ignore it. My answer to patients and doctors who question the role of nerves in a particular case is to say that they play a definite role in many skin eruptions, but rarely are "nerves" the precipitating cause of a dermatosis. If a patient has an emotional problem and also has an itching dermatitis, a flare-up of the problem will intensify his itch as it would aggravate another patient's duodenal ulcer or migraine headache.

Therapy of patients with skin disease where "nerves" are thought to play a dominant part can well be handled by the calm, receptive, attentive, interested general physician. Simple local therapy prescribed with the confidence of a competent physician will often establish in the patient the necessary faith that will cure his complaint. Occasionally, these patients will not respond to such therapy, and a rare case might benefit from special psychiatric care.

The following list will divide the psychocutaneous diseases into those thought to be (1) related to psychoses, (2) related to neuroses, and (3) those with questionable psychic relationship.

1. DERMATOSES RELATED TO PSYCHOSES.

Factitial dermatitis (Fig. 93 B). The patient denies that he is producing the skin disease. This is not to be confused with neurotic excoriations.

Skin lesions due to compulsive movements. An example is the chronic biting of an arm in a feeble-minded patient.

Delusions of parasitism, cancer, syphilis, etc. Various "proofs" are often presented by the patient to substantiate his existing belief.

Trichotillomania in adults. A rare cause of hair loss.

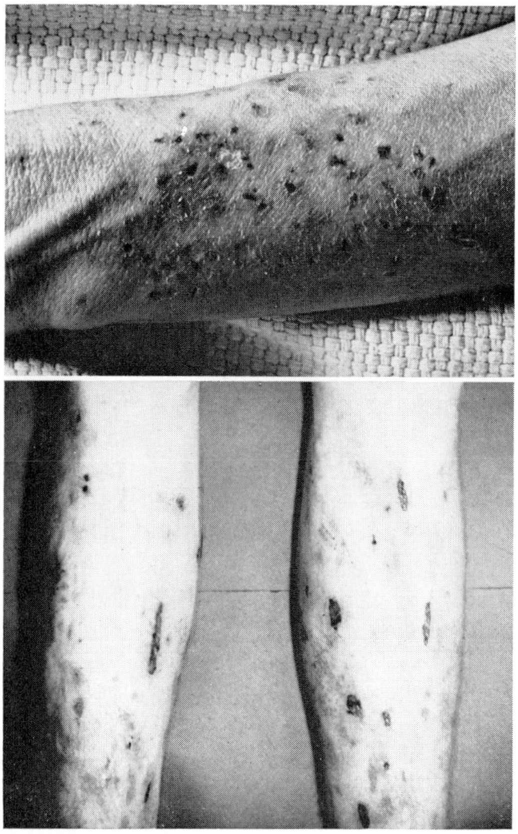

Fig. 93. Skin manifestations of nervous disorders.

(*Top*) Neurotic excoriations on the forearm. (K.U.M.C.)
(*Bottom*) Factitial dermatitis on the legs. (Dr. David Morgan)

2. Dermatoses Related to Neuroses

Neurotic excoriations (Fig. 93 A). The patient admits picking or scratching the lesions.

Phobias. A fear that the patient will contract a disease, i.e., syphilophobia, acarophobia, cancerophobia, bacteriophobia, etc.

Trichotillomania of children. Not as serious as in adults. The physician's index of suspicion must be high to diagnose this disease.

Neurodermatitis (Fig. 31). The primary cause can be an insect bite, contact dermatitis due to a permanent wave, psoriasis, stasis dermatitis, or many other conditions that can initiate the scratching habit. The habit then outlives the disease, and the neurodermatitis cycle develops.

3. Dermatoses of Questionable Psychic Cause

- Hyperhidrosis of palms and soles
- Dyshidrosis
- Alopecia areata
- Lichen planus
- Chronic urticaria
- Rosacea
- Atopic eczema
- Psoriasis
- Aphthous stomatitis
- Primary pruritus, local or generalized

INTERNAL MANIFESTATIONS OF SKIN DISEASE

The purpose of the author in this section is to list some of the internal phenomena that occur with certain diseases that primarily involve the skin. The collagen diseases belong in this group, particularly lupus erythematosus and scleroderma, but they have been discussed earlier in this book.

Rosacea. Eye lesions, such as keratitis, conjunctivitis and blepharitis, are seen rather commonly. Stomach achlorhydria or hypoacidity is of doubtful significance.

Atopic Eczema. This is one manifestation of a triad of atopic conditions, the other two being bronchial asthma and hayfever. Eye cataracts are seen with severe forms of atopic eczema but only rarely. Blood eosinophilia is common.

Urticaria Pigmentosa. This rare maculopapular disease, mainly of children, is characterized by urtication of the lesions following scratching. The skin lesions are composed of mast cells, and mast cell infiltrates are found in bone, liver, lymph nodes and the thymus. The disease usually disappears spontaneously after a few years.

Psoriasis. This chronic papulosquamous eruption is associated with arthritis in a small number of cases. The psoriasis usually exists as one of the more severe forms of the disease, such as the exfoliative type, and frequently precedes the development of the arthritis. Most observers believe that the joint lesions are a form of rheumatoid arthritis.

Pseudoxanthoma Elasticum. This rare but characteristic skin disease of yellowish papules or plaques, mainly of the body folds, is a degeneration of the elastic tissue. Systemically, angioid streaks of the retina are seen in 25% of cases and result in a slowly progressive loss of visual acuity.

Diseases Affecting the Hair

CHAPTER 22

THE HAIR on an individual's scalp and body is a personal mark. Care of the scalp hair receives more attention, from both men and women, than any other part of the human anatomy. Thus it is easy to understand the psychological problems caused by a disease of the hair. Unfortunately, however, two of the commonest diseases of the hair, hereditary hair loss on the scalp and excessive growth on the face, cannot be prevented, contrary to magazine and newspaper ads.

There are many rare diseases of the hair that will be defined in the Dictionary-Index under "Hair Diseases."

GRAY HAIR

The congenital presence of completely gray or white hair (albinism) or patches of gray hair is quite rare. More commonly, grayness of the scalp hair is a slowly progressive process. Hereditary factors determine whether such grayness will begin in early or late adulthood or not at all. There is no proof that worry hurries this graying process.

Patchy gray hair can develop following nerve injuries. The new hair that grows in during the healing of alopecia areata is usually white or gray.

Treatment. The desirability of eliminating gray hair is confined mainly to the women. Vegetable and chemical dyes and rinses (and bleaches to reverse the process) are used in fantastic quantities throughout the world and are safe if the individual is not irritated by or allergic to the agent used. When an allergy or irritation develops it is to be treated as contact dermatitis, usually with mild shampoos, 2% boric acid solution wet dressings and an appropriate water washable salve.

HYPERTRICHOSIS

Excessive growth of hair (hypertrichosis or hirsutism) can be a definite psychological problem when it occurs on the face or the legs of women. It would be a mistake for a physician to underestimate the seriousness attached to a woman's request for information regarding the treatment of such a problem. This form of hypertrichosis is called the *essential type,* but other less common forms exist.

Congenital hypertrichosis is very rare and is characterized by the "dog-faced boys" seen in circus sideshows. This is a form of congenital ectodermal defect that is hereditary. The lanugo hairs of infancy are not replaced with the coarser adult hairs, and this results in a continuing growth of the long silken lanugo hairs.

Localized hypertrichosis is ordinarily seen in association with pigmented or nonpigmented intradermal nevi. This may consist of only 2 or 3 hairs, or the hairy growth may cover a large part of the body.

After a small hairy nevus is removed by electrosurgery and the site healed, it is often necessary to remove the remaining excess long hairs by an electrosurgical method.

Endocrinopathic hypertrichosis is rare but must be ruled out when recently acquired hirsutism is noted. The menstrual history in a female can give valuable information. If menstruation is completely normal, it can be assumed that the patient does not have a pituitary, adrenal or ovarian tumor causing the excessive hair growth. If menstruation is abnormal and other findings are noted, such as obesity, deepening of the voice, enlargement of the clitoris, etc., then further clinical and laboratory studies are indicated.

Treatment of essential hypertrichosis in a 35-year-old attractive female. Examination reveals long dark hairs of the upper lip, the chin and the jaw areas.

1. Obtain a menstrual history. If it is completely normal, as we shall assume that it is in this patient, she can be assured that she has no abnormal internal reason for this excessive growth. If the menstrual history is not normal, proceed with further studies as indicated.

2. Question the patient regarding similar excess hair growth (do not use the word "beard") in her family. Other female members will usually be found to have this condition. This unalterable hereditary influence should be stressed.

3. Attempt to talk the patient into the fact that the excess hair she has is normal for her, is more noticeable to herself than others, and that treatment is not very satisfactory. If this cannot be accomplished, and it usually cannot be, then proceed to a discussion of the forms of treatment. The following suggested types of therapy begin with the easiest, the least expensive and the least injurious.

4. Bleaching the hairs. This can be done by using any of the many available proprietary preparations; it is not permanent but is simple, effective and seldom irritating.

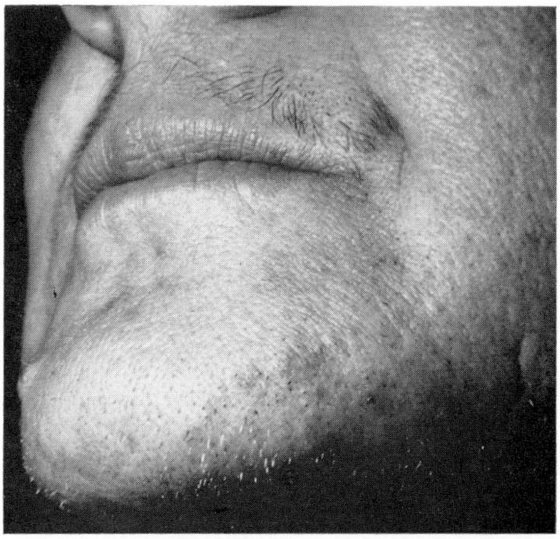

Fig. 94. Hypertrichosis of chin and upper lip in a 50-year-old woman.

5. Plucking the hair. If the area of excess hair growth is not too large this is a temporary, not too simple, but effective method which can result in a folliculitis. Plucking the hair does not increase hair growth.

6. Depilatories dissolve the hair shaft and offer a temporary, simple, effective and somewhat irritating method.

7. Epilating waxes produce a mass plucking effect, and offer a temporary though somewhat painful, effective form of hair removal. Folliculitis can follow.

8. Electrosurgical removal of the hairs is the only permanent method. (X-rays can also cause permanent removal of hairs but adequate dosage seriously damages the skin. The use of x-rays to epilate hair permanently is a form of malpractice.) Electrosurgical treatments can be carried out by electrolysis or by electrocoagulation (see p. 40). This latter method is faster but can result in scarring if not done carefully. Either procedure should be done by a skilled technician, who can be found in any large city. This form of hair removal is effective, slightly painful, very

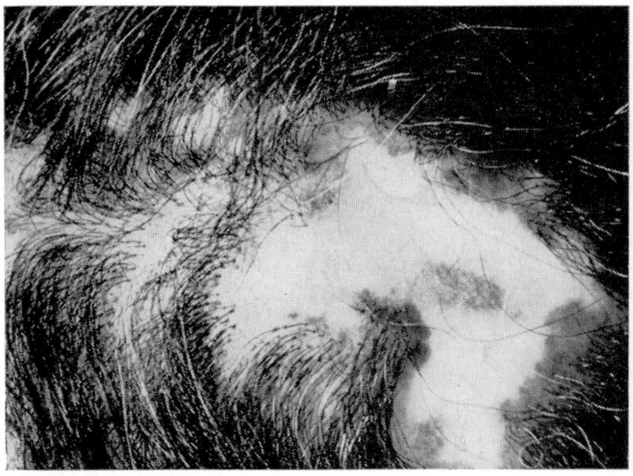

Chronic Discoid L. E. (Negro)

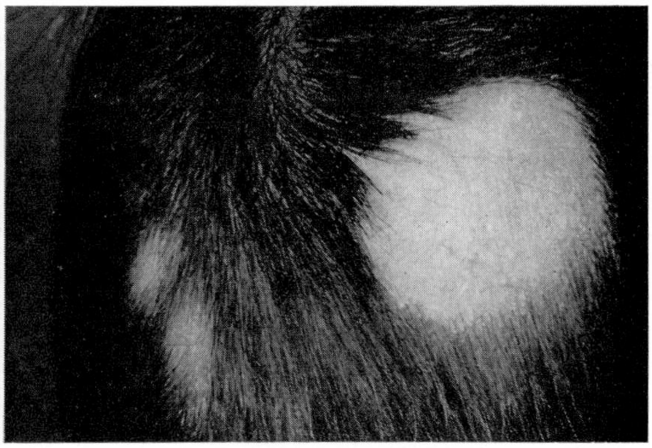

Tinea of the Scalp

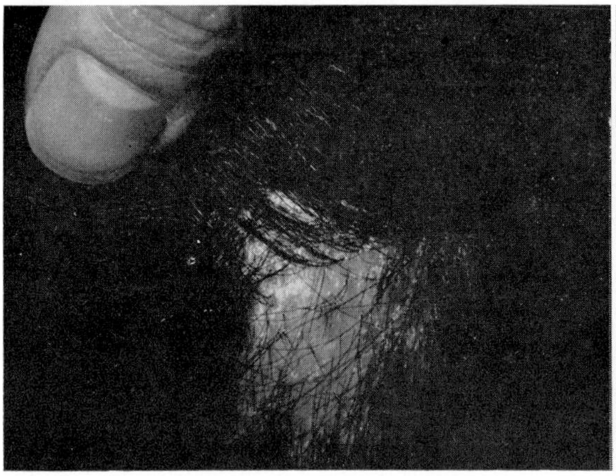

Alopecia Cicatrisata

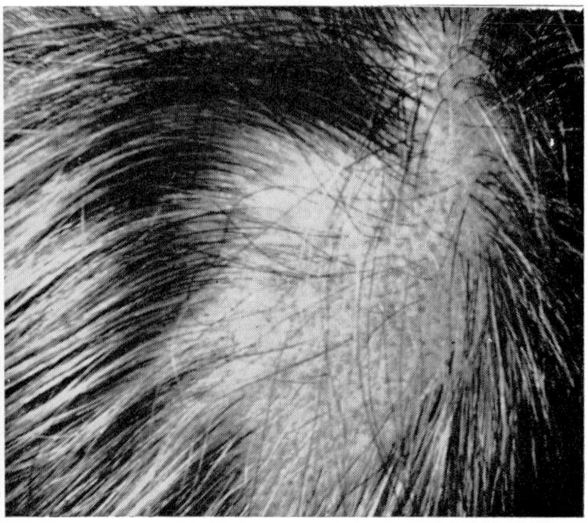

Traumatic Alopecia

Fig. 95. Hair loss due to various causes.

The case of traumatic alopecia was caused by the accidental catching of the scalp hair in a rotary massaging instrument used on the patient's back.

FACTS REGARDING HAIR

1. Shaving, cutting or plucking the hair does not affect the hair growth.

2. Frequent shampooing does not damage normal scalp hair.

3. Excessive brushing of the hair can be harmful.

4. Hair growth or loss in normal individuals is a physiologic process that cannot be altered by cosmetic applications.

5. Graying of the hair cannot occur overnight.

time-consuming if large areas are to be treated, and quite expensive. Scarring should be minimal or nonexistent when the procedure is done by a skilled technician. All of these facts should be stated to the patient.

HAIR LOSS

Hair loss (alopecia) in the scalp is important mainly because it is so obvious (Fig. 95). Hair loss on other parts of the body is unusual, but when present it is commonly associated with scalp alopecia.

There are two types of scalp hair loss, *diffuse* and *patchy*. Patchy alopecias can be of the nonscarring or of the scarring variety. In the scarring variety the hair cannot regrow because of a destroyed follicle. A complete classification follows, but only the more common alopecias will be discussed.

CLASSIFICATION

Diffuse Hair Loss

1. Male-pattern hair loss
2. Female-pattern hair loss
3. Temporary hair loss in females
4. Hair loss due to infection: pneumonia, exanthems and typhoid
5. Hair loss due to chemicals and drugs: severe reactions to locally applied chemicals, oral ingestion of thallium, nitrogen mustard, heparin and excess vitamin A
6. Hair loss due to endocrinopathy: hypothyroid and hypopituitary states
7. Hair loss associated with other diseases: exfoliative dermatitis, systemic lupus erythematosus, dermatomyositis, lymphomas, etc.
8. Congenital ectodermal defects: hair loss only, or associated with congenital loss of nails, teeth and cutaneous glands

Patchy Nonscarring Hair Loss

1. Alopecia areata
2. Tinea of the scalp
3. Trichotillomania
4. Secondary syphilis
5. Traumatic marginal alopecia

Patchy Scarring Hair Loss

1. Tinea infection of the scalp of the rare severely infected form
2. Bacterial infection of the scalp
3. Alopecia cicatrisata
4. Hair loss associated with other diseases: chronic discoid lupus erythematosus, scleroderma, lichen planus, neoplasms, zoster, etc.
5. Hair loss due to physical and chemical agents: overdose of x-rays, third-degree burns, trauma, caustics

DIFFUSE HAIR LOSS

1. **Male-Pattern Hair Loss.** This very common condition results in the expenditure of hundreds of thousands of dollars every year for medicines that promise the presumably unfortunate male a head of thick, luxuriant hair. Contrary to the statements in the most convincing "hair-restoring" ads, there is no "cure" for this hereditary disease.

Clinically, the earliest hair loss extends back on both sides of the forehead in an M-shape to meet a slowly enlarging area of similar hair loss on the vertex of the scalp. The degree of hair loss varies with the individual, as does the age at which it begins.

ETIOLOGY: The dominant factors are heredity, age of the individual, and hormones. The heredity and the age, of course, cannot be altered. Hormonal therapy in safe dosage has no beneficial effect. Castrated males do not have this male-pattern hair loss, but castration is not recommended as a form of treatment.

DIFFERENTIAL DIAGNOSIS

Alopecia areata: patchy hair loss with exclamation point hairs (see below)

Trichotillomania: patchy and bizarre areas of hair loss (see below)

TREATMENT: A 27-year-old male with

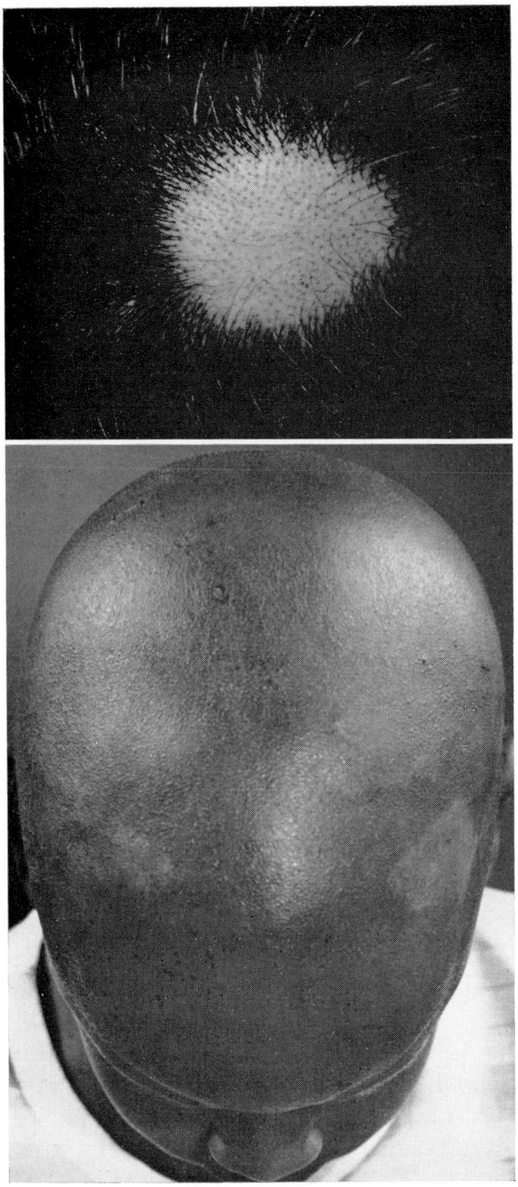

Fig. 96. Alopecia areata.
(*Top*) Single area on vertix of scalp. Exclamation point hairs are barely visible.
(*Bottom*) Total alopecia of 4-year-old Negro girl.

receding hairline and a slight amount of scaling on his scalp.

1. Question the patient about his heredity. Usually there is a history that the father began to lose his scalp hair when he also was in his twenties. Explain about this unalterable factor of heredity.

2. Tell the patient that treatment is of no value, contrary to the hair-restoring ads.

3. Suggest the use of a dandruff-removing shampoo such as Selsun Suspension to keep the scalp as healthy as possible. *Dandruff, unless it becomes severely secondarily infected, does not cause hair loss.*

2. **Female-Pattern Hair Loss.** This mild diffuse hair loss occurs in a small percentage of women, most commonly after the age of 50. The loss begins on the vertex of the scalp and is never complete. It probably is related to a relative increase in the male hormone. There is no effective form of therapy.

3. **Temporary Hair Loss in Females.** A moderately common complaint from a young female patient is that for 6 months her hair has been "falling out in handfuls." Examination reveals a good head of hair but some diffuse thinning. The patient is otherwise healthy.

ETIOLOGY: This temporary hair loss can follow the use of an anesthetic, the birth of a baby, a nervous upset, or from no apparent cause. During pregnancy the hair growth is often increased, but this fact is not obvious to the patient. However, when the patient returns to the unpregnant state and the luxuriant hair growth begins to shed she becomes alarmed. This cycle of events should be explained to the patient.

TREATMENT consists of pointing out the causative factor and reassuring the patient that she will not become bald. Usually the hair loss will slowly cease. and the normal hair pattern, though somewhat less thick, will be re-established.

PATCHY NONSCARRING HAIR LOSS

1. **Alopecia Areata.** This common

disease of unknown cause results in serious psychological problems when it occurs over large areas of the scalp (Fig. 96).

PRIMARY LESION. See loss of hair in a slowly enlarging area or areas. *No scaling or evidence of infection is present.* The hair breaks off at a point approximately 2 to 3 mm. above the scalp surface. The broken hairs are aptly called "exclamation-point hairs" because they appear to be thicker at the top and thin at the base like the top part of an exclamation point (!). These "exclamation-point hairs" are pathognomonic of alopecia areata and are found in all active cases, usually at the periphery of the bald patch. When healing begins the new hairs are commonly white but eventually they regain their normal color.

DISTRIBUTION. Any hairy area of the body can be affected. The commonest areas are the scalp, the eyebrows, the eyelashes and the beard.

PROGNOSIS. The great majority of cases of alopecia areata that have one or several small patches will regrow their hair in 6 to 12 months time with no treatment. Recurrences are quite common. Prepubertal cases have a poorer prognosis for permanent "cure." Total loss of the scalp hair and/or the body hair (alopecia totalis) carries with it a very poor prognosis for eventual return of the hair.

AGE GROUP. This disease occurs most commonly in children and young adults.

ETIOLOGY. The cause is unknown. Some cases appear to be due to a focus of infection (teeth, prostate, sinuses, gallbladder, genito-urinary tract, etc.), and some may be due to emotional problems.

DIFFERENTIAL DIAGNOSIS

Tinea of the Scalp: no exclamation-point hairs, mainly in children, see scaliness, usually some infection; Wood's light usually shows fluorescence; fungi found on KOH slide preparation of hair or culture media (p. 144).

Trichotillomania: no exclamation-point hairs, irregular areas of hair loss, "nervous" child (see below).

Secondary Syphilis: no exclamation-point hairs, see other secondary skin lesions, serologic test for syphilis is positive (p. 113).

Chronic Discoid Lupus Erythematosus: no exclamation-point hairs, in the active lesions see redness, enlarged hair follicle opening and scaliness, but in the healed stage see atrophic hyperpigmented or depigmented patches with absent hair follicles (p. 172).

Alopecia Cicatrisata: no exclamation-point hairs; find small area of hair loss with no inflammation and no change over many years time; hair follicles are atrophic (p. 191).

Folliculitis Decalvans: no exclamation-point hairs; see folliculitis and eventual destruction of the hair follicle (p. 191).

TREATMENT. A young female patient presents herself in your office with two 3 x 2 cm. sized areas of hair loss of 2-weeks' duration. Her father died 1 week prior to onset of the disease. Examination reveals exclamation-point hairs at the periphery of both lesions. She is able to comb her hair so as to cover the bald areas.

1. Reassure the patient (1) that it would be exceedingly rare for her to lose all of her hair; and (2) that the lesions might enlarge some but that within 6 to 8 months' time all of her hair will be back. Tell her that the new hair may come in white at the beginning, but the natural color will soon return.

2. Treat her dandruff, if she has any, with Fostex Cream Shampoo or Selsun Suspension Shampoo. (Selsun Suspension rarely, if ever, causes hair loss.)

3. Have her return if necessary for reassurance.

Subsequent visit with considerable ex-

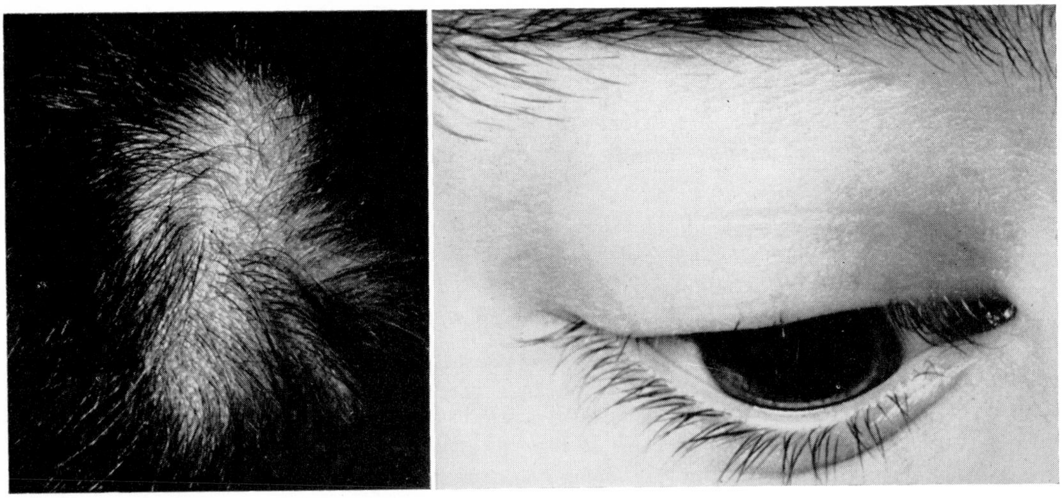

Fig. 97. Trichotillomania.
(*Left*) Of the scalp of a 9-year-old boy.
(*Right*) Of the eyelashes of a 10-year-old girl.

tension of the bald areas. No specific therapy is known. Injections of vitamins or Pituitary Liquid (Armour) (1 cc. subcutaneously at weekly or less frequent intervals) might satisfy the patient and allow you to follow her more closely until the hair begins to regrow.

Treatment of recurrent severe cases or cases of alopecia totalis

1. The prognosis is poor for return of hair in these severe cases, and the patient should be told this. A statement of the truth can prevent useless migration of the patient from one physician to another.

2. A wig may be desired by the patient, and this purchase can be encouraged.

3. Oral corticosteroid therapy. This therapy causes regrowth of hair in some of the severe cases but should not be initiated without careful examination of the patient and a thorough discussion with the patient regarding the side-effects and the expense of months of therapy. An accepted course of therapy would be hydrocortisone (20 mg.) or methylprednisolone (Medrol) (4 mg.) q.i.d. for 1 week, then one tablet b.i.d. for 4 weeks, then 1 a day for several months. If the hair begins to regrow, this will be noticed within 1 to 2 months after the onset of therapy. Treatment may have to be maintained for months and years and adjusted up or down as the response indicates. Most cases relapse when the drug is stopped completely. This questionable therapeutic modality is indicated for some patients and not indicated for others.

2. **Tinea of the Scalp.** This is characterized by broken-off hairs, scaliness and occasionally infection, fluorescence under Wood's light, the finding of the organism in KOH preparations of the hair and growths on Sabouraud's media; usually it is seen in children. (See p. 144 and Figs. 95 and 73.)

3. **Trichotillomania.** This rare form of hair loss must be thought of when exclamation-point hairs, scaliness and infection are not seen (Fig. 97). Children are usually affected. It can occur in the

scalp, the eyebrows and the eyelids. The emotional problems of the patient and the parents are responsible for this disease, and these problems may be simple or serious. The patient and the parents may or may not be aware of the "pulling tendency." These cases should be handled by a dermatologist and, in severe cases, by a psychiatrist.

4. **Secondary Syphilis.** Alopecia due to secondary syphilis is uncommon. The usual form of hair loss due to syphilis is the patchy moth-eaten form (Fig. 58 A), but very rarely a diffuse hair loss occurs. The absence of exclamation-point hairs differentiates it from alopecia areata, which it resembles closely.

Patchy Scarring Hair Loss

1. **Tinea of the Scalp.** The rarer forms of tinea that are accompanied by severe kerion formation may result in small spots of permanent hair loss as a result of destruction of the hair follicles. The organisms *Microsporum canis, M. gypseum, Trichophyton mentagrophytes* and *T. tonsurans* are the ones most frequently responsible for scarring (see p. 144).

2. **Bacterial Infection of the Scalp.** Any deep bacterial process can destroy the hair follicle and produce patches of permanent hair loss. These deep infections can be due to pyogenic bacteria, tuberculosis, leprosy and syphilis, but all of these are rare causes of hair loss.

Folliculitis decalvans is the name given to a rare form of hair loss apparently due to bacterial infection that progresses slowly for many years with recurrent crops of infection at the spreading border. Atrophic scarring remains in the center. This diagnosis should not be made until at least two attempts have failed to grow a fungus on culture media. Favus of the scalp due to *Trichophyton schoenleini* can mimic this disease.

3. **Alopecia Cicatrisata.** This very rare form of permanent hair loss is characterized by no history or evidence of scaling or infection (Fig. 95). The cause is unknown, and treatment is ineffective.

Diseases Affecting the Nails

CHAPTER 23

THE NAILS are affected by (1) primary nail diseases, (2) by any dermatitis that involves the surrounding skin and (3) by many internal diseases.

A frequent misconception among patients is that nutrition plays an important part in the production of nail disorders. Lack of calcium and vitamins is mentioned most by patients. No little amount of verbal persuasion is necessary to correct this assumption. The questionable role of gelatin therapy for the improvement of fragile nails will be considered under that disorder.

PRIMARY NAIL DISEASES

Only the most common primary nail diseases will be included in this chapter. The terminology for the rare primary conditions is very complex and will be found in the Dictionary-Index under "Nail Disorders" (Fig. 98).

Contact Reactions

Changes in the nails, mainly the fingernails, from cosmetic applications are related to the constant attempts by manufacturers to discover a nail polish or covering that will adhere to and become a part of the nail for the life of the individual, or at least for the duration of a certain fad. Several years ago such a cosmetic panacea was discovered in the form of a base coat, but the nail bed rebelled with the development of thickening and loosening of the nail plate. More recently, the use of artificial nails and a press-on type covering resulted in splitting of the distal ends of the nail.

These nail-bed reactions are not related to, and should be differentiated from, the allergic sensitivity manifested by some women to chemicals in the nail polish. The fingernails, interestingly enough, do not react to this allergy, but the sensitivity shows up on the eyelids and the neck as a contact dermatitis (see p. 42).

Nail-Biting

This common nervous habit of some children and fewer adults is very difficult to stop. Often the less attention that is paid to this tic the better, with the resulting cessation of the biting. The local application of distasteful chemicals to the nails seldom helps.

Ingrown Nails

The mechanism of this disorder is the growth of the lateral edge of the nail plate, usually of the big toe, into the adjacent skin groove. Tight-fitting shoes and improper nail-trimming initiate the process. The result is a foreign-body type reaction with pain, redness, swelling and infection.

Prophylactic management is simple: the toenail never should be trimmed in a semilunar manner but should be trimmed

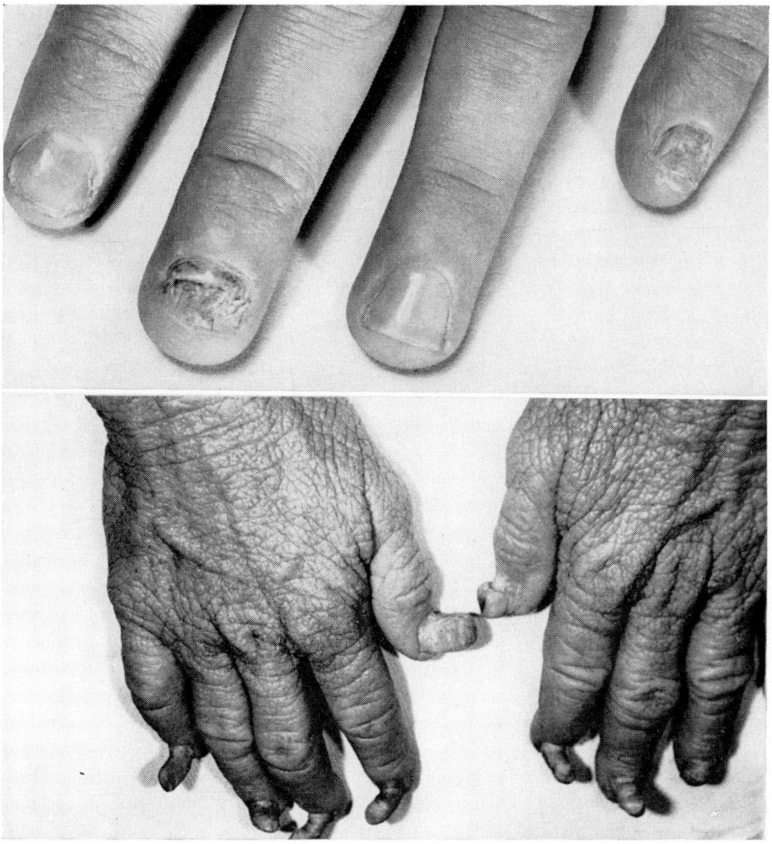

Fig. 98. Primary nail diseases.

(*Top*) Tinea of the nails due to *T. rubrum*.
(*Bottom*) Onychogryphosis of unknown cause. (Dr. Chester Lessenden)

straight across so the corner lies above the skin groove.

Active treatment of an acute process consists of hot soaks and local application of an antiseptic tincture. After the pain has lessened, the placement of a pledget of cotton gently under the nail may be sufficient to raise the pointed corner up above the skin surface. More resistant cases are treated by removing the overlying skin by excision and suture, or by removing the lateral section of the nail back to the nail base with or without destruction of the base by electrosurgery.

Hang Nails

Some patients are prone to develop small cutaneous tags from the lateral and posterior skin folds. Accidental or intentional pulling on these skin flaps tears into the deeper skin with resultant bleeding and a painful raw area that is susceptible to bacterial infection. This can be prevented by removal of the hang nail with scissors.

Treatment of the infection, which may develop into a *bacterial paronychia,* is with hot soaks, local application of antiseptic tinctures or ointments, avoidance of covering dressings, and in severe cases systemic antibiotics.

Leukonychia

The common "white spots" of the nail plate have been responsible for many interesting homespun etiologic labels. Medically speaking, we cannot do much better regarding the cause. (I've always thought they followed the telling of white lies.) The histogenesis is also not known, but current theories propose that the white spots are due to tiny air bubbles in the

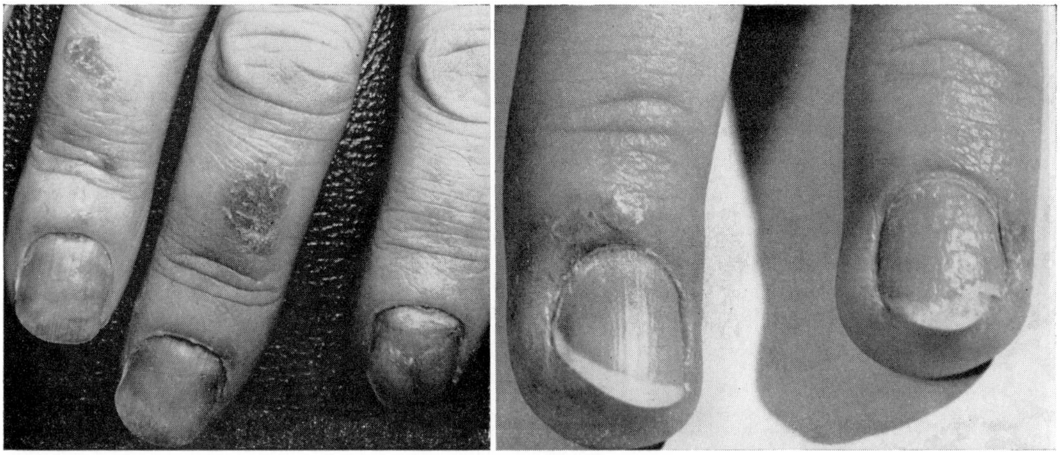

Psoriasis

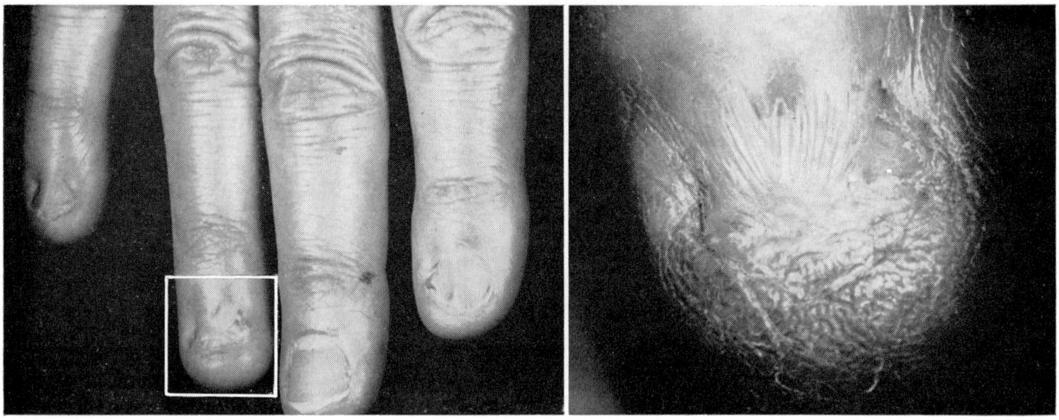

Lichen Planus

Fig. 99. Nail disease secondary to other dermatoses.

nail or due to the presence of incompletely keratinized cells. No treatment is indicated.

Fragile Nails

The distal splitting of fingernails is a common complaint of women. In most instances the cause cannot be determined, but some cases are due to the "permanent" type of nail polishes or the solvents used in removing the polish.

The only therapy that appears to be beneficial is the daily oral ingestion of one envelope of Knox Gelatin mixed with fruit juices or water. This treatment should be kept up for at least 3 months to receive benefit, since it takes that long for the nail to grow out to the fragile end.

NAIL DISEASE SECONDARY TO OTHER DERMATOSES

The nail, as one of the skin appendages, is susceptible to diseases of the skin adjacent to the nail or dermatoses on distant areas. It is important to remember that a dermatitis of the skin can be made to heal rather rapidly, but that any concurrent nail involvement will take approximately 3 months to grow out with the nail. The "scar" remains on the nail much longer than on the skin.

Tinea of the Nails

Disturbance of nail growth due to fungi is the most commonly observed nail problem (Fig. 98). A major per cent of the male population have one or more thickened toenails which almost invariably are caused by fungi. Females have onychomycosis of the toenails less frequently, and both sexes have fingernail involvement only rarely. Tinea of the nails is discussed in detail on page 140.

Warts

Verrucae can occur anywhere on the body, but one of the most difficult warts to treat is the type that grows around the nail and under the nail plate. If the wart is large and extends rather far under the nail, a deformed nail may result from the removal. The patient should be told about this possibility in advance. The management of these problem warts is discussed on page 128.

Eczematous Eruptions of the Fingers

These eczematous skin eruptions include contact dermatitis, atopic eczema and nummular eczema. The nail becomes involved when these dermatoses affect the adjacent skin. When the skin dermatitis heals the nail will heal also, but, as stated previously, the mark of the dermatitis on the nail will take 3 months to disappear completely.

An unusual reaction of the nail is the development of a highly polished nail surface in some patients with severely itching atopic eczema. This is due to the habit of some atopics of constantly rubbing the skin with the flat nail surface instead of scratching with the distal end of the nail.

Psoriasis

An astute clinician can occasionally diagnose psoriasis by merely examining the nails. Often the only sign of psoriasis will be the nail changes for which the patient seeks medical advice. Psoriasis can cause any and all of the dystrophic changes of the nails (Fig. 99). The commonest changes are small pinpoint pits, with or without distal detachment of the nail. A proximal red halo frequently is present around the distal detachment. In severe psoriatic nail involvement there is complete disintegration of the plate surface with massive subungual proliferation. Even these severe changes are usually asymptomatic. Treatment of the nails is very unsatisfactory. If psoriasis is present on other areas and responds to therapy, the nails may also clear up. Superficial x-ray therapy to the nails is sometimes beneficial.

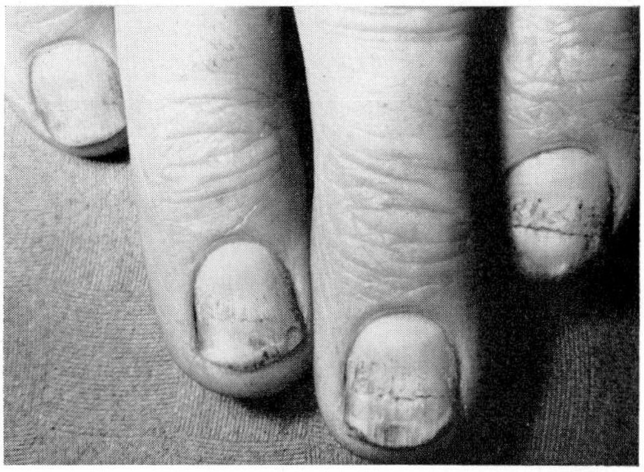

Fig. 100. Beau's lines following exfoliative dermatitis due to arsenic in Fowler's solution.

Other Dermatoses

Nonspecific nail changes can occur along with lichen planus (Fig. 99), alopecia areata, Darier's disease, epidermolysis bullosa, ichthyosis, pityriasis rubra pilaris and other dermatoses.

NAIL DISEASE SECONDARY TO INTERNAL DISEASE

Changes in the nails can reflect internal

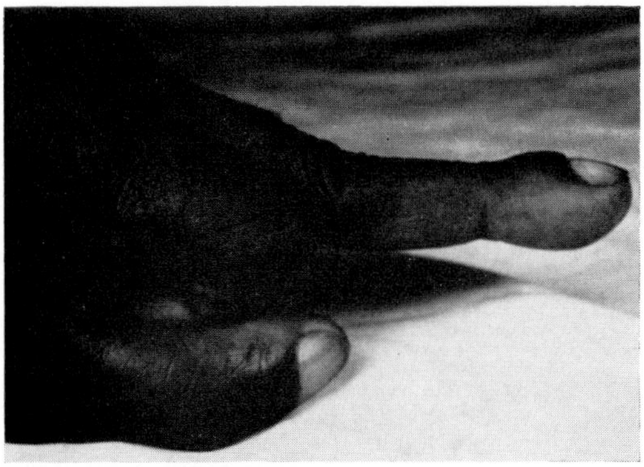

Fig. 101. Hippocratic or clubbed nails and fingers in Negro male with cardiovascular syphilis.

disease. The greatest majority of these changes are nonspecific.

Beau's Lines

Beau's lines, or transverse furrows of the nails, may develop with any of a large group of cutaneous and systemic disturbances (Fig. 100). The latter include many of the acute infectious febrile diseases, such as malaria, syphilis and pulmonary tuberculosis, and coronary disease, pregnancy, collagen diseases and emotional shock.

Beau's lines are due to a temporary growth disturbance in the nail plate. A simile is the alteration in the annual growth rings of trees when affected by drought, fire, or pestilence. The width of Beau's lines varies directly with the duration of the internal disease. As stated before, the "scar" of this nail alteration will take approximately 3 months to grow out. Many are the awesome, astute, detective-like, laity impressive deductions made by the clever physician when these lines are noted. A proper and impressive statement on finding Beau's lines approximately halfway down all of the fingernails is, "I see that you had a rather severe illness about 6 weeks ago."

Hippocratic Nails

Clubbed nails and fingers are classically associated with chronic lung and heart disorders (Fig. 101). These changes apparently are due to the prolonged anoxemia present. Equally common is a congenital and hereditary form of hippocratic nails seen in healthy individuals.

Dermatoses Due to Physical Agents

CHAPTER 24

PHYSICAL AGENTS, such as heat, cold, pressure and radiant energy (x-rays, ultraviolet, gamma rays), can produce both irritative reactions and allergic reactions on the skin. The two common physical irritations of the skin are *sunburn,* due to ultraviolet radiation, and *radiodermatitis* due to ionizing radiation. Allergic reactions can also develop from these two physical agents and from the other agents listed above.

SUNBURN

A sunburn can be mild and desired, or severe and feared. The most severe reactions come from prolonged exposure at swimming areas or when the unfortunate individual falls asleep under an ultraviolet lamp. The degree of reaction depends on several factors, including length and intensity of exposure, the individual's complexion and previous conditioning of the skin.

Primary Lesions. Varying degrees of redness develop within 2 to 12 hours after exposure to the ultraviolet radiation and reach maximum intensity within 24 hours. Vesiculation occurs in severe cases along with systemic weakness, chills, malaise and local pain.

Secondary Lesions or Reactions. Scaling or peeling, though not desired by the sun devotee, is the aftermath of any overexposure. Vesiculation can be complicated by secondary infection. An increase in pigmentation is usually the desired end result, but this tanning is not accomplished by overzealous exposure.

Lupus erythematosus of either the acute disseminated or chronic discoid type may be triggered by sun exposure in a susceptible person (p. 172). Latent *sun allergy (actinic dermatitis)* also needs activation to become manifest.

Late Reactions to Sunlight. *Actinic or senile keratoses* appear mainly after the age of 50 but are seen in highly susceptible individuals in their 30's. Chronic sun and wind exposure on the part of a light-complexioned farmer, sailor, or gardener

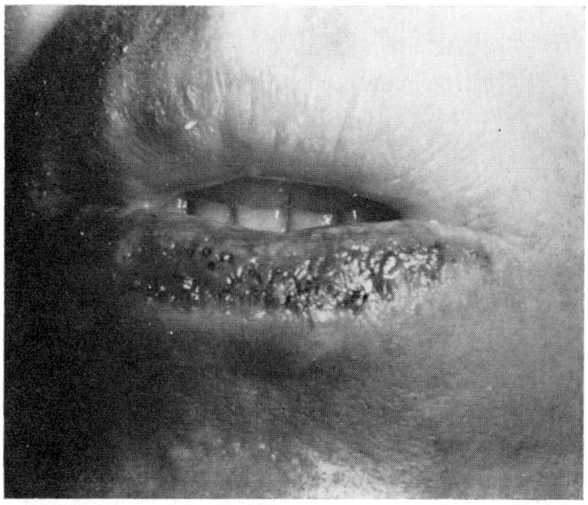

Fig. 102. Cheilitis due to sunlight sensitivity.

will lead to the development of these superficial, red, scaling keratoses on exposed surfaces of the face, the lips (actinic cheilitis, Fig. 102), the ears, the neck and the dorsum of the hands. *Prickle cell epitheliomas* arise in an appreciable percentage of these actinic keratoses (see pp. 210 and 218).

Prophylactic Treatment. The ultraviolet rays from the sun or from other sources can be either completely blocked or partially blocked from the skin surface.

1. Complete blocking of the sun rays is desired for prevention of actinic keratoses, a flare-up of lupus erythematosus, or a sun allergy reaction. Application of A-fil Cream (Texas Pharmacal) or Skolex Cream (Williams) will accomplish this for 4 to 6 hours after a single application.

2. Partial blocking can be accomplished by the use of any of the many available proprietary "suntan" oils, lotions and creams. It is best to avoid the use of oily or greasy preparations, since a pustular or acnelike eruption can ensue in susceptible individuals. Sensible and gradual sun exposure of the skin is the best preventative for sunburn, but most people learn this the hard way.

Active Treatment. A young woman presents herself with a painful, erythematous, vesicular skin reaction on her face, back and thighs of 24-hours' duration following a Decoration Day trip to the beach (first- and second-degree burns).

1. Boric acid crystals 60.0
   Sig: 1 tablespoon to 1 quart of cool water. Apply cloths wet with the cool solution to the affected areas for as long a time as necessary to keep comfortable.
2. Menthol 0.25%
   Nonalcoholic white shake lotion q.s. 120.0
   Sig: Apply locally t.i.d. to affected areas.

3. Blisters can be drained but should not be débrided.

Subsequent Care. A day or two later to soften the scales and to prevent secondary infection prescribe:

1. Menthol 0.25%
   Neosporin or other antibiotic ointment 15.0
   White petrolatum 15.0
   Sig: Apply locally t.i.d.

2. Warn the patient to resume cautiously sun exposure to the now very sensitive skin.

RADIODERMATITIS

The hazards of ionizing radiation have reached the front page of the newspapers and the feature articles of most magazines. This is the Atomic Age. Some of the publicity is good, but it has made the pendulum swing to the side of general criticism of all forms of ionizing therapy as used in medicine. X-rays and other forms of such therapy are established as unique therapeutic modalities, but, as with all potent medicinal agents, they must be administered intelligently. When they are not so administered the result is varying degrees of damage to the skin and the underlying organs. We shall be concerned here with the skin changes, radiodermatitis.

Clinical Lesions. *Acute radiodermatitis* is divided into 3 degrees of severity similar to the reactions from thermal burns. The first degree is manifested by the slow development of erythema, hyperpigmentation and usually hair loss. A single dose of x-rays necessary to produce these changes is called an "erythema dose." All of the changes in the first degree are reversible.

The second degree is characterized by vesicle formation, erosions, hair loss, secondary infection and delayed healing. Atrophy and telangiectasis are the end-results.

The third degree of radiodermatitis includes ulceration, infection and greatly delayed healing. Epitheliomatous changes

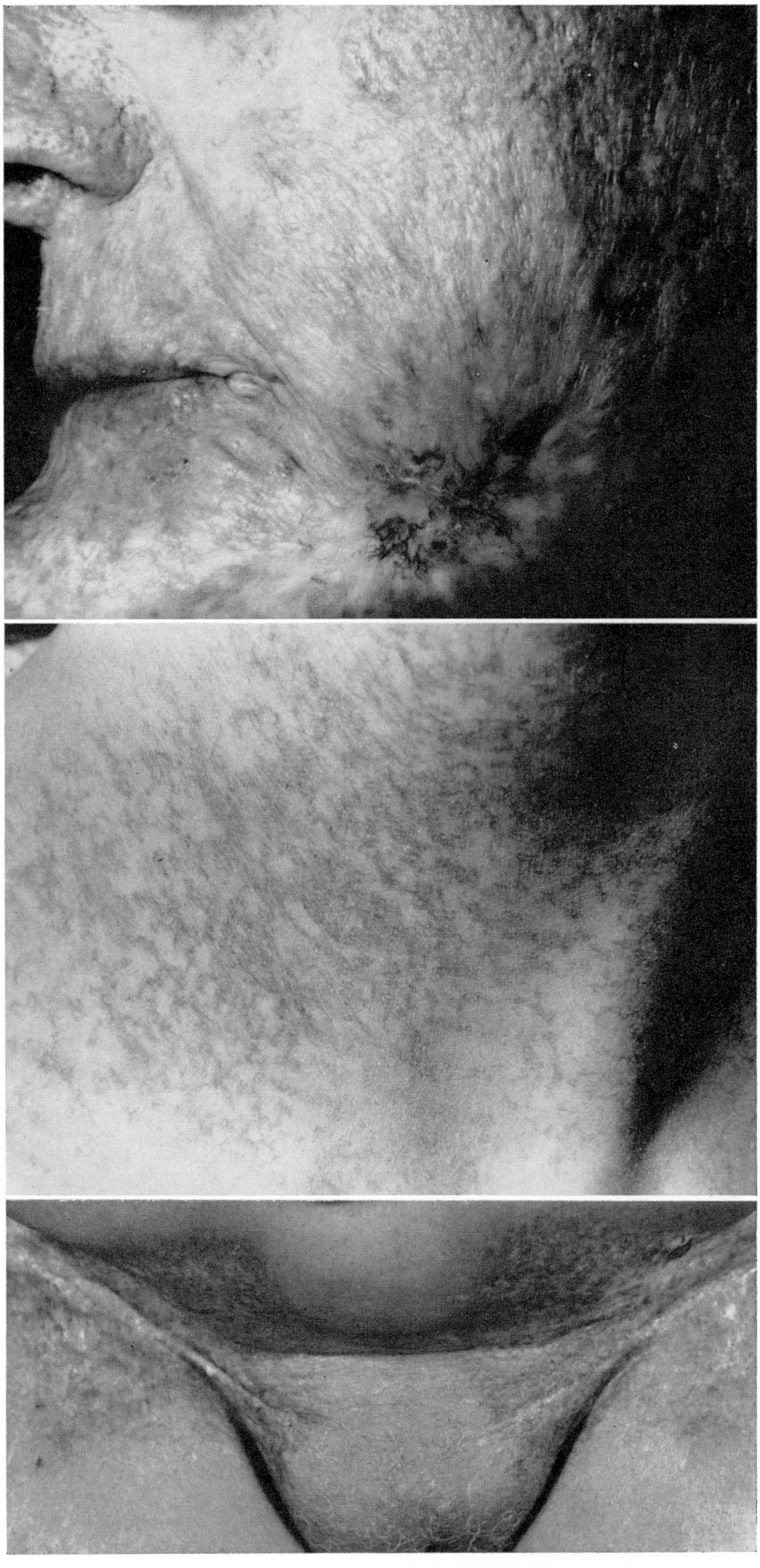

Fig. 103. Chronic radiodermatitis.

(*Top*) Atrophy and scarring of face following permanent epilation of hypertrichosis by x-ray therapy given 30 years previously.

(*Center*) Telangiectasia on neck due to excessive x-ray dosage for acne with improper shielding.

(*Bottom*) On groin areas. This is the expected and normal atrophic reaction from x-ray therapy directed toward a uterine malignancy in a Negro woman. (K.U.M.C.)

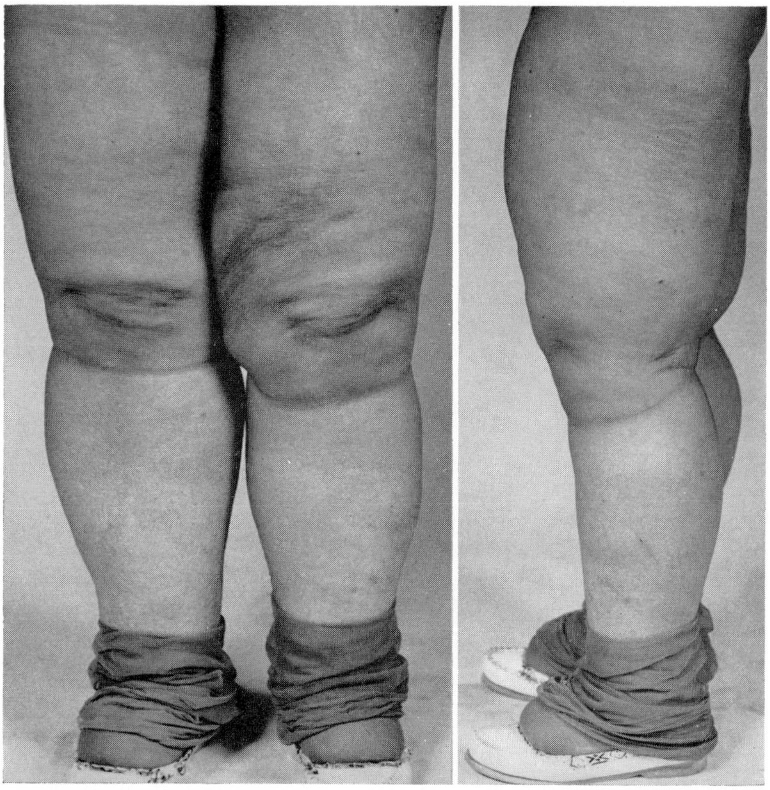

Fig. 104. Elephantiasis type of lymphedema following x-ray therapy of uterine malignancy.

are very common in the chronic ulcer or scar.

Chronic radiodermatitis can follow acute radiation injury or develop slowly following repeated small radiation exposures (Figs. 103 and 104). *The dosage of ionizing radiation on the skin is cumulative; the effect of previous radiation therapy is never erased by the passage of time.*

Etiology. Many factors influence the development of radiodermatitis. These include the physical factors of kilovoltage, milliamperage, distance, filters and the half-value layer; the individual's factors of health, age, complexion, type of lesion, and size and depth of the area to be treated, and the treatment factors of dosage, number of treatments and interval between treatments.

Prophylactic Treatment. If all of the above etiologic factors are remembered, acute and chronic radiodermatitis will not develop following radiation therapy for benign conditions. However, certain degenerative changes are unavoidable when therapy must be directed toward the removal of a malignant condition. Ionizing therapy should be administered only by competently trained dermatologists or radiologists. It is most important for all concerned to remember that when a so-called complete course of radiation therapy has been given to a particular body area, no further radiation should be administered to this area at *any* future time.

Active Treatment. The acute cases of radiodermatitis can be treated symptomatically with bland local measures. Therapy of chronic radiodermatitis should be carried out by a dermatologist, a surgeon or a plastic surgeon. The damaged skin is markedly sensitive to other forms of irritation, such as wind, sunlight, injury, harsh cosmetics and local therapy.

Geographical Skin Diseases in North America

CHAPTER 25

Most common skin diseases of North America are universal in geographic distribution, but a few are confined to, or more prevalent in, certain sections of the country. In my attempt to cover completely the common skin diseases, I have called upon other dermatologists from representative areas of the United States and Canada to list their geographic skin diseases (Fig. 105). A list of the dermatologists consulted follows. I am taking the liberty of quoting certain parts of their letters because they add interest to this question of geographic dermatoses.

CANADA

Vancouver, British Columbia—Dr. Stuart Maddin. "It was quite generally

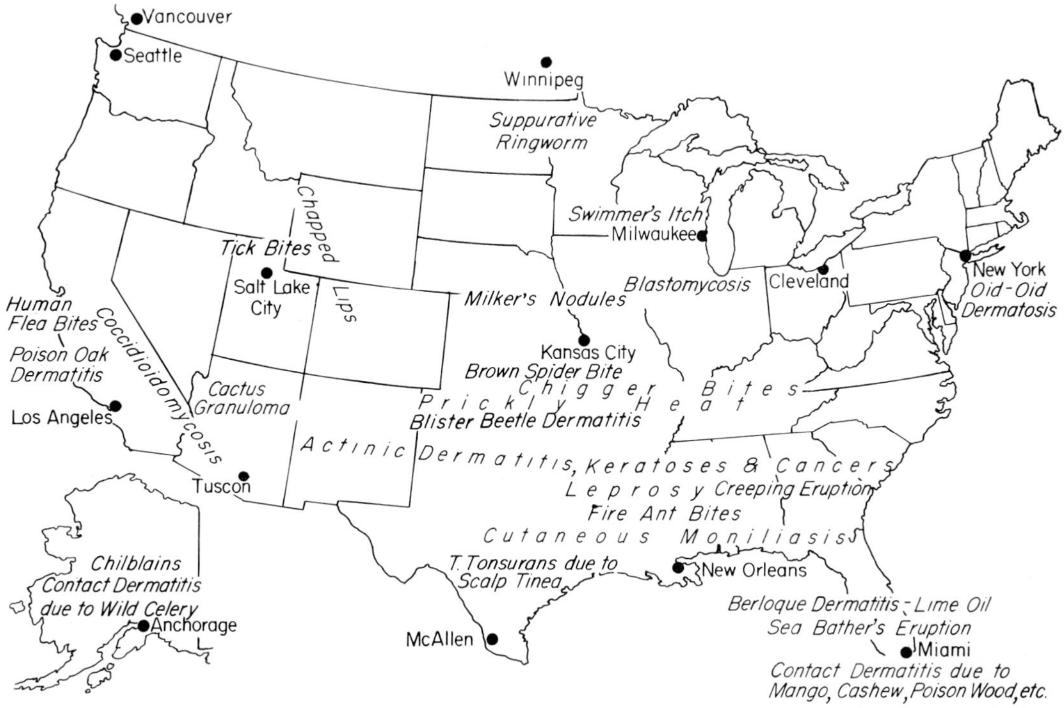

PREDOMINANT LOCALIZATION of GEOGRAPHICAL DERMATOSES

Figure 105.

agreed that we did not have any important or common dermatologic problem out here that was unusual due to our geographic location."

Winnipeg, Manitoba—Dr. Saul Berger. "We do have a fungus condition here which is called *suppurative ringworm.* It is contracted from cattle and is a common infection in rural Manitoba." Dr. Berger enclosed a reprint of an article on the subject by A. R. Birt and J. C. Wilt (A.M.A. Arch. Dermat. and Syph. **69**: 441, 1954). They concluded that the majority of cases of *suppurative ringworm* seen in rural areas of Manitoba are due to *Trichophyton faviforme.*

UNITED STATES

Anchorage, Alaska—Dr. Thomas McGowan. In a long informative letter Dr. McGowan stated that the data he had gathered in Alaska had not yet been completely tabulated or evaluated and should be considered as his personal clinical impression based on examination and interviews of several thousand natives. ". . . these impressions actually apply only to the Aleuts, resident in the Aleutian Islands and Alaska Peninsula, and to the Indians resident in Southeastern Alaska. Among these two groups I found that the only skin diseases seen with any frequency were impetigo, scabies, pediculosis capitis, and pruritus ani associated with pinworms, and all of these were almost completely limited to children. Acne vulgaris was quite common in the Indian but very rare in the Aleut. Very rare in both groups were allergic infantile eczema, vesicular eczematoid dermatoses of the hands, and fungus infections of the nails and of the scalp. I found no cases of fungus infection of the skin, of psoriasis, of skin malignancy or of tuberculosis cutis (other than old healed scars of scrofuloderma), nor did I find any active venereal disease. One condition of interest, common among children of both groups in the springtime, was an acute *dermatitis venenata,* similar to poison ivy, occurring on the face and hands after contact with the juice of the outer skin of the local 'wild celery.' "

Seattle, Washington—Dr. Harvey Roys. "I know of no skin disease that is peculiar to the Northwest."

Milwaukee, Wisconsin—Dr. Daniel Hackbarth. "*Swimmer's itch* is seen occasionally and possibly you could also list *milker's nodules.*"

New York, New York—Dr. A. I. Weidman. ". . . there is no specific regional dermatologic condition present in New York City. Perhaps conditions having their origin primarily in tension could be listed." (From my limited experience in New York City I feel that *exudative discoid and lichenoid chronic dermatosis* should be listed. It will be discussed later in this chapter.)

Los Angeles, California—Dr. Samuel Ayres, III. In addition to *human flea bites* which will be discussed more fully later, Dr. Ayres listed *actinic keratoses* and *skin cancers,* and as an uncommon condition, *coccidioidomycosis* of the San Joaquin Valley. "On the negative side, we do not have *chiggers, chilblains,* or *miliaria.*"

Salt Lake City, Utah—Dr. Arthur M. Burton. "The exanthem of Rocky Mountain spotted fever is characteristic and well documented. The tic bite itself, however, does not leave a characteristic cutaneous lesion. This I have observed from personal observation on myself. The tic burrows into the skin with its head, engorges itself with blood, then withdraws and drops off the body. There is actually very little if any evidence remaining at the site of the tic bite."

Kansas City, Missouri—Author. The two commonest geographic dermatoses of the Midwest are *chigger bites* and *prickly heat.* These will be referred to later in the chapter. *Milker's nodules, grain itch* and *bites from the brown spider* (Fig. 106 C) are peculiar to this area but not common.

Cleveland, Ohio—Dr. George H.

Curtis. "I know of no common skin disease endemic to this area." Dr. Curtis proceeded to list the most common skin conditions seen and treated at the Cleveland Clinic. At the top of the list were neurodermatitis circumscripta (including pruritus ani), superficial fungus infections and pyogenic infections.

Tucson, Arizona—Dr. Otis Miller. I requested information concerning *atopic eczema,* since so many of these patients improve when in Tucson or Phoenix. Dr. Miller's reply was, "There is little question that the warm climate of Arizona is beneficial to many, but not all, cases of atopic dermatitis. In the acute and angry stage, sunlight and heat make the condition considerably worse. There are many children who are born in Arizona with familial histories of allergies, who develop atopic dermatitis right here in Tucson. Many of these are highly allergic to pollens which are peculiar to this neck-of-the-woods. One of the most common troublemakers is Bermuda grass."

He continued with a discussion of *cactus granuloma.* "This is a tissue reaction which is found principally on the exposed areas of the body, due to the penetration of the sticker-weed into the skin. It's conceivable that the same type of reaction is produced by small thorns found on various cacti.

"*Coccidioidomycosis* is of more vital concern to Arizonians. This respiratory disease occurs with varying degrees of severity in humans and about 20% of cases require the services of a physician. Nearly every long-time resident of the southwestern region is exposed to this disease. It also occurs in desert rodents, sheep, cattle and most severely in dogs. As far as the skin manifestations of this disease, contrary to what is written in the textbooks, erythema multiforme is much more commonly seen than erythema nodosum. The primary involvement of the skin is an extremely rare condition. I think the frequency of *vitiligo* is higher here in

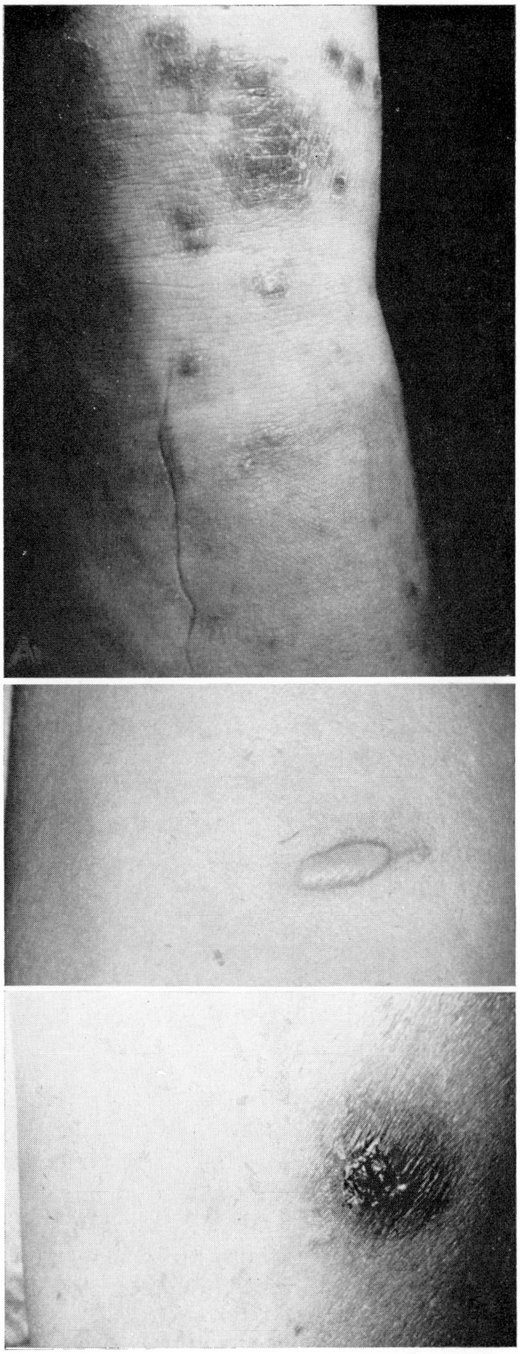

Fig. 106. Geographic dermatoses of the Midwestern and Southern states.

(A, *top*) Excoriated chigger bites on the dorsum of the ankle.
(B, *center*) Blister beetle vesicle on the arm.
(C, *bottom*) Brown spider bite on leg. (Dr. Thomas Burns)

the land of the sun than elsewhere. I don't believe that there is actually a greater frequency, but I do believe that it is more apparent here because of the fact that sun exposure magnifies the difference between the normal skin and that which is involved by the vitiligo."

McAllen, Texas—Dr. Ivan Kuhl. Dr. Kuhl listed *tinea capitis* due to *T. tonsurans, keratoses* and *skin cancers, leprosy, contact dermatitis* due to Mango fruit, *moniliasis* of all forms and *fleabites.* "Tineas and other fungus infections plus keratoses and skin cancers probably constitute about 60% of my practice. The biggest single problem is the tinea capitis due to *T. tonsurans* and *T. violaceum.*"

New Orleans, Louisiana—Dr. Leslie K. Mundt. "I can think of only two skin diseases endemic to this part of the country: *Hansen's disease (leprosy)* and *fire ant bites.*"

Miami, Florida—Dr. Harvey Blank. Dr. Blank listed *creeping eruption, cutaneous moniliasis, Portuguese Man-of-War stings, contact dermatitis* due to various members of the Anacardiaceae, not only Rhus, but Mango, Cashew and Poison wood *(Metopium toxiferum),* and Brazilian pepper tree *(Schinus terebinthifolius), eczema solare, berlock dermatitis* due to lime oil, and *actinic skin with keratoses and carcinomas.*

These letters corroborated my feeling that in addition to certain skin diseases we as dermatologists know to be endemic to a particular area, such as swimmer's itch in Wisconsin and creeping eruption in the Gulf States, there are a few other common but less well-known geographic dermatoses.

The accompanying map (Fig. 105) lists these geographic skin diseases. A few will be discussed in greater detail.

BITES DUE TO THE HUMAN FLEA

The following is quoted from Dr. Ayres's letter regarding dermatoses localized to the California area, "I would first list human fleabites, that is, those due to *Pulex irritans.* These seem to be more or less limited to the Pacific coast and more particularly to San Francisco. They are not to be confused with dog or cat fleas which may occasionally bite humans but prefer their natural hosts. Inhabitants of the area frequently are immune to the effect of the bites so that only newcomers are aware of the infestation. Interestingly enough this was my own experience when I went to medical school in San Francisco (Stanford). I had grown up in Southern California and had never known anything about human fleas bites but I was nearly eaten alive by them during my years in San Francisco, while those of my fellow students who were native San Franciscans had no trouble at all. This is a widely recognized phenomenon in these areas. The manifestations are typically grouped, highly pruritic papules with central punctae, more prevalent over the covered portion of the body."

Certain cases of *papular urticaria* have been found to be due to the bites of insects such as fleas, bedbugs, chiggers (a mite larva), flies and mosquitoes. This form of urticaria represents an allergic reaction to such bites which develops in children who have not been previously sensitized.

Treatment of fleabites consists of preventive measures to destroy the insects. This is done best by spraying the home environment with a powder containing D.D.T. The powder can also be used directly on the patient and his clothing.

CHIGGER BITES

Chigger bites, or trombidiosis, is a very common summer eruption of inhabitants of the southern United States (Fig. 106). The small urticarial papule is caused by the bite of the larva of the Chigger. The larva does not burrow into the skin but drops off after engorging itself on blood.

Due to its almost microscopic size it is rarely seen on the skin.

Clinically, the markedly pruritic papules occur where the larva meets resistance as it climbs up the legs, such as around the tops of the socks, the beltline and the neckband area. Excoriation of the lesions leads to secondary infection. An allergic papulovesicular eruption is seen occasionally in sensitive individuals following extensive generalized chigger bites. Papular urticaria has been mentioned above. In children particularly, chigger bites are a common cause of secondary impetigo, especially in the scalp. For the first two summers that we lived in Kansas City my two youngest children developed recurrent crops of impetiginous lesions on the scalp from the chigger bites. It was difficult to eradicate the lesions because of continued reinfestation and recurrent secondary infection. In recent summers the bites have been milder. This may be another example of the development of immunity following repeated exposure, similar to that seen from the fleabites of the San Francisco area.

Treatment. Preventive measures that are partially successful consist of applying Flowers of Sulfur powder to the feet and the stockings, and, if desired, spraying of the infested lawn with insecticide. Active therapy includes the use of the alcoholic white shake lotion for the pruritus, with the addition of sulfur 3%, or Aureomycin 250 mg. per ounce if secondary infection is present. For infected scalp lesions, sulfur 5% in an antibiotic ointment is beneficial.

SWIMMER'S ITCH

Bathers in the fresh-water lakes of Wisconsin, Michigan and Minnesota are prone to periodic attacks of inflammatory papular, urticarial and vesicular eruptions on the uncovered areas of the body, mainly the legs. This pruritic eruption, which usually subsides within a week, is caused by the invasion of the skin by the cercariae of the schistosomes of ducks and mammals. The life cycle of these various species of schistosomes includes the snail as an intermediate host. Upon invasion of the abnormal definitive host, the human skin, the cercariae dies, and the resulting skin eruption is the skin's reaction in ridding itself of the foreign bodies. Repeated attacks are met with stronger resistance, and the dermatitis becomes increasingly more severe. Secondary infection, edema and lymphangitis can occur.

Seabather's eruption is a similar clinical entity but of unknown etiology. Two main differences separate it from swimmer's itch: the predominance of the seabather's eruption on the bathing suit area, and the limitation of this dermatosis to salt-water areas, particularly around the Florida coast.

Treatment. Prevention of swimmer's itch is accomplished best by destruction of the snails, with careful addition to the lake water of a combination of copper sulfate and hydrated lime. Rapid drying of the swimmer with a towel apparently prevents penetration of the cercariae. Active therapy is directed toward the relief of the itching and secondary infection.

CREEPING ERUPTION

Larva migrans is a dermatosis of the southeastern United States characterized by the presence of a serpiginous, advancing, ridge overlying the tunnel of a migrating *Ancylostoma* larva. The advancing ridge is slightly behind the larva and is the skin's reaction to the foreign body. Itching and secondary infection is common.

The larva most commonly is derived from the roundworms of the genus Ancylostoma but occasionally from various species of botflies. The natural reservoir of the ancylostoma hookworm is the intestines of dogs and cats. Infected feces on sand provide an excellent source for the passage of the larvae to the unsuspecting sunbather or barefoot child. Man is not the natural host, so the parasite remains in the skin until destroyed.

Treatment. Destruction of the larva is not easy but can be accomplished with patience. The problem is to find the burrowing parasite. Cleaning the skin with immersion oil and using a hand lens helps. Dry ice, ethyl chloride, Freon 114 or electrosurgery can be applied to the intraepidermal larva.

PRICKLY HEAT

Prickly heat, or miliaria rubra, is a common disease of hot and humid climate. The physiologic pathology of the disease is the constant maceration of the skin which leads to a blockage of the sweat duct opening. Continued exercise and further maceration of the skin results in dilatation of the epidermal portion of the sweat duct and rupture into the mid-epidermis. The result is a tiny vesicular papule that itches and burns. Pustular and deep forms of miliaria are observed mainly in the tropics and in particularly susceptible individuals.

The distribution of the eruption is predominately on the neck, the back, the chest, the sides of the trunk, the abdomen and the folds of the body. Babies commonly show prickly heat confined to the diaper area. The eruption under adhesive tape is a form of localized miliaria due to blockage of the sweat pores.

Treatment. Prevention is of paramount importance. If the cycle of maceration and heat can be broken for a few hours out of each day, the eruption will not develop. Rest under fans or air-conditioning for some hours of the day or the night is of great value. When these conditions are not available, application of a mild lotion or powder gives relief from the itching and may eliminate some of the skin maceration. A good example is:

Alcoholic white shake lotion q.s. 120.0

EXUDATIVE DISCOID AND LICHENOID CHRONIC DERMATOSIS

Oid-oid disease of Sulzberger and Garbe is probably a variant of atopic eczema, but with several important additional characteristics. It is seen predominantly among Jewish males in the New York City area and is a very chronic, disabling, markedly pruritic, lichenoid and exudative dermatitis. Characteristic penile lesions are a diagnostic feature.

Treatment. Similar to that for a severe case of atopic eczema. A vacation or permanent removal of the patient to the southwestern part of the United States is quite often beneficial.

Tumors of the Skin

CHAPTER **26**

CLASSIFICATION

A PATIENT comes into your office for care of a tumor on his skin. What kind is it? What is the best treatment? This complex problem of diagnosing and managing skin tumors is not learned easily. As an aid to the establishment of the correct diagnosis, all skin tumors (excluding warts which are due to a virus) will be classified (1) as to their *histologic origin,* (2) according to the patient's *age group,* and (3) on the basis of *clinical appearance.*

A complete histologic classification will be found in the Dictionary-Index under "Tumors." The more common tumors will be classified and discussed in this chapter. The histologic classification is divided into epidermal tumors, mesodermal tumors, nevus cell tumors, lymphomas and myeloses. In making a clinical diagnosis of any skin tumor, a histopathologic label should be applied. Whether the label is correct or not depends on the clinical acumen of the physician and whether the tumor, or a part of it, has been examined microscopically. *A histologic examination should be performed on any malignant skin tumor or on any tumor where a malignancy cannot be ruled out clinically.*

Histologic Classification*

Epidermal Tumors

I. **Tumors of the Surface Epidermis**

1. Nevoid tumors. Defined as benign neoplasms which probably arise from arrested embryonal cells.
   A. Cysts
      (a) Epidermal cyst
      (b) Sebaceous cyst
      (c) Milium
      (d) Dermoid cyst
      (e) Mucous retention cyst
2. Precancerous tumors
   A. Senile or actinic keratosis and cutaneous horn
   B. Arsenical keratosis
   C. Leukoplakia
3. Epitheliomas
   A. Basal cell epithelioma
   B. Prickle cell epithelioma
4. Seborrheic keratosis and dermatosis papulosa nigra
5. Pedunculated fibromas

Mesodermal Tumors

I. **Tumors of Fibrous Tissue**

1. Histiocytoma and dermatofibroma
2. Keloid

II. **Tumors of Vascular Tissue:** Hemangiomas

Nevus Cell Tumors

I. **Nevi**

1. Junction (active) nevus
2. Intradermal (resting) nevus

II. **Malignant Melanoma**

* This partial classification and the complete one in the Dictionary-Index are modified from the one listed by Walter F. Lever: Histopathology of the Skin, ed. 2. Philadelphia, Lippincott, 1954.

Lymphomas

I. **Monomorphous Group**
II. **Polymorphous Group:** Granuloma fungoides

Classification by Age Groups

An age-group classification is helpful from a differential diagnostic viewpoint. Viral warts will be considered in this classification because of the frequent necessity of differentiating them from other skin tumors. The most common tumors are listed first.

I. **Tumors of Children**
   1. Warts (viral), very common
   2. Nevi, junction type common
   3. Hemangiomas
   4. Granuloma pyogenicum
   5. Molluscum contagiosum (viral)
   6. Mongolian spot
   7. Xanthogranuloma

II. **Tumors of Adults**
   1. Warts (viral), plantar type common
   2. Nevi
   3. Cysts
   4. Pedunculated fibromas
   5. Histiocytomas
   6. Keloids
   7. Lipomas
   8. Granuloma pyogenicum

III. **Additional Tumors of Older Adults**
   1. Seborrheic keratoses
   2. Senile keratoses
   3. Papillary hemangiomas
   4. Leukoplakia
   5. Basal cell epitheliomas
   6. Prickle cell epitheliomas

Classification Based on Clinical Appearance

The clinical appearance of any tumor is a most important diagnostic factor. Some tumors have a characteristic color and growth that is readily distinguishable from any other tumor, but a large number, unfortunately, have clinical characteristics common to several similar tumors. A further hindrance to making a correct diagnosis is that the same histopathologic lesion may vary in clinical appearance. The following generalizing classification should be helpful, but, if in doubt, the lesion should be examined histologically.

I. **Flat, skin-colored tumors**
   1. Flat warts (viral)
   2. Histiocytomas
   3. Leukoplakia

II. **Flat, pigmented tumors**
   1. Nevi, usually junction type
   2. Lentigo
   3. Histiocytoma
   4. Mongolian spot

III. **Raised, skin-colored tumors**
   1. Warts (viral)
   2. Nevi, usually intradermal type
   3. Cysts
   4. Lipomas
   5. Keloids
   6. Basal cell epitheliomas
   7. Prickle cell epitheliomas
   8. Molluscum contagiosum (viral)
   9. Xanthogranuloma (yellowish)

IV. **Raised, brownish tumors**
   1. Warts (viral)
   2. Nevi
   3. Senile keratoses
   4. Seborrheic keratoses
   5. Pedunculated fibromas
   6. Basal cell epitheliomas
   7. Prickle cell epitheliomas
   8. Malignant melanoma
   9. Granuloma pyogenicum
   10. Keratoacanthomas

V. **Raised, reddish tumors**
   1. Hemangiomas
   2. Granuloma pyogenicum
   3. Glomus tumors

VI. **Raised, blackish tumors**
   1. Seborrheic keratoses
   2. Nevi
   3. Granuloma pyogenicum
   4. Malignant melanomas
   5. Blue nevi

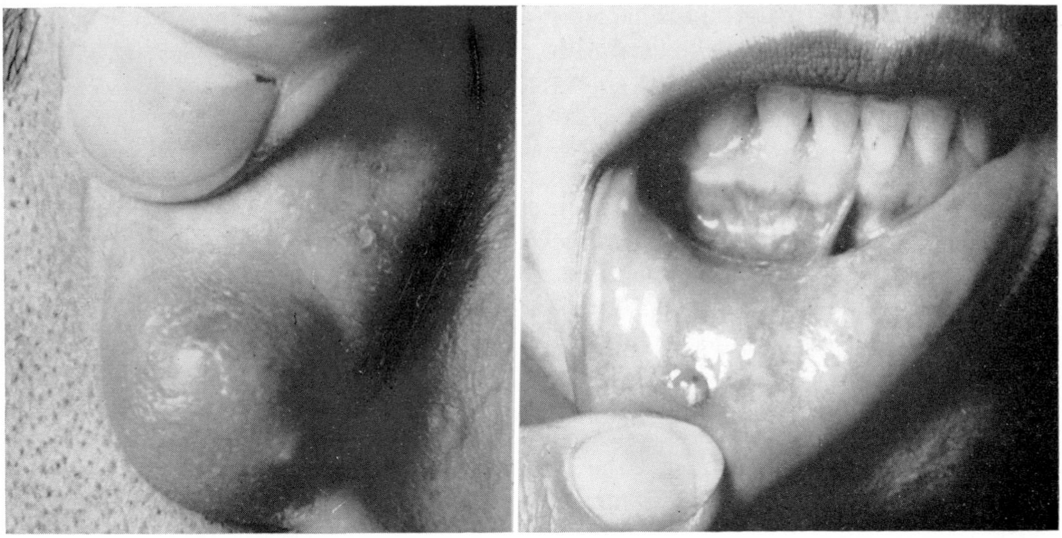

Fig. 107. Cysts.
(A, *left*) Infected epidermal cyst of ear lobe.
(B, *right*) Mucous retention cyst of lower lip.

CYSTS

1. Epidermal cyst
2. Sebaceous cyst
3. Milium

The common skin cyst or wen that is clinically labeled a "sebaceous" cyst will turn out to be an epidermal cyst in 99.5% of cases when studied histologically.* A true *sebaceous cyst,* from arrested embryonal cells or from a plugged sebaceous gland, is relatively uncommon. An *epidermal cyst* has a wall composed of true epidermis and probably originates from an invagination of the epidermis into the dermis and subsequent detachment from the epidermis (Fig. 107 A). The most common location for epidermal cysts is the scalp, where many such tumors of varying size can be found.

Milia are very common, white pinhead-sized, firm lesions that are seen on the face. They are formed by proliferation of epithelial buds following trauma to the skin (dermabrasion for acne scars), following certain dermatoses (pemphigus, epidermolysis bullosa, and acute contact dermatitis) or from no apparent cause.

* Warvi, W. N., and Gates, O.: Epithelial cysts and cystic tumors of the skin, Am. J. Path. **19**:765, 1943.

Differential Diagnosis of Epidermal and Sebaceous Cysts

Lipoma: rather difficult to differentiate clinically, more firm, lobulated, no cheesy material extrudes on incision, removal is by complete excision, clinically similar to *hibernoma.*

Dermoid Cyst: clinically similar, can also be found internally; usually a solitary skin tumor; histologically, contains hairs, eccrine glands, sebaceous glands, etc.

Mucous Retention Cysts (Fig. 107 B): translucent pea-sized or smaller lesions on the lips, treated by cutting off top of the lesion and carefully lightly cauterizing the base with a silver nitrate stick.

Synovial Cysts of the Skin (Fig. 108 A): globoid, translucent, pea-sized swellings around the joints of fingers and toes.

Treatment of Epidermal and Sebaceous Cysts. Several methods can be used with success. The choice depends on the ability of the operator, and the site and the number of cysts. Cysts can regrow following even the best surgical care, because of incomplete removal of the sac.

1. A single 3-cm.-diameter cyst on the back should be removed by surgical excision and suturing. This can be done in two ways: either by incising the skin and skillfully removing the intact cyst sac, or by cutting straight into the sac with a small incision, shelling out the evacuated lining and suturing the skin. The latter procedure is simpler, requires a smaller incision and is quite successful.

2. A patient with several cysts in the scalp or a small cyst on an exposed area of the body can be treated in another simple way. A 2-to-3-mm. incision can be made directly over and into the cyst. Then the contents can be evacuated by gentle pressure and the use of a small curette. In many instances the entire sac can be grasped firmly with a small hemostat and pulled out of the opening. If the entire sac is not removed at this time, a repeated attempt in one week, aided by the development of a mild infection, will usually be successful. No suturing or only a single suture is necessary. The resulting scar will be imperceptible in a short time.

3. If, during incision by any technic, a solid tumor is found instead of a cyst, the lesion should be excised completely and the material studied histologically. This diagnostic error is very common because of the clinical similarity of cysts, lipomas and other related tumors.

Treatment of Milia

1. Simple incision of the small tumors with a scalpel or a Hagedorn needle and expression of the contents by a comedone extractor is sufficient.

2. Another procedure is to remove the top of the milia lightly with electrodesiccation.

PRECANCEROUS TUMORS

1. Senile keratosis and cutaneous horn
2. Arsenical keratosis
3. Leukoplakia

SENILE KERATOSIS

This common skin lesion of light-complexioned, older persons occurs on the skin surfaces exposed to sunlight (Fig. 109). A small percentage of these lesions

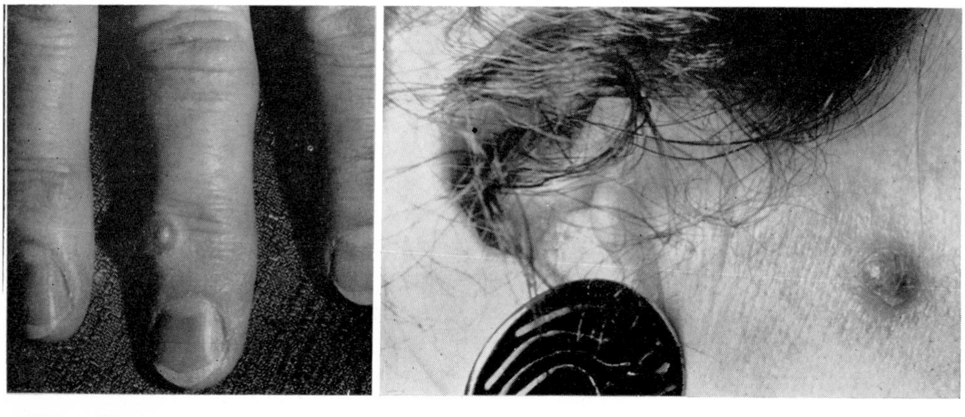

Fig. 108. Cysts.

(A, *left*) Synovial cyst of finger. (Dr. Chester Lessenden)
(B, *right*) Foreign body inclusion cyst on the cheek.

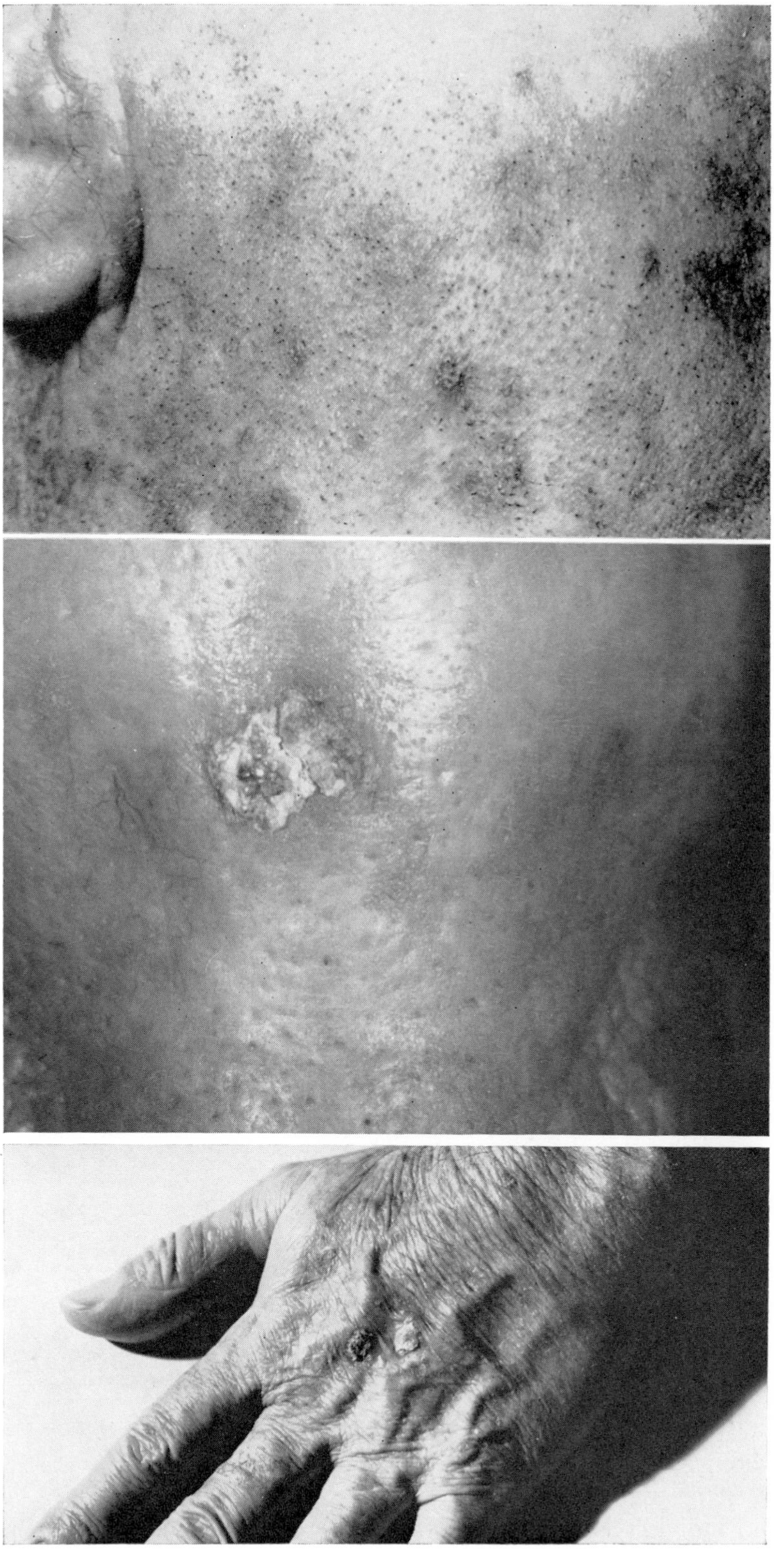

Fig. 109. Senile or actinic keratoses.

(*Top*) Multiple lesions on the cheek of a farmer.

(*Center*) Close-up of a nose lesion. (Dr. Lawrence Hyde)

(*Bottom*) Two lesions on the dorsum of the hand. (K.U.M.C.)

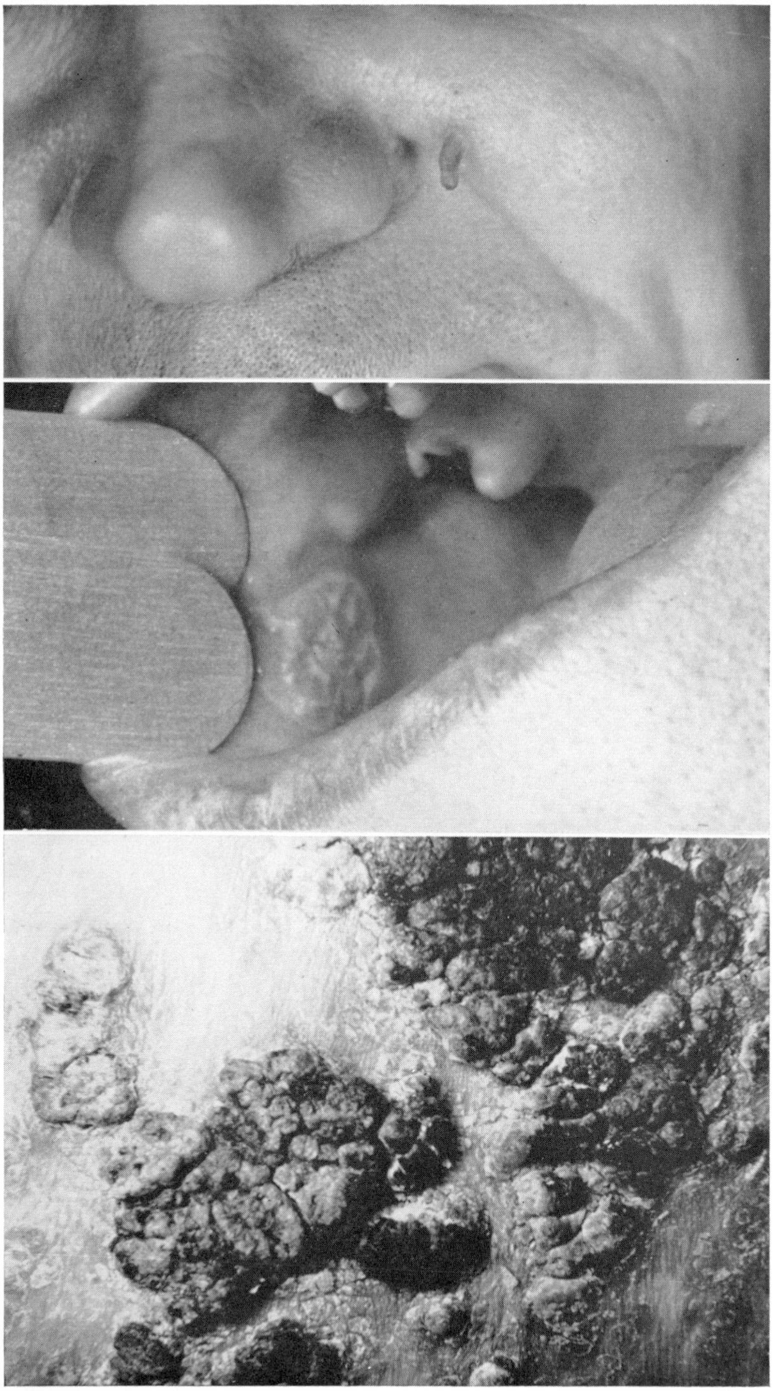

Fig. 110. Precanceroses.

(A, *top*) Cutaneous horn on the cheek. There was no epithelioma at the base of this lesion.

(B, *center*) Biopsy-proved leukoplakia on the mucous membrane of the cheek. This was erroneously diagnosed clinically as lichen planus.

(C, *bottom*) Bowen's disease covering extensive areas on the abdomen. (Patient of Dr. M. D. Marcus)

slowly develop into prickle cell epitheliomas. Another term, *actinic keratosis,* can be used when these tumors are seen in individuals in the 30-to-50 age group.

Description. Usually multiple, flat or slightly elevated, brownish or tan colored, scaly, adherent lesions measuring up to 1.5 cm. in diameter. Individual lesions may become confluent. A *cutaneous horn* is a very proliferative, hyperkeratotic form of senile keratosis that resembles a horn (Fig. 110 A).

Distribution. Areas of skin exposed to sunlight, such as face, ears, neck, and dorsum of hands.

Course. Lesion begins as a faint-red, slightly scaly patch that enlarges slowly peripherally and deeply over many years. A sudden spurt of growth would indicate a change to a prickle cell epithelioma.

Subjective Complaints. Patients often complain that these lesions burn and sting.

Etiology. Heredity and sun exposure are the two main causative factors. The blue-eyed, thin-skinned, light-haired farmer or sailor with a family history of such lesions is the best subject for multiple senile keratoses. Excessive sun exposure is important but not necessary.

Sex Incidence. Most commonly seen in men.

Differential Diagnosis

Seborrheic Keratosis (see chart)

Prickle Cell Epithelioma: any thickened lesion that has grown rapidly should be biopsied (p. 218).

Arsenical Keratosis: mainly on palms and soles.

Treatment. A 60-year-old farmer has 3 small senile keratoses on his face.

1. Examine the lesions carefully. *If there is any evidence of induration or marked inflammation, the lesion should be biopsied.* (See scissors technic, p. 10.)

2. Curettement followed by destruction of the base by acid or electrosurgery is a very satisfactory way to remove early small keratoses. The technic is as follows. Local anesthesia is usually not necessary unless electrosurgery is used. Firmly scrape the lesion with the dermal curette, which will remove the mushy, scaly keratosis and bring you down to the more fibrous normal skin. Experience will provide the necessary "feel" of the abnormal versus the normal tissue. Some of the bleeding can be controlled by pressure or use of either one of the two following procedures: (1) apply saturated solution of trichloracetic acid with caution to the bleeding site, using a cotton applicator; or (2) the bleeding base may be electrocoagulated. I prefer the acid technic because local anesthesia is not necessary for most patients, and healing is faster. Small lesions will heal in 7 to 14 days. No bandage is required; in fact, bandaging promotes infection.

3. Request the patient to return every 6 months for a checkup and treatment of new lesions as they develop.

4. For younger patients with these keratoses a sun screen cream (Skolex Cream or A-fil Cream) should be prescribed for prevention of future lesions.

Treatment of a Cutaneous Horn. The same technic as for senile keratosis. *To rule out cancer, every cutaneous horn should be sent with intact base for histopathologic examination.* The incidence of

	Senile Keratosis	Seborrheic Keratosis
Appearance	Flat, brownish or tan, scale firmly attached to skin	Greasy, elevated, brown or black, scale is warty and can be easily scratched away
Location	Sun-exposed areas	Face, back and chest
Complexion	Blue eyes, light hair, dry skin	Brown eyes, dark hair, oily skin
Subjective Complaints	Some burning and stinging	None
Precancerous	Yes	No

prickle cell epitheliomatous change in the base of a cutaneous horn is appreciable.

Arsenical Keratosis

Prolonged ingestion of inorganic arsenic (Fowler's Solution, Asiatic Pills) can result in the formation many years later of small puntate keratotic lesions mainly seen on the palms and the soles. Progression to a prickle cell epithelioma can occur but is unusual.

Treatment. Small arsenical keratoses can be removed by electrosurgery; larger lesions can be excised and skin grafted if necessary. Vitamin A orally may be helpful.

Leukoplakia

Leukoplakia is a senile keratosis of the mucous membrane (Fig. 110 B).

Description. A flat, whitish plaque localized to the mucous membranes of lips, mouth, vulva and vagina. Single or multiple lesions may be present.

Course. Progression to prickle cell epithelioma occurs in 20 to 30% of chronic cases.

Etiology. Smoking, sunlight and chronic irritation are the important factors in the development of leukoplakia. Recurrent actinic cheilitis may precede leukoplakia of the lips. The vulvar form may develop from presenile or senile atrophy of this area.

Differential Diagnosis

Lichen Planus: see a lacy network of whitish lesions mainly on the sides of the buccal cavity; when on lips, it may clinically resemble leukoplakia; see lichen planus elsewhere on body (p. 92).

Pressure Calluses From Teeth or Dentures: see evidence of irritation; differentiation may be possible only by biopsy.

On the vulva, *lichen sclerosis et atrophicus* or *kraurosis vulvae:* see no induration as in leukoplakia of this area; can extend onto skin of inguinal folds and perianal region; pruritus may or may not be present.

Treatment. Small patch of leukoplakia on lower lip of man who smokes considerably.

1. Examine lesion carefully. Biopsy any questionable area that shows inflammation and induration. If a prickle cell epithelioma is present the patient should receive surgical or radiation therapy by a physician expert in this form of treatment.
2. Advise against smoking. The seriousness of continued smoking or other use of tobacco must be pointed out to the patient. Many early cases of leukoplakia disappear when smoking is stopped.
3. Eliminate any chronic irritation from teeth or dentures.
4. Protect the lips from sunlight with a sun screen cream such as Skolex, A-fil Cream or A-fil Sunstick.
5. Electrosurgery preceded by local anesthesia is excellent for small persistent areas of leukoplakia. The coagulating current is effective. Healing is usually rapid.

EPITHELIOMAS

1. Basal cell epithelioma
2. Prickle cell epithelioma

Basal Cell Epithelioma
(Plates 1 C and 3 A)

This is the commonest malignancy of the skin. Very fortunately, a basal cell epithelioma is not a metastasizing tumor, and the cure rate can be 100% if these lesions are treated early and adequately (Figs. 111 and 112). Death from a basal cell epithelioma results from neglected cases, either by the patient or by the therapist.

Description. There are 4 clinical types of basal cell epithelioma: (1) nodulo-ulcerative, (2) pigmented, (3) fibrosing and (4) superficial.

The *nodulo-ulcerative basal cell epithelioma* is the commonest type. It begins

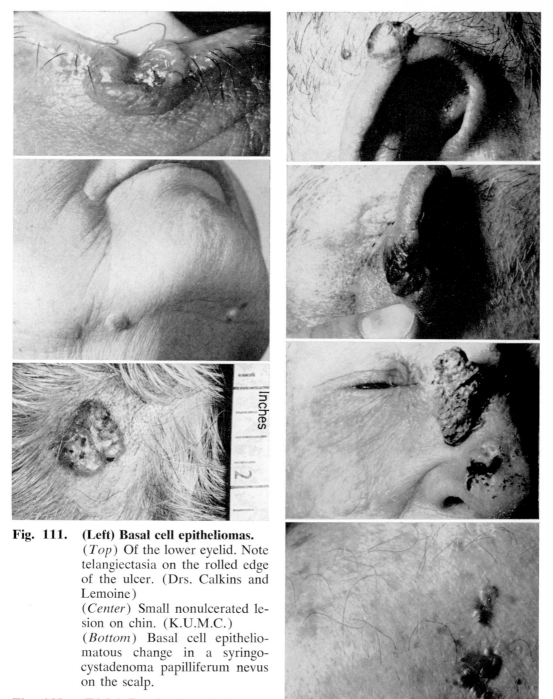

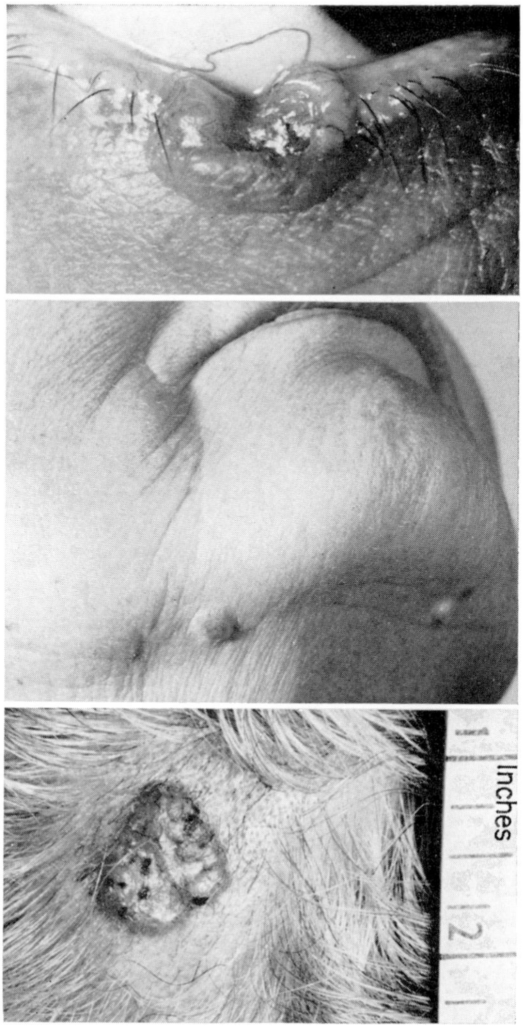

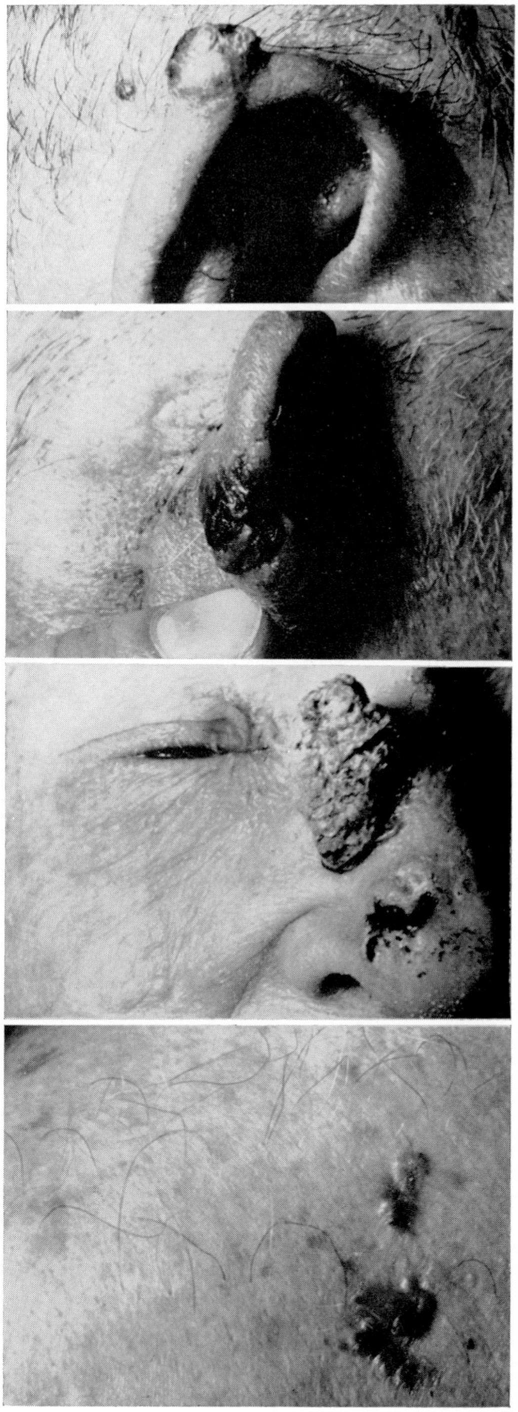

Fig. 111. (Left) Basal cell epitheliomas.
(*Top*) Of the lower eyelid. Note telangiectasia on the rolled edge of the ulcer. (Drs. Calkins and Lemoine)
(*Center*) Small nonulcerated lesion on chin. (K.U.M.C.)
(*Bottom*) Basal cell epitheliomatous change in a syringocystadenoma papilliferum nevus on the scalp.

Fig. 112. (Right) Basal cell epitheliomas.
(*Top to bottom*)
A. On helix of ear.
B. Hemorrhagic lesion on helix of ear.
C. Cutaneous horn with basal cell epitheliomatous degeneration of the base.
D. Superficial basal cell epithelioma on posterior aspect of shoulder. Patient took arsenic (Fowler's solution) for 3 months 30 years previously for psoriasis.

as a small waxy nodule that enlarges slowly over the years. A central depression forms that eventually progresses into an ulcer surrounded by the pearly or waxy border. The surface of the nodular component has a few telangiectatic vessels which are highly characteristic.

The *pigmented type* is similar to the nodulo-ulcerative form, with the addition of brown or black pigmentation.

The *fibrosing type* is extremely slow growing, usually seen on the face, and consists of a whitish scarred plaque with an ill-defined border which rarely becomes ulcerated.

The *superficial form* may be single or multiple, usually seen on the back and the chest, and is characterized by slowly enlarging red scaly areas that on careful examination reveal a nodular border with telangiectatic vessels. A healed atrophic center may be present. Ulceration is superficial when it develops.

Distribution. Over 90% of the basal cell epitheliomas occur on the head and the neck, with the trunk next in frequency. These tumors are rarely found on the palms and the soles.

Course. Very slow growing, but sudden rapid growth periods do occur. Destructive forms of this tumor can invade cartilage, bone, blood vessels, large areas of skin surface, and result in death. The very rare cases of metastasizing basal cell epitheliomas probably represent wrong diagnoses.

Etiology. Basal cell epitheliomas develop most frequently on the areas of the skin exposed to sunlight and in blond or red-haired individuals. Trauma and overexposure to radium and x-radiation can cause basal cell epitheliomas. Long-term ingestion of inorganic arsenic can lead to formation of superficial basal cell epitheliomas. Most authors believe that a basal cell epithelioma is a carcinoma of the basal cells of the epidermis. Lever and others believe it not to be a carcinoma but a nevoid tumor derived from incompletely differentiated embryonal cells.

Age Group. Can occur from childhood to old age but is seen most frequently in male patients above the age of 50.

Differential Diagnosis. *Whenever the clinical appearance of a skin tumor suggests a basal cell epithelioma, the lesion should be studied histologically.*

Prickle Cell Epithelioma: see more rapid growth, firm scaly papule or nodule, more inflammation, no pearly telangiectatic border; biopsy may be necessary to differentiate.

Other lesions that can mimic a basal cell epithelioma are *keratoacanthomas, sebaceous adenomas, large comedones, warts, nevi, small cysts, and scarring from injury or radiation.*

Superficial basal cell epitheliomas can resemble lesions of *psoriasis, seborrheic dermatitis, lupus vulgaris* and *Bowen's disease* (Fig. 110 C).

Treatment. A 48-year-old female has an 8 x 8 mm. basal cell epithelioma on her forehead.

1. Inform the patient that she has a tumor of the skin that needs to be removed. (If the patient asks if the tumor is a cancer, I say that it is, and add that it is not like the cancer that develops inside the body.) Tell the patient that this tumor cannot spread into the body, but if it is not treated it can spread on the skin. State that removal of the lesion is almost 100% effective, but that periodic examinations will be necessary to check for any regrowth. If this tumor would come back it would regrow only at its previous site. Tell the patient that a slight scar will result from the treatment.

2. If the diagnosis of the lesion is not definite clinically, a scissors biopsy, as described on page 10, may be done safely. Further treatment will depend on the laboratory report.

3. Surgical excision of a basal cell epi-

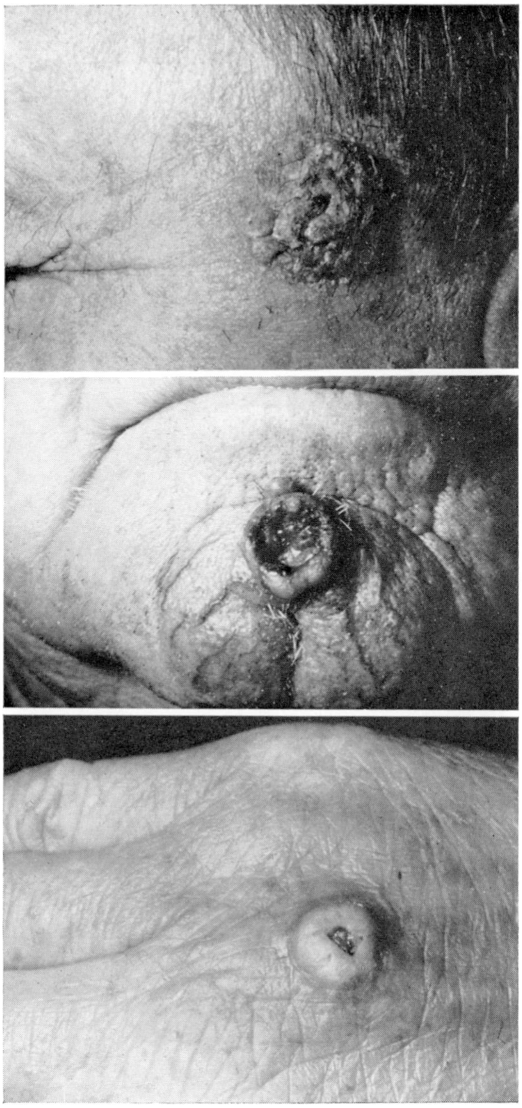

Fig. 113. (Left) Prickle cell epitheliomas.

(*Top*) On temple area.
(*Center*) On chin with marked ulceration.
(*Bottom*) On the dorsum of the hand.

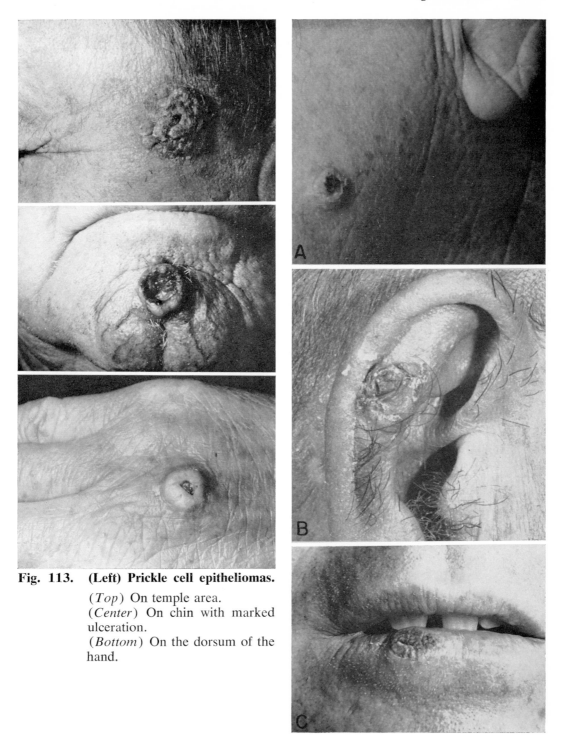

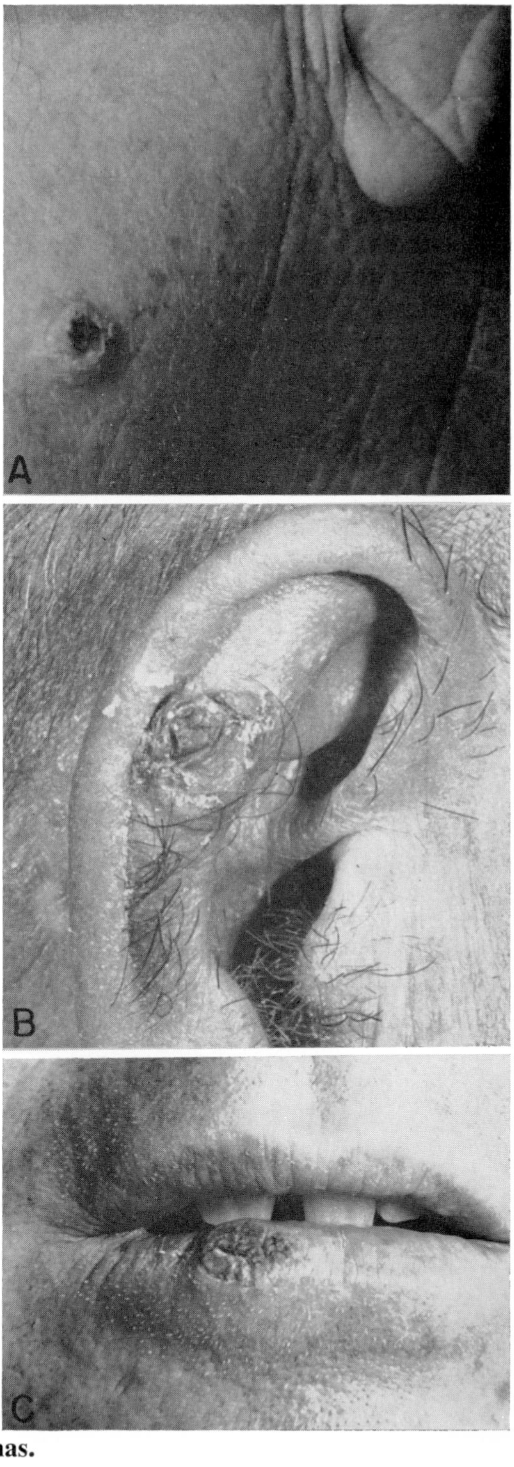

Fig. 114. (Right) Prickle cell epitheliomas.

A. On the cheek.
B. On the ear resembling a senile keratosis. (K.C.G.H.)
C. On the lower lip of a 36-year-old male.

thelioma is the only method of treatment that should be attempted by the physician who only occasionally is confronted with these tumors. (Some criticism will arise from this statement, but it is my belief that a great amount of experience is necessary to remove these tumors adequately by curettement, chemocautery, electrosurgery, radiation or any combination of these methods. If the operator feels that he is qualified in these procedures, then this statement was not meant for him.) To excise the lesion, anesthetize the area, make an elliptical incision with a scalpel to include a border of 3 to 4 mm. around the tumor, tag one side of the excised skin with a piece of suture, close the incision and submit the specimen for careful histologic examination. If the pathologist states that the tumor extends up to the edge of the excision, a further more radical excision should be performed.

4. Have the patient return for a checkup in 1 month, then 2, then 3, then 6 months, then yearly for 3 to 5 years.

Treatment of deeply ulcerated, fibrosing, or superficial basal cell epitheliomas should be in the domain of the competent dermatologist, surgeon, or radiologist.

Prickle Cell Epithelioma

This rather common skin malignancy can arise primarily or from a senile keratosis or leukoplakia. The grade of malignancy and metastasizing ability varies from Grade I (low) to Grade IV (high). Other terms for this tumor include squamous cell carcinoma and epidermoid carcinoma (Figs. 113 and 114).

Description. The commonest clinical picture is a rather rapidly growing nodule which soon develops a central ulcer and an indurated raised border with some surrounding redness. This type of lesion is the most malignant. The least malignant form has the clinical appearance of a warty, piled-up growth which may not ulcerate. However, it is important to realize that the grade of malignancy can vary in the same tumor from one section to another, particularly in the larger lesions. This variation demonstrates the value of multiple histologic sections.

Distribution. Can occur on any area of the skin and mucous membrane, but most commonly on the face, particularly lower lip and ears, tongue, and dorsum of the hands. Chronic trauma associated with certain occupations can lead to formation of this cancer on unusual sites, such as mule skinners' cancer of the scrotum from machinery oils, chimney sweeps' cancer, etc.

Course. This varies with the grade of malignancy of the tumor. Lymph node metastases may occur early in the development of the tumor or never. The cure rate can be very high when the lesions are treated early and with the best indicated modality.

Etiology. As with basal cell epitheliomas, many factors contribute to provide the soil for growth of a prickle cell epithelioma. A simple listing of factors will be sufficient: hereditarily determined type of skin; age of patient; trauma from chemicals (tars, oils), heat, wind, sunlight, x-radiation and severe burns; skin diseases that form scars such as chronic discoid lupus erythematosus, lupus vulgaris and chronic ulcers; ingestion of inorganic arsenic; and in the natural course of xeroderma pigmentosum.

Age and Sex Incidence. Most usually seen in elderly males, but exceptions are not rare.

Differential Diagnosis. *Whenever the clinical appearance of a skin tumor suggests a prickle cell epithelioma, the lesion should be studied histologically.*

Basal Cell Epithelioma: see slower growth, pearly border with telangiectasis, less inflammation; biopsy may be necessary to differentiate (p. 214).

Fig. 115. Keratoacanthomas.

A. Single lesion on dorsum of the hand.
B. Multiple lesions on leg of 4 years' duration.
C. Close-up of lesions in B.

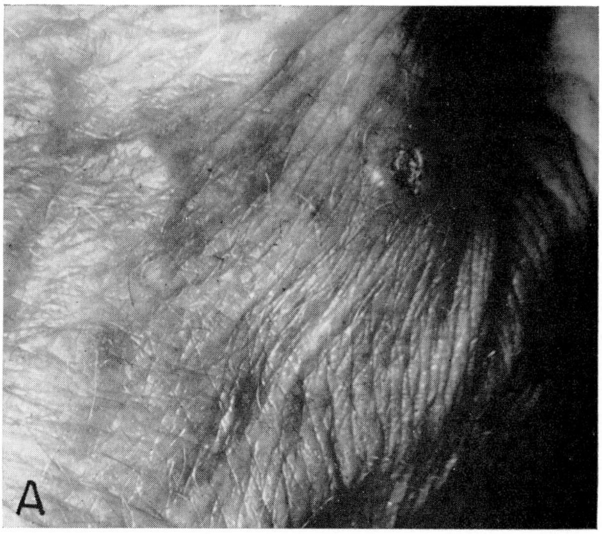

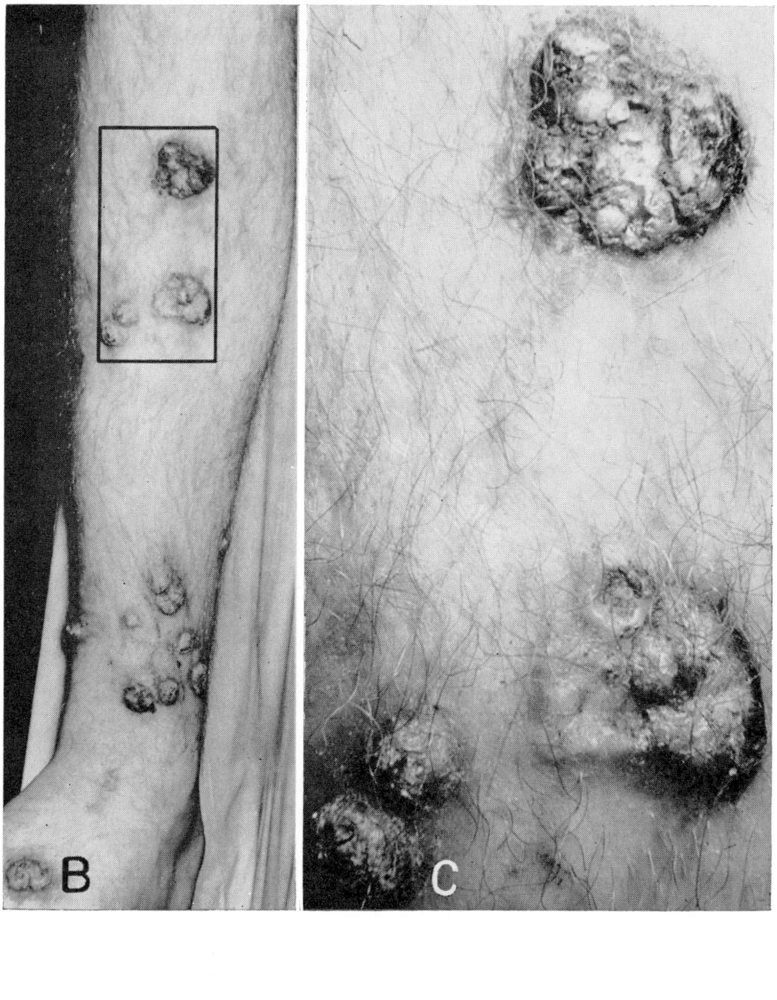

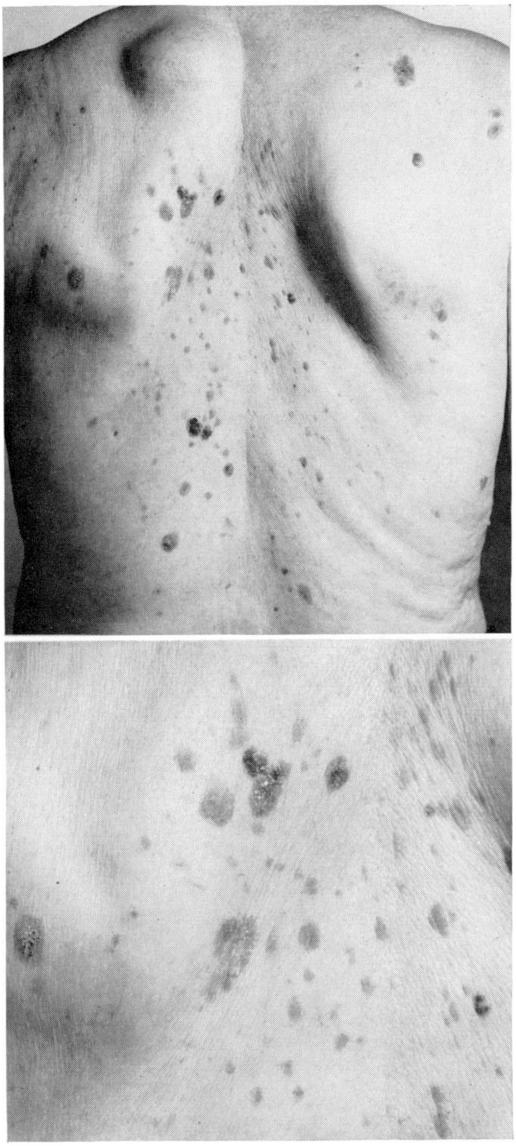

Fig. 116. Seborrheic keratoses.

Photograph of the entire back and a close-up of multiple lesions. Note lipoma over the left scapula in the top photograph.

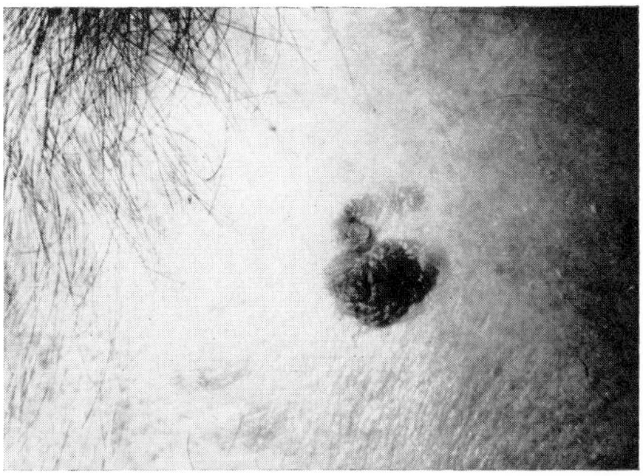

Fig. 117. Seborrheic keratosis on the forehead.

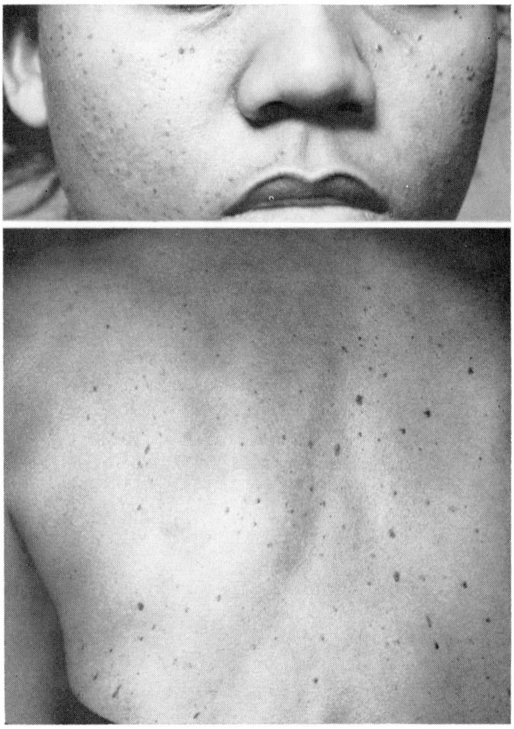

Fig. 118. Dermatosis papulosa nigra.

On the face and the back of a Negress. (K.U.M.C.)

Senile or Actinic Keratosis: see slow-growing flat scaly lesions, no induration, little surrounding erythema (p. 210).

Pseudoepitheliomatous Hyperplasia: see primary chronic lesion, such as old stasis ulcer, bromoderma, deep mycotic infection, syphilitic gumma, lupus vulgaris, basal cell epithelioma and pyoderma gangrenosum; differentiation often impossible clinically and very difficult histologically.

Keratoacanthoma (Fig. 115): see very

fast-growing single or, more rarely, multiple type of keratoacanthoma; clinically this is a firm, raised nodule with a central crater; it should be studied histologically; it may disappear spontaneously.

Treatment. Because of the invasive nature of prickle cell epitheliomas, intensive surgical and/or radiation therapy is indicated. Such procedures are beyond the scope of this text.

SEBORRHEIC KERATOSIS

It is a rare elderly patient that does not have any seborrheic keratoses. These are the unattractive "moles" or "warts" that perturb the elderly patient, occasionally become irritated but are otherwise benign (Figs. 116 and 117).

Dermatosis papulosa nigra is a form of seborrheic keratosis of Negroes that occurs on the face, mainly in women (Fig. 118). These small, multiple tumors should not be removed, because of the possibility of causing keloids.

Description. The size of seborrheic keratoses varies up to 3 cm. for the largest, but the average diameter is 1 cm. The color may be flesh-colored, tan, brown, or coal black. They are usually elevated and have a greasy, warty sensation to touch.

Distribution. On face, neck, scalp, back and upper chest, less frequently on arms, legs and lower part of trunk.

Course. They become darker in color and enlarge slowly. Trauma from clothing occasionally results in infection, and this prompts the patient to come to your office. Any inflammatory dermatitis around these lesions causes them to enlarge temporarily and become more evident, so much so that many patients suddenly note them for the first time. Malignant degeneration of seborrheic keratoses is doubted.

Etiology. Heredity is the biggest factor, along with old age. They are seen more commonly in patients with an oily, acne-seborrhea type of skin.

Differential Diagnosis

Actinic or Senile Keratoses (see p. 213 for chart).

Pigmented Nevi: longer duration, smoother surface, softer to touch, may not be able to differentiate clinically (p. 227).

Flat Warts: in younger patients, acute onset with rapid development of new lesions (p. 127).

Malignant Melanoma: very rare, usually rapid growth, indurated, examine histologically.

Treatment. A 58-year-old female patient requests the removal of a warty, tannish, slightly elevated 2 by 2 cm. lesion on the right side of her forehead.

1. Examine the lesion carefully. The diagnosis usually can be made clinically, but if there is any question a scissors biopsy (p. 10) can be performed. It would be ideal if all of these seborrheic keratoses could be examined histologically, but this is not economically feasible or necessary.

2. A very adequate form of therapy is curettement, with or without local anesthesia, followed by a light application of trichloracetic acid as outlined under senile keratosis (p. 213). The resulting fine atrophic scar will hardly be noticeable in several months. Electrosurgery can be used, but this requires anesthesia. Surgical excision is an unnecessary and more expensive form of removal.

PEDUNCULATED FIBROMAS

Multiple skin tags are very common on the neck and the axillae of middle-aged, usually obese, men and women (Fig. 119). The indications for removal are twofold: cosmetic as desired and requested by the patient, and to prevent the irritation and the secondary infection of the pedicle that frequently develops from trauma of a collar, a scarf, etc.

Description. Pedunculated pinhead-sized to pea-sized soft tumors of normal skin color or darker. The base may be inflamed from injury.

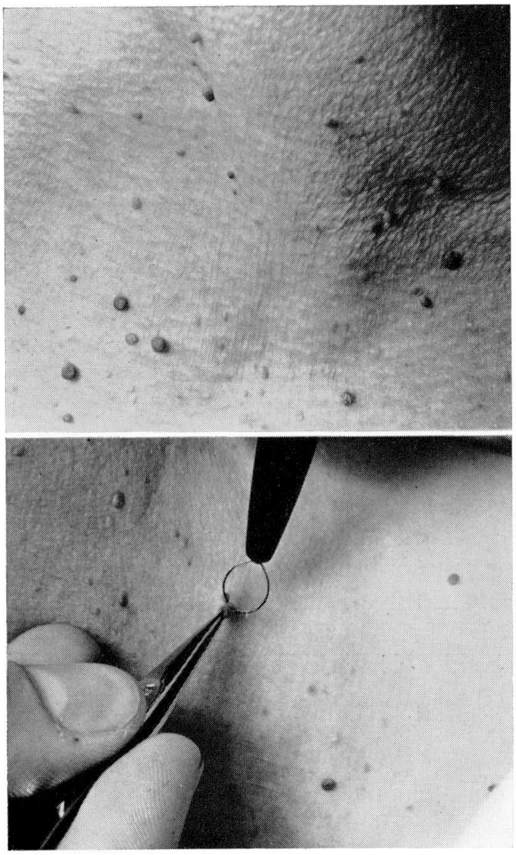

Fig. 119. Pedunculated fibromas.
(A, *top*) On the neck of a woman.
(B, *bottom*) A method of removal by grasping the skin tag with thumb forceps and applying a coagulating current to the base.

Distribution. Neck, axillae, groin, or less frequently on any area.

Course. Grow very slowly. May increase in size during pregnancy. Some become infected and drop off.

Differential Diagnosis

Filiform Wart: see digitate projections, more horny, also seen on chin area (p. 128).

Pedunculated Seborrheic Keratosis: see larger lesion, darker color, warty or velvety appearance (p. 221).

Neurofibromatosis: see lesions elsewhere, larger; can be pushed back into skin; also see café-au-lait spots, hereditary.

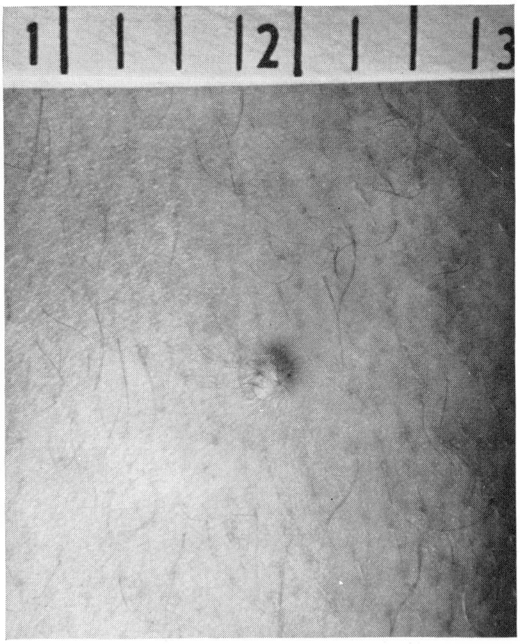

Fig. 120. Histiocytoma on the anterior tibial area of the leg.

Treatment. A 42-year-old woman with 20 small pedunculated fibromas of her neck and axillae which she desires removed. This should be done by electrosurgery. Without anesthesia gently grab the small tumor in a thumb forceps and stretch the pedicle (Fig. 119 B). Touch this pedicle with the electrosurgery needle and turn on the current for a split second. The tumor separates from the skin, and no bleeding occurs. The site will heal in 4 to 7 days.

HISTIOCYTOMA AND DERMATOFIBROMA

These are common, single, flat or very slightly elevated, tannish, reddish or brownish nodules, less than 1 cm. in size that occur mainly on the anterior tibial area of the leg (Fig. 120). This tumor has a characteristic clinical appearance and firm buttonlike feel that establishes the diagnosis. It occurs in adults, is nonsymptomatic and unchanging.

The histologic picture varies with the

age of the lesion. The younger lesions are called histiocytomas, and the older ones dermatofibromas. If the nodule contains many blood vessels it is histologically labeled a *sclerosing hemangioma.*

Differential Diagnosis. *Fibrosarcoma:* see active growth with invasion of subcutaneous fat; any questionable lesion should be excised and examined histologically.

Treatment: None indicated. If there is any doubt as to the diagnosis, surgical excision and histologic examination are indicated.

KELOID
(Plate 3 B)

A keloid is a tumor resulting from an abnormal overgrowth of fibrous tissue following injury in certain predisposed individuals (Fig. 121). Very unusual configurations can occur, depending on the site, the extent and the variety of the trauma. This tendency occurs so commonly in Negroes that one should think twice before attempting a cosmetic procedure on a Negro or on any other person with a history of keloids. The face and the upper chest areas are especially prone to this proliferation.

Treatment. Very unsatisfactory. Certain combined procedures utilizing excision, x-rays and hyaluronidase injections have been used with varying success.

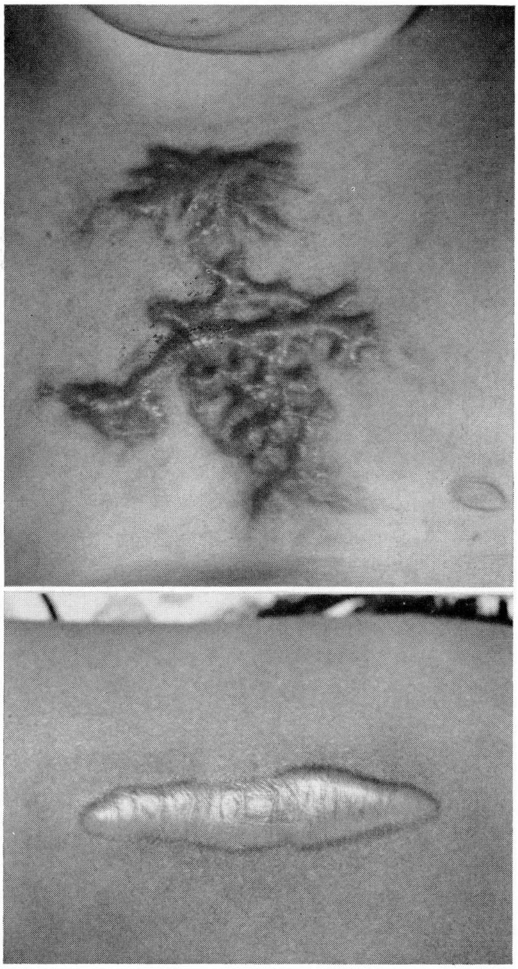

Fig. 121. Keloids.
(*Top*) On the chest of a baby girl following a burn.
(*Bottom*) On the forearm.
(K.C.G.H.)

HEMANGIOMAS
(Plates 1 A and D)

Hemangiomas are vascular abnormalities of the skin. Heredity is not a factor in the development of these lesions. There are 8 types of hemangiomas, which vary as to depth, clinical appearance and location.

1. Superficial hemangioma
2. Cavernous hemangioma
3. Mixed hemangioma (when both superficial and cavernous elements are present)
4. Spider hemangioma
5. Port-wine stain
6. Nuchal hemangioma
7. Papillary hemangioma
8. Angiokeratoma

Superficial Hemangiomas

The familiar bright-red, raised "strawberry" tumor has been seen by all physicians (Fig. 122). Strawberries have to grow, and they start from a small beginning. The parents are usually the first to

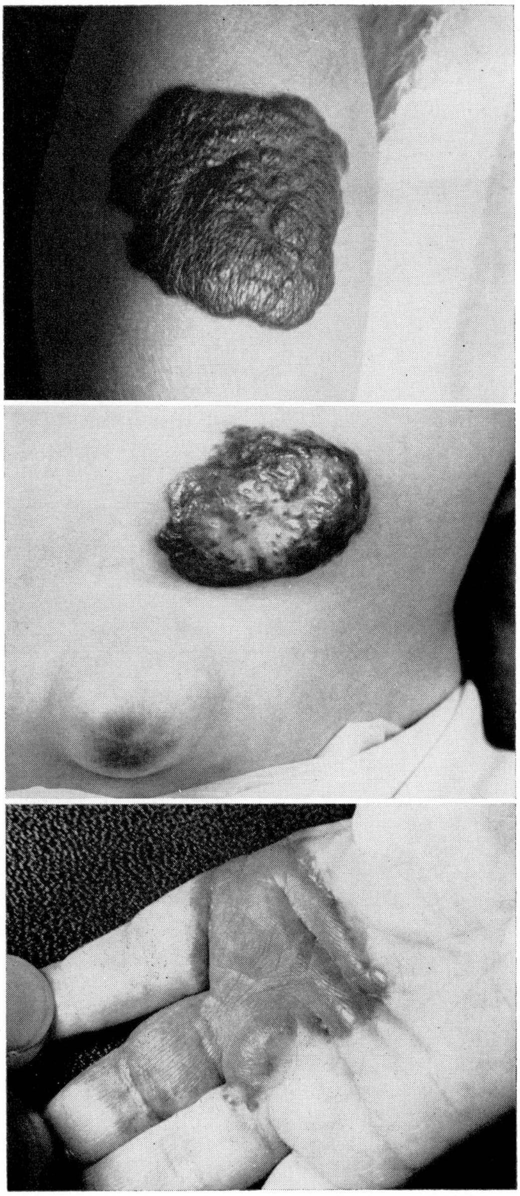

Fig. 122. Hemangiomas.

(*Top*) Superficial hemangioma on calf of the leg of a child. (*Center*) Mixed hemangioma on the abdomen above an umbilical hernia. (See Color Plate 1.) (*Bottom*) Cavernous hemangioma on the palm of the hand.

notice the small red, pinhead sized, flat lesion on 3-week-old Sarah Sue's cheek. For purposes of illustration and as an attempt to solve the problem of whether or not to treat these small lesions, let us transport Sarah Sue first to one physician and then, hypothetically, start over again with another physician.

Sarah Sue is rushed to Dr. A because of the "birthmark." Dr. A examines the lesion and advises the mother, "This birthmark will probably go away. The majority of them do. Let's just watch it."

At the age of 6 weeks the previously flat lesion is slightly raised and measures 4 x 4 mm. The doctor says, "Let's just watch it some more."

At the age of 3 months the strawberry has developed further; it is raised, bright red and measures 12 x 12 x 5 mm. A bluish mass is evident at the base of the red tumor. Dr. A's advice, "I am sure this will still go away, but if you would like to see Dr. D, a skin specialist, it might be a good idea."

Sarah Sue's mother says humbly, "We have faith in what you say, Dr. A, so we will wait a little longer. Sarah Sue has a cold anyway and I'm sure the doctor would not want to do anything now."

Sarah Sue's father had an appendectomy the next week, and before Dr. A saw Sarah Sue again, at the age of 5 months, the tumor was twice the size it was 2 months previously. Dr. A's advice was, "I definitely want you to see Dr. D." Sarah Sue's father asks, "Dr. A, is this going to cause a scar on Sarah Sue's cheek?" Dr. A's reply was, "You ask Dr. D about that."

Dr. D saw Sarah Sue the next week and treated her with dry ice and x-rays, which caused the tumor to flatten down gradually over a period of 6 months. The residual effect was a quarter-sized red and white, mottled, concave scar on Sarah Sue's cheek.

Let's begin again, hypothetically. Sarah Sue is rushed to Dr. B because of this "birthmark." She is 4 weeks old. Dr. B examines the lesion and says, "This is a very small blood vessel tumor on Sarah Sue's cheek. It may turn out to be nothing, but I have seen these grow and end up causing a large scar. It is so simple to treat now, right here in my office, if you are willing. I will apply dry ice to it for about 4 seconds. One treatment should do it. Sarah Sue will cry for a minute but then in a week or two the birthmark will be gone."

Sarah Sue's mother replies, "We have faith in what you say, Dr. B, so let's do it now. Will this treatment leave a scar?"

"I am almost sure it won't, but if it gets bigger, then I'm sure a scar will result," was Dr. B's reply. The birthmark was treated with dry ice and never seen again.

To recapitulate, in a 2-month-old baby the treatment of a superficial hemangioma that measures 4 x 4 mm. on her cheek is as follows:

1. Reassure the parents that this birthmark is not hereditary, and that it will not turn into a cancer.

2. Apply a solid dry ice "pencil" directly to the lesion for 4 to 8 seconds with firm pressure. The "pencil" tip should be shaped to conform exactly to, or 1 millimeter larger than, the size of the tumor. Unusually a second or third treatment is necessary in 3 to 6 weeks. Tell the parents that a blister will form within 24 hours at the site of the treatment but, if left alone, it will heal in 6 to 14 days. If any infection develops, have them contact you.

Dry ice can be purchased in blocks from any ice cream manufacturer and shaped to fit the lesion, or it can be made in a Kidde Dry Ice Kit (see p. 236).

Mixed and Cavernous Hemangiomas

Treatment of a *mixed hemangioma* on the forearm of a 1-year-old boy. The tumor has been growing slowly. The lesion measures 2 cm. in diameter, and the bright-red surface (the superficial part) is elevated. A deeper bluish mass (the cavernous part) extends for 5 mm. around the superficial part.

1. Reassure the parents that it is not hereditary, and that it will not turn into a cancer. The end result of treatment will be a scar.

2. Apply solid dry ice to the lesion as directed under "Superficial Hemangioma." The entire tumor should not be treated on the first visit. The patient should return in 3 weeks. Three or 4 treatments may be necessary. These treatments will essentially eliminate the red superficial part of the hemangioma and occasionally the deeper cavernous part. If the deeper part remains and is objectionable, the patient should be referred to a dermatologist or a radiologist for radiation therapy. It might be advisable to refer these deeper cases to a dermatologist for the entire care.

Spider Hemangioma

A spider hemangioma consists of a small pinpoint to a pinhead-sized central red arteriole with radiating smaller vessels like the spokes of a wheel or the legs of a spider (Fig. 123 A). These lesions develop for no apparent reason or may develop in association with pregnancy or chronic liver disease. The commonest location is on the face. The reason for removal is cosmetic.

Differential Diagnosis

Venous Stars: small bluish, telangiectatic veins, usually seen on the legs and the face but may appear anywhere on the body; these can be removed if desired by the same method as for spider hemangioma.

Hereditary Hemorrhagic Telangiectasis (Rendu-Osler-Weber): small red lesions on any organ of the body that can hemorrhage; get familial history.

Treatment of a spider hemangioma on the cheek of a young woman who is postpartum 6 months. This lesion developed

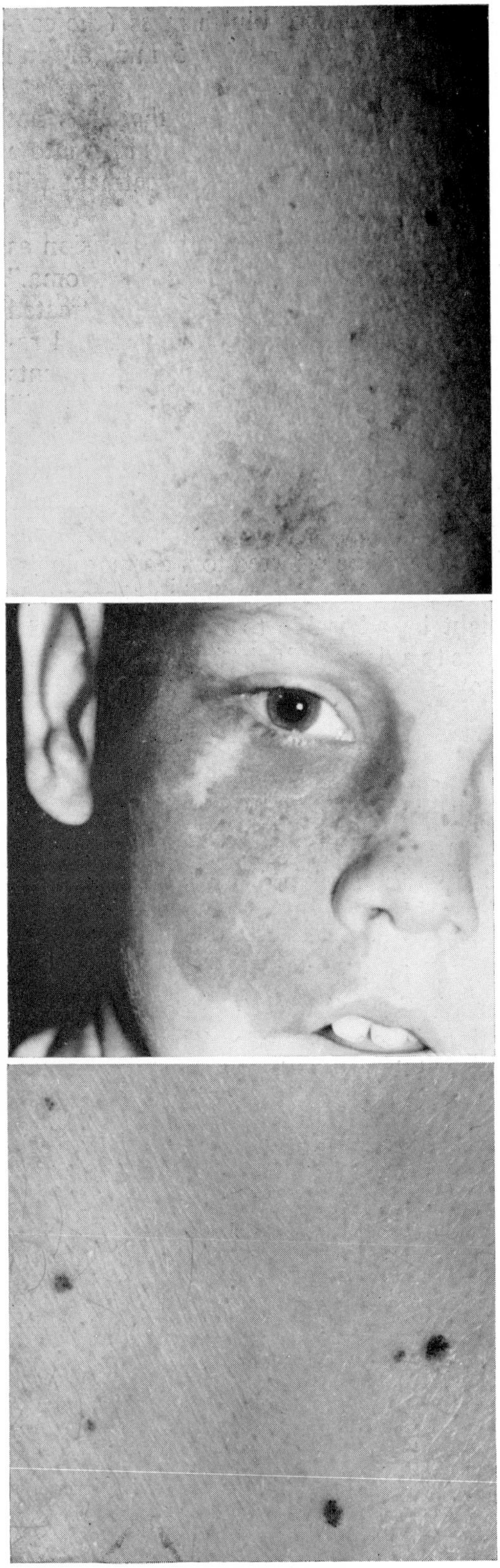

Fig. 123. Hemangiomas.

(A, *top*) Two spider hemangiomas on the arm of an adult.
(B, *center*) Port-wine stain on the face of a boy.
(C, *bottom*) Papillary (senile) hemangiomas on the back.

during her pregnancy and has persisted unchanged.

Treat by electrosurgery. Use the fine epilating needle with either a very low coagulating sparking current or a low cutting current. Stick the needle into the central vessel and turn on the current for 1 or 2 seconds until the vessel blanches. No anesthetic is necessary in most patients. The area will form a scab and heal in about 4 days leaving an imperceptible scar. Rarely, a second treatment is necessary to eliminate the central vessel. If the radiating vessels are large and persistent, they can be treated in the same manner as the central vessel.

Port-wine Stain

The port-wine stain is commonly seen on the face as a reddish purple, flat, disfiguring facial mark (Fig. 123 B). It can occur elsewhere in a less extensive form. Faint reddish lesions are often found on infants on the sides of the face, the forehead, the eyelids and the extremities. The color increases with crying, alarms the mother, but most of these faint lesions disappear shortly after birth.

Treatment of an extensive port-wine stain on the left side of the face of an adult male.

1. There is no satisfactory treatment for this defect. Tattooing and dermabrasion have been used by some with minimal success.

2. Cosmetics, such as "Covermark" or any good pancake type of make-up, are effective to a certain degree.

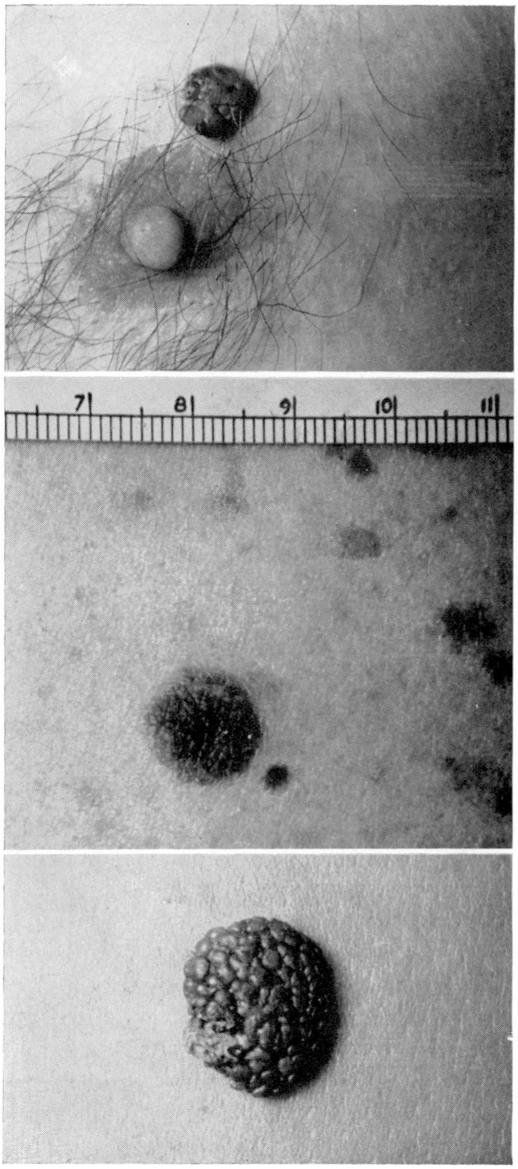

Fig. 124. Nevi.

(*Top*) Compound nevus above the nipple.
(*Center*) Compound nevus on the back.
(*Bottom*) Verrucous compound nevus on the back.

Nuchal Hemangioma

This is a common, persistent, faint-red patch on the posterior neck region at or below the scalp margin. It does not disappear with aging, and treatment is not effective or necessary. Since the posterior neck area is also the site of the common neurodermatitis, it is well to remember that following the cure of the neurodermatitis a redness that persists could be a nuchal hemangioma that was present for years and not noticed previously.

Papillary Hemangioma

These are also called *senile hemangiomas,* but this term obviously should not be used in discussing the lesion with the patient who is in the 30-to-60-year-old group. These pinhead or slightly larger, bright-red, flat or raised tumors are present in many young adults and in practically all elderly persons (Fig. 123 C). They cause no disability except when they are injured and bleed. Treatment is usually not desired but, if it is, light electrosurgery is effective.

Angiokeratomas

Three forms of this condition are known. The Mibelli form occurs on the dorsum of the fingers, the toes and the knees; the Fabry form occurs over the entire trunk in an extensive pattern; and the Fordyce form occurs on the scrotum. The lesions are dark-red pinhead-sized papules with a somewhat warty appearance. Treatment is not indicated.

NEVUS CELL TUMORS

Classification

I. **Nevi**
  1. Junction or active nevus
  2. Intradermal or resting nevus

II. **Malignant Melanoma**

Nevi

Nevi are pigmented or nonpigmented tumors of the skin that contain nevus cells (Figs. 124 and 125). Nevi are present on every adult, but some individuals have more than others. There are two main

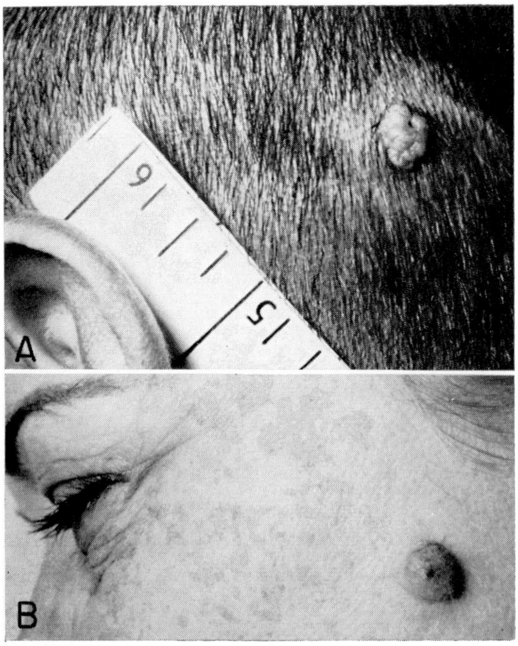

Fig. 125. Intradermal nevi.

A. On the scalp.
B. On the cheek.

questions concerning nevi or moles. When and how should they be removed? What is the relationship between nevi and malignant melanomas?

Histologically, it is possible to divide nevi into *junction or active nevi* and *intradermal or resting nevi*. Combinations of these two forms commonly exist and are labeled *compound nevi*. Clinically, one never can be positive with which histopathologic type one is dealing, but certain criteria are helpful in establishing a differentiation between the two forms.

Description. Clinically, nevi can be pigmented or nonpigmented, flat or elevated, hairy or nonhairy, warty, papillomatous, or pedunculated, and with a small or a wide base. The brown or black pigmented, flat or slightly elevated, nonhairy nevi are usually junction nevi. The nonpigmented or pigmented, elevated, hairy nevi are more likely to be the intradermal nevi.

Distribution. Very prevalent on the head and the neck but may be on any part of the body. The nevi on the palms, the soles and the genitalia are usually junction nevi.

Course. A baby is born with no, or relatively few, nevi; but with increasing age, particularly after puberty, nevi slowly become larger, can remain flat or become elevated, and may become hairy and darker. A change is also seen histologically with age. A junction-type active nevus, while it may remain as such throughout the life of the individual, more commonly changes slowly into an intradermal or resting nevus. Some nevi do not become evident until adult or later life, but the precursor cells for the nevus were present at birth. A malignant melanoma can originate in a junction nevus. Histologically, a benign junction nevus in a child can look like a malignant melanoma. This poses a difficult problem.

Histogenesis. The origin of the nevus cell is disputed, but the most commonly accepted theory is that it originates from cutaneous nerve cells.

Differential Diagnosis. IN CHILDHOOD, *warts:* flat or common warts not on the hands or the feet may be difficult to differentiate clinically, should see warty growth with black "seeds" (the capillary loops), rather acute onset and rapid growth (p. 127).

Freckles: see on exposed areas of the body, many lesions, fade in winter, not raised.

Lentigo (Fig. 126): see flat, tan or brown spot, usually on exposed skin surfaces; histologically, this is an early junction nevus.

Blue Nevus: see flat or elevated, soft, dark-bluish or black nodule.

Granuloma Pyogenicum (Fig. 127): rapid onset of reddish or blackish vascular tumor, usually at site of injury.

Molluscum Contagiosum: see one, or usually more, cratershaped, waxy tumors (p. 130).

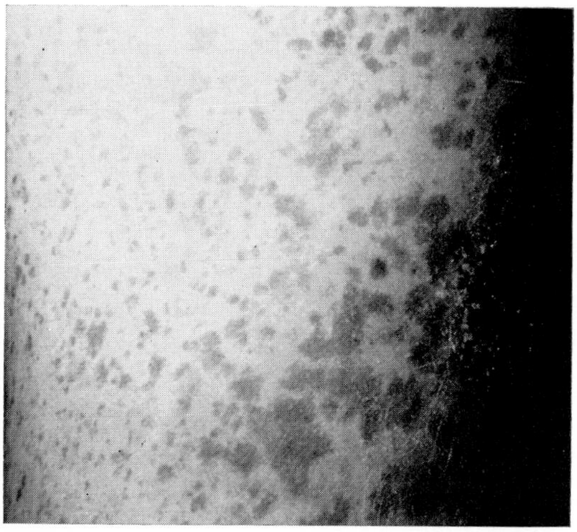

Fig. 126. Lentigines on the arm of the patient with the superficial melanoma in Figure 128 (Bottom).

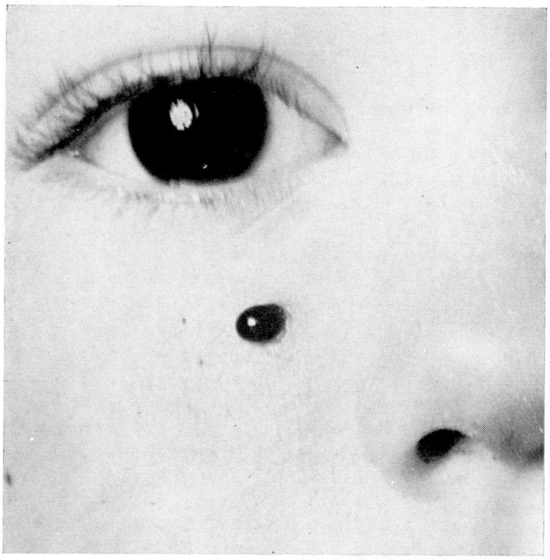

Fig. 127. Granuloma pyogenicum on the cheek of a 2-year-old boy.

Urticaria Pigmentosa: see single but more commonly multiple, slightly elevated, yellowish to brown papules, that urticate with trauma.

IN ADULTHOOD, *warts:* usually rather obvious, see black "seeds" (p. 127).

Pedunculated Fibromas: see on neck and axillae (p. 221).

Histiocytoma: see on anterior tibial

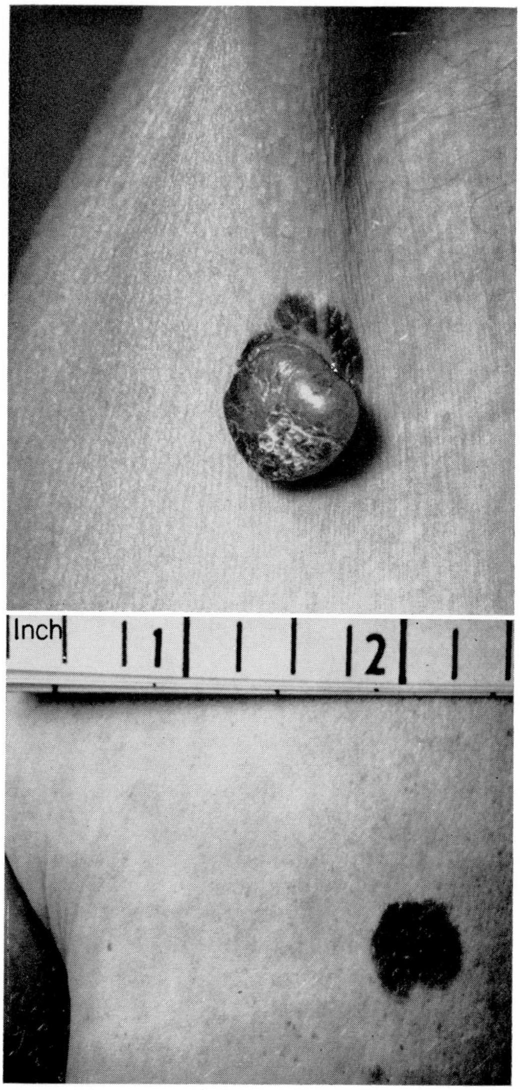

Fig. 128. Malignant melanomas.

(*Top*) On posterior axillary fold. (K.C.G.H.)

(*Bottom*) Superficial melanoma on the upper part of the arm of patient with lentigines (Fig. 126).

area of leg, flat, buttonlike in consistency (p. 222).

Other *epidermal and mesodermal tumors* are differentiated histologically.

IN OLDER ADULTS, *senile keratosis:* on exposed areas, scaly surrounding skin usually thin and dry, not a sharply demarcated lesion (p. 210).

Seborrheic Keratosis: see greasy, waxy, warty tumor, "stuck on" the skin; however some are very difficult to differentiate clinically from nevus or malignant melanoma (p. 221).

Malignant Melanoma (Fig. 128): see at site of junction nevus or can arise from normal-appearing skin, shows a change in pigmentation either by spreading, becoming spotty, or turning darker; may bleed, form a crust or ulcerate; partial or complete excision biopsy is indicated with a more radical excision being performed later if the histologic report is of a malignant melanoma.

Basal Cell and Prickle Cell Epitheliomas: if there is any question of malignancy, a biopsy is indicated (pp. 214 and 218).

Treatment

1. A mother comes into your office with her 5-year-old son, who has an 8 x 8 mm. flat brown nevus on the forehead. She wants to know if this "mole" is dangerous and if it should be removed.

A. Examine the lesion carefully. This lesion shows no sign of recent growth or change in pigmentation. (If it did, it should be excised and examined histologically.)

B. Reassure the mother that this mole does not appear to be dangerous and that it would be very unusual for it to become dangerous. If any change in the color or growth would appear, the lesion should be examined again.

C. Tell the mother that it is best to leave this nevus alone at this time. The *only* treatment would be surgical excision, and you are quite sure that her boy would not sit tight for this procedure unless he was given a general anesthetic. When the boy is 16 years of age or older the lesion can be examined again and possibly removed at that time by a simpler method under local anesthesia.

2. A 25-year-old attractive female desires a brown raised hairy nevus on her upper lip removed. There has been no recent change in the tumor.

A. Examine the lesion carefully for induration, scaling, ulceration and bleeding. None of these signs is present. (If the diagnosis is not definite, a scissors

DO'S AND DON'TS REGARDING NEVI

1. Don't remove a nevus in a child by electrosurgery; remove only by surgical excision.

2. Do remember that in a child a benign junction nevus may resemble a malignant melanoma histologically. Don't alarm the parents unnecessarily, since these nevi are usually no threat to life.

3. Don't remove a flat pigmented nevus, particularly on the palm, the sole or the genitalia by electrosurgery. These should be excised surgically if indicated.

4. Do tell the patient that a small slightly depressed scar will result from electrosurgery.

5. Don't remove a suspicious nevus by electrosurgery. Excise it and examine it histologically.

6. Don't perform a radical deforming surgical procedure on a possible malignant melanoma until the biopsy report has been returned. Many of these tumors will turn out to be seborrheic keratoses, granuloma pyogenicum, etc.

biopsy may be performed safely, and the base gently coagulated by electrosurgery. Further treatment will depend on the biopsy report.)

B. Tell the patient that you can remove the mole safely, but that there will be a residual, very slightly depressed scar, and that probably the hairs will have to be removed separately after the first surgery has healed.

C. Surgical excision is the best method of removal. However, hairy raised pigmented nevi have been removed by electrosurgery for years with no real proof that this form of removal has caused a malignant melanoma. If a malignant melanoma became evident later, it undoubtedly was there prior to the treatment. Again, if there is any question of malignancy the lesion should be biopsied or excised!

Electrosurgery, following local anesthesia, can be performed with the coagulating or cutting current or with cautery. The site should not be covered and will heal in 7 to 14 days, depending on the size. If the hairs regrow they can be removed later by electrosurgical epilation (p. 40).

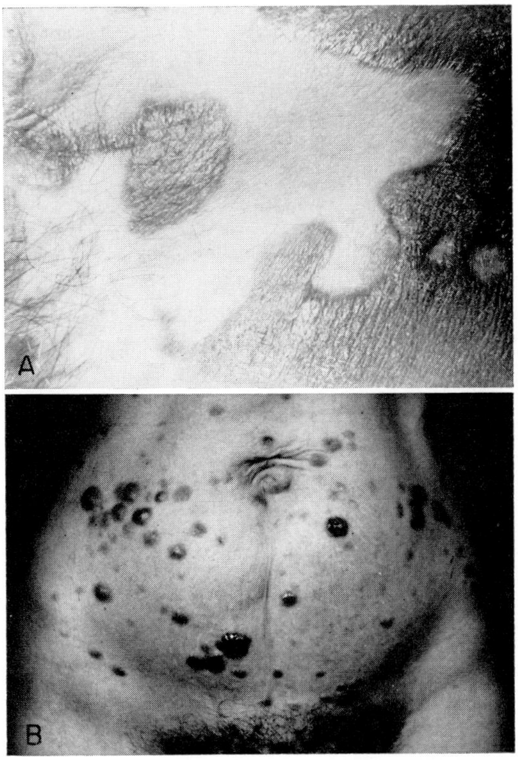

Fig. 129. Lymphoblastomas involving the skin.

A. Granuloma fungoides of 10-years' duration on abdomen near pubic area.
B. Nodules of acute monocytic leukemia. (Dr. Sloan Wilson)

LYMPHOMAS

Granuloma Fungoides

Also known as *mycosis fungoides,* this polymorphous lymphoma involves the skin only, except in some rare cases that terminally invade the lymph nodes and the visceral organs (Fig. 129). As is true with most lymphomas, the histology may change gradually to another form of lymphoma with progression of the disease. However, most cases of granuloma fungoides began as such and terminate unchanged.

Description. The clinical picture of this disease is quite classic and is divided into 3 stages: the erythematous stage, the plaque stage and the tumor stage. The course usually proceeds in order, but all stages may be evident at the same time, or the first two stages may be by-passed.

Erythematous Stage: Commonly seen are scaly, red, rather sharply defined patches that resemble atopic eczema, psoriasis, or parapsoriasis. The eruption may become diffuse as an exfoliative dermatitis. Itching is usually quite severe.

Plaque Stage: The red scaly patches develop induration and some elevation with central healing that results in ring-shaped lesions. This stage is to be differentiated from tertiary syphilis, psoriasis, erythema multiforme perstans, mycotic infections and other lymphomas.

Tumor Stage: This terminal stage is characterized by nodular and tumor growths of the plaques, often with ulceration and secondary bacterial infection. These tumors are to be differentiated from any of the granulomas (see index).

Course. The early stages may progress slowly, with exacerbations and remissions over many years, or the disease may be rapidly fulminating. Once the tumor stage is reached, the eventual fatal outcome is imminent.

Treatment. The combined services of a dermatologist, a radiologist and an internist or a hematologist are required for the management of this ultimately fatal disease. Corticosteroid therapy systemically is helpful during the early stages of the disease to relieve itching and scaling. X-ray therapy in small doses melts away the early lesions, but since the skin tolerance to radiation may be soon exceeded, it is advisable to withhold this form of therapy as long as possible. Nitrogen mustard and triethylmelamine have been used systemically with some palliative effect. Antimony is of value in some cases.

Basic Dermatologic Equipment

CHAPTER 27

THOSE of us engaged in the practice of medicine can well recall the opening of our first office and the many decisions that had to be made concerning purchase of equipment. Certain mistakes were made; some were avoidable. I can remember wishing that I had a list of necessary materials to guide me in making my selection. With this in mind, the following is a compilation of basic equipment used in my office. This is not the most complete list, and some will find that they can perform with less. For the physician already in practice much of this equipment will be on hand, particularly that in the Biopsy Setup, but the list can serve as a guide for organization and completeness in treating dermatologic patients.

The use of a definite manufacturer's name has been done for only one reason—to aid you and your supply dealer in the selection of the equipment. I have been told that almost every dealer has these manufacturer's catalogs on hand and therefore can supply the equipment of this manufacturer, or similar equipment from any of the many other reliable surgical supply manufacturers. The manufacturers mentioned on the following list are not necessarily those used in my office.

I am indebted to Mr. Robert Goetze for supplying the catalog numbers which we hope will be available for reference at your supply dealer.

BASIC DERMATOLOGIC TRAY

(Fig. 130)

(Numbers in Parentheses Refer to the Illustration)

(1) 1—Comedone extractor, Sklar, #115-52, or Millers Forge

(2) 1—Hagedorn needle, straight, cutting edge, flat body, 3 in., Torrington #719 (can use eye end as comedone extractor)

(3) 1—Thumb forceps, 4 in., Sklar, #160-115

(4) 1—Tweezers, eyebrow, sharp points, 3½ in., Sklar, #320-65

(5) 1—Scissors, iris, straight S/S, 4½ in., Sklar, #320-415

(6) 1—Scissors, bandage, 5½ in., Sklar, #130-05

(7) 1—Knife handle, Bard-Parker, #3

(8) 2—Knife blades, Bard-Parker, #15

(9) 2—Knife blades, Bard-Parker, #11 (to obtain skin scrapings for fungus culture)

(10) 1—Piffard dermal curette, #2 size, Kny-Scheerer, #R2941-I

(11) 1—Nail clipper, Millers Forge, #701

(12) 1—2 cc. syringe, Becton-Dickinson, #2YL

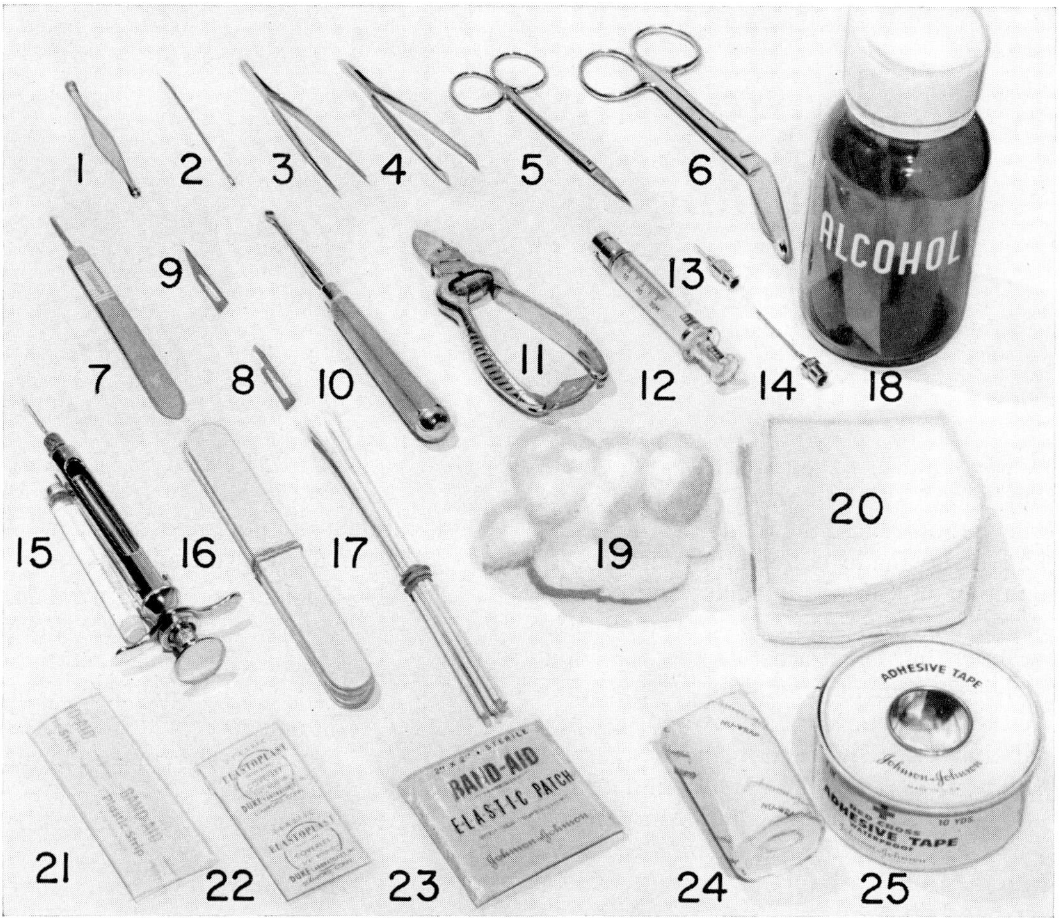

Fig. 130. Basic dermatologic tray.

(13) 2—Hypodermic needles, #25, 3/8 in., Becton-Dickinson, #LNR

(14) 2—Hypodermic needles, #21, 1 1/4 in., Becton-Dickinson, #LNR

(15) A good substitute for the above syringe and needles is the following: Cook-Waite Carpule Syringe, with carpules of Ravocaine 0.4%, Novocain 2%, and Levophed 1:30,000, 2.2 cc., with 26 gauge dental needles, 1 5/8 inches.

1—25% Podophyllum resin in alcohol, 30 cc.

1—Saturated soln. trichloracetic acid, 30 cc.

1—Powdered soda bicarbonate, 30 Gm. (to neutralize locally applied acids)

1—20% Potassium hydroxide soln., 30 cc. (for mycologic slide preparations)

1—Cover slips, box, 7/8 in., #1 thickness, Glasco, #2980

1—Microscopic slides, box, 1 in. x 3 in., Glasco #2950

1—Zephirin Solution diluted 1:1,000, with 16 Anti-rust Tablets, one gallon

1—9 in. x 5 in. x 2 in. tray with lid, enamel (for cold steriliz-

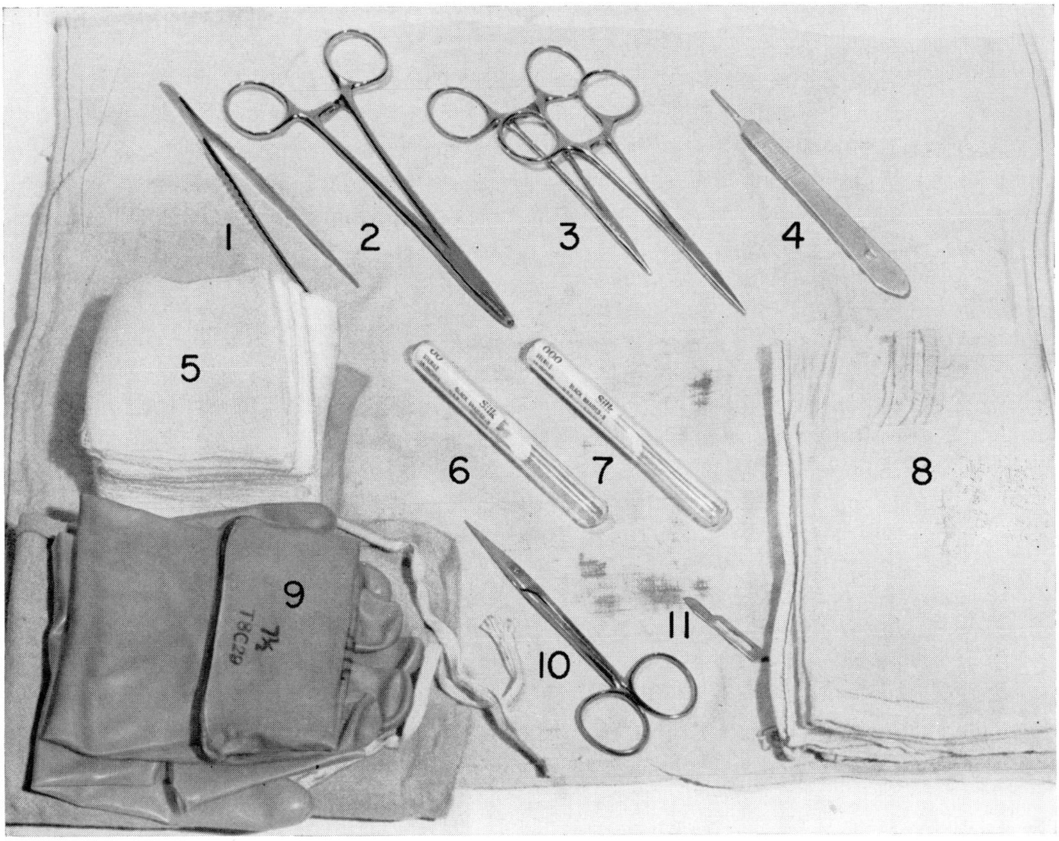

Fig. 131. Skin biopsy setup.

ing liquid in which the above surgical instruments should be placed)

(16) 12—Tongue blades, adult

(17) 12—Cotton-tipped applicators, 6 in.

(18) 1—Alcohol dispenser, Menda, #608

(19) 24—Cotton balls, Johnson and Johnson, medium, 6101

(20) 12—3 in. x 3 in., 12 ply gauze sponges, Johnson and Johnson

(21) 12—Band-aid plastic strips, 1 in. x 3 in., Johnson and Johnson #5644

(22) 12—Elastoplast Coverlets, Duke, #305

(23) 12—Band-aid 2 in. x 2 in. elastic patch, Johnson and Johnson, #5712

100—Elastopatch, large, Duke, #71 (for patch tests)

1—Gauze roll, 1 in. wide

(24) 1—Gauze roll, 2 in. wide

1—Tape roll, ½ in. wide

(25) 1—Tape roll, 1 in. wide

1—Tape roll, 3 in. wide

SKIN BIOPSY SETUP
(Fig. 131)
(Numbers in Parentheses Refer to the Illustration)

A. *Sterilized in Wrapper:*

(1) 1—Thumb forceps, delicate pattern, 5 in., Sklar, #160-05

(2) 1—Needle holder, Mayo-Hegar, 6 in., Sklar, #170-30

(3) 2—Halsted mosquito hemostats, straight, 5 in., Sklar, #150-70

(4) 1—Bard-Parker #3 knife handle

(5) 10—Gauze sponges, 3 in. x 3 in., 12 ply, Johnson and Johnson

(6) 1—Cuticular silk suture, with cutting needle, 00, Ethicon, B 685

(7) 1—Cuticular silk suture, with cutting needle, 000, Ethicon, B 684

(8) 1—12 in. x 12 in. piece of cloth with square 3 in. x 3 in. hole in center

(9) B. *Rubber Gloves, Powdered, Sterilized, in Separate Wrapper.*

C. *In Cold Sterilizing Liquid:*

(10) 1—Scissors, iris, 4½ in., Sklar, #320-415

(11) 2—Bard-Parker knife blades, #15

1—Biopsy punch, sizes 2, 4, 6, 8 and 10 mm. Keyes, 105-985

After use, remove the scissors, the blades and the biopsy punches from the dirty setup, clean them and put them back in the cold sterilizing liquid. This prevents rusting.

OPTIONAL EQUIPMENT

Wood's light, Burton Fluorescing Ultra-Violet Light, #1910 with #1911 bulb, around $25 (for diagnosing tinea of the scalp)

Dry Ice Kit, Kidde Manufacturing Company, Bloomfield, N. J., #60-5052, around $40 (for treating hemangiomas)

Moto-Tool Hand Drill, Dremel Manufacturing Company, Racine, Wisconsin, Model 1, around $13, with steel carving cutters #HS-413 and HS-89 (for débriding tinea of nails)

Dictionary-Index

THE PURPOSE of the author in this section, as stated in the Preface, is to add to the usefulness of this book by defining and classifying some of the rarer dermatologic terms not covered in the main section. Very few tropical and parasitic diseases have been included. Some very rare or unimportant terms have purposely been omitted, but undoubtedly some terms that are *not* rare and *are* important have also been omitted. Suggestions or corrections from the reader will be appreciated.

Please note especially the following groupings and classifications in this Dictionary-Index: Atrophies of the skin, Hair diseases, Hereditary skin diseases, Ichthyosis, Mucous membrane disorders, Nail disorders, Pigmentary disorders, Primary chancre-type diseases, Tuberculosis of the skin, and Tumors.

Boldface numbers refer to the main discussion.

Italicized numbers refer to important illustrations.

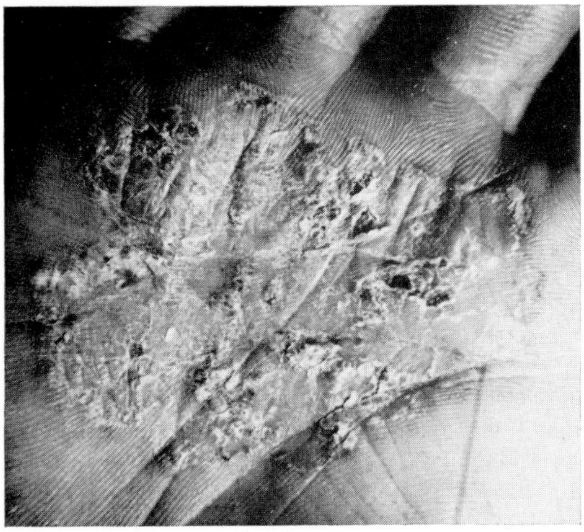

Fig. 132. Acrodermatitis perstans.

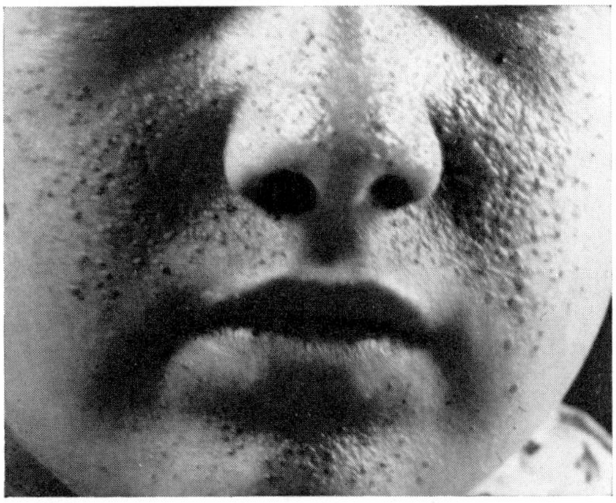

Fig. 133. Adenoma sebaceum with epiloia.
(*Dr. A. Theodore Steegmann*)

Acrodynia (*Cont.*)
orexia, painful hands and feet. The disease is most common in infants, who may die from secondary infection.

Acrokeratosis verruciformis. A rare disease affecting the dorsum of the hands and the feet characterized by flat warty papules. Probably hereditary. Differentiate from flat warts and from *epidermodysplasia verruciformis*.

Adenoma sebaceum (Pringle) (Fig. 133). A familial disease characterized by small yellowish papules distributed over the nose, the cheeks and the nasolabial folds. *Epiloia* is a syndrome consisting of mental deficiency, epilepsy and adenoma sebaceum. This can be differentiated from *epithelioma adenoides cysticum* by a biopsy.

Adiposis dolorosa (Dercum's disease). A lipomalike disorder characterized by irregular and painful deposits of fat in the subcutaneous tissue of the trunk and the limbs, more common in women than in men.

Ainhum. Essentially a tropical disease of Negroes that results in the amputation of a toe or toes due to constricting bands.

Albinism. A rare congenital and hereditary disease characterized by partial or universal loss of skin pigmentation. The partial type is to be differentiated from *vitiligo*.

Allergic granulomatosis. The combination of transitory pulmonary infiltrations of Loeffler's syndrome, blood eosinophilia and nodular, purpuric, or erythema multiformelike skin lesions.

Allergy. An altered state of reactivity by a first contact and made manifest by subsequent specific contacts.

Alopecia. From the Greek *alopekia* meaning hair loss.

Amyloidosis: Cutaneous amyloidosis is a rare condition which can be suspected clinically but should be proved by histologic examination. Amyloid is a protein-carbohydrate complex which on histologic section assumes a diagnostic stain when treated with certain chemicals. Three forms of cutaneous amyloidosis are known.

A. Localized amyloidosis. The skin only is involved. Clinically, this dermatosis appears as a patch of lichenified papules seen most commonly on the anterior tibial area of the legs. These pruritic lesions can be differentiated from neurodermatitis or hypertrophic lichen planus by biopsy.

B. Secondary amyloidosis. Secondary amyloid deposits are very rare in the skin, but are less rare in the liver, the spleen and the kidney, where they occur as a result of certain chronic infectious diseases, and in association with multiple myeloma.

C. Primary systemic amyloidosis. This peculiar and serious form of amyloidosis commonly involves the skin along with the tongue, the heart, and the musculature of the viscera. The skin lesions appear as transparent-looking, yellowish papules or nodules which are occasionally hemorrhagic.

Angioma serpiginosum. Characterized by multiple telangiectases which may start from a

congenital vascular nevus but often arise spontaneously. This rare vascular condition is to be differentiated from *Schamberg's disease, Majocchi's disease* and *pigmented purpuric dermatitis* (*Gougerot and Blum*).
Angioneurotic edema, 67
Anhidrosis. The partial or complete absence of sweating, seen in ichthyosis, extensive psoriasis, scleroderma, prickly heat, vitamin A deficiency and other diseases. Partial anhidrosis is produced by many antiperspirants.
Anhidrotic asthenia, tropical. Described in the South Pacific and in the desert in World War II. Soldiers showed increased sweating of neck and face and anhidrosis (lack of sweating) below the neck. It was accompanied by weakness, headaches and subjective warmth and was considered as a chronic phase of prickly heat.
Anthralin. A proprietary name for dihydroxyanthranol, which is a strong reducing agent useful in the treatment of chronic cases of psoriasis. Its action is similar to chrysarobin.
Anthrax. A primary chancre-type disease caused by *Bacillus anthracis,* occurring in people who work with the hides and the hair of infected sheep, horses or cattle. A pulmonary form is known.
Antimalarial agents. Dermatologically active agents include quinacrine (Atabrine), chloroquine (Aralen) and hydroxychloroquine (Plaquenil). Their mode of action is unknown, but these agents are used in the treatment of chronic discoid lupus erythematosus and the polymorphic actinic dermatoses.
Aphthae, recurring painful scarring. An extremely painful form of aphthae (ulcers) that result in rather deep ulcerations of the mucous membranes that heal with scar formation.
Aphthous stomatitis, 121
recurrent. "Canker sores" are single or multiple acute painful superficial ulcers of the mucous membranes of the mouth which last from 10 to 14 days. Differentiate from herpes simplex, Vincent's stomatitis and secondary syphilis.
Apocrine sweat glands, 6
Apocrinitis, 101
Apresoline drug eruption, 174
Arachnids, 155
Argyll Robertson pupils. Small irregular pupils which fail to react to light but react to accommodation. This is a late manifestation of neurosyphilis, particularly tabes.
Arizona dermatoses, 203
Arsenic. Inorganic arsenic preparations include Fowler's solution and Asiatic pills and are used in the treatment of resistant cases of psoriasis but can cause arsenical pigmentation and keratoses. Organic arsenic agents include neoarsphenamine and Mapharsen, used formerly in the treatment of syphilis.
and superficial basal cell epithelioma, *215*
Arsenical keratoses, 214
Arterial spiders. *See* Hemangioma, spider
Arthritis, rheumatoid, 176
Arthropod dermatoses, 155
Arthus phenomenon. Characterized by local anaphylaxis in a site that has been injected repeatedly with a foreign protein.
Ascorbic acid deficiency, 181
Atopic eczema, **51.** *See also* Eczema, atopic
Atopy. *See* Allergy
Atrophies of the skin
A. Congenital atrophies. Associated with other congenital ectodermal defects.
B. Acquired atrophies
1. Noninflammatory.
a. *Senile atrophy.* Often associated with senile pruritus and winter itch.
b. *Linear atrophy* (*striae albicantes or distensae*). On abdomen, thighs and breasts associated with pregnancy and obesity.
c. *Secondary atrophy* from sunlight x-radiation, injury, and nerve diseases.
d. *Macular atrophy* (*anetoderma of Schweninger-Buzzi*). Characterized by the presence of small, oval, whitish, depressions or slightly elevated papules which can be pressed back into the underlying tissue. This may be an early form of von Recklinghausen's disease.
2. Inflammatory.
a. *Acrodermatitis chronica atrophicans.* A moderately rare idiopathic atrophy in older adults, particularly females, characterized by the presence of thickened skin at the onset, with ulnar bands on the forearm, changing into atrophy of the legs below the knee and of the forearms. In the early stages this is to be differentiated from scleroderma. High doses of penicillin may be effective.
b. *Folliculitis ulerythematosa reticulata.* A very rare reticulated atrophic condition localized to the cheeks of the face; seen mainly in young adults.
c. *Ulerythema ophryogenes.* A rare atrophic dermatitis that affects the outer part of the eyebrows, resulting in redness, scaling, and permanent loss of the involved hair.

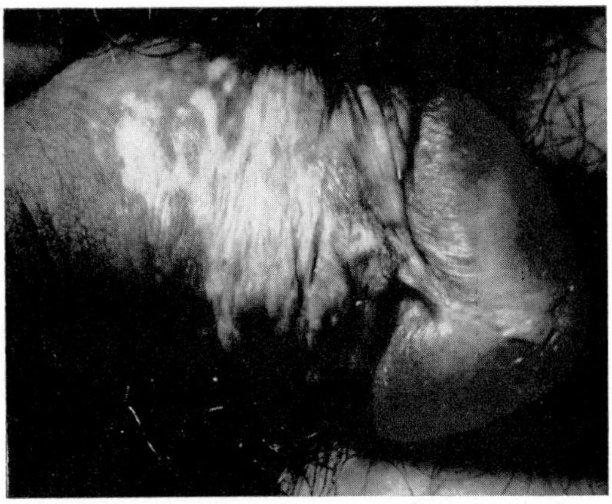

Fig. 134. Balanitis xerotica obliterans.
(*Dr. David Morgan*)

Atrophies of the skin, inflammatory (*Cont.*)

d. *Macular atrophy* (*anetoderma of Jadassohn*). A very rare condition characterized by the appearance of circumscribed reddish macules which develop an atrophic center that progresses toward the edge of the lesion, seen mainly on the extremities.

e. *Lichen sclerosus et atrophicus* (*kraurosis vulvae, kraurosis penis and balanitis xerotica obliterans*) (Fig. 134). An uncommon atrophic process, mainly of women, which begins as a small whitish lesion that contains a central hyperkeratotic pinpoint-sized dell. These 0.5 cm. size or less whitish macules commonly coalesce to form whitish atrophic plaques. The commonest localizations are on the neck, shoulders, arms, axillae, vulva and perineum. Many consider kraurosis vulvae, kraurosis penis and balanitis xerotica obliterans to be variants of this condition.

f. *Poikiloderma atrophicans vasculare* (*Jacobi*). This rare atrophic process of adults is characterized by the development of patches of telangiectasia, atrophy and mottled pigmentation on any area of the body. This resembles chronic radiodermatitis clinically and may be associated with dermatomyositis or scleroderma. May precede the development of a lymphoma.

g. *Hemiatrophy*. May be localized to one side of the face or may cover the entire half of the body. Vascular and neurogenic etiologies have been propounded, but most cases appear to be a form of localized scleroderma.

h. *Atrophie blanche en plaque*. A rare form of cutaneous atrophy characterized by scarlike plaques with a border of telangiectasia and hyperpigmentation that cover large areas of the legs and the ankles, mainly of middle-aged or older women.

i. *Secondary atrophy*. From inflammatory diseases such as syphilis, chronic discoid lupus erythematosus, leprosy, tuberclosis, scleroderma, etc.

Autoeczematization. *See* Id reaction

Autohemotherapy. A form of nonspecific protein therapy, administered by removing 10 cc. of venous blood from the arm and then immediately injecting that blood intramuscularly into the buttocks. It has been shown to produce a fall in circulating eosinophils presumably due to a mild increase in the adrenal steroid hormones.

Ayres, Dr. Samuel, III, 202, 204

Babinski's reflex. Extension of the toes instead of flexion following stimulation of the sole of the foot, due to lesions of the pyramidal tract from syphilis infection or other causes.

Bacterial infection(s), 96-111
  primary, 96-102
  of scalp, 191
  secondary, 102-106
  systemic, 106-111
  See also Pyodermas

Bacterial paronychia, 193

Bacterid, pustular, 139
  See also Acrodermatitis perstans

Balanitis, fusospirochetal (Fig. 140). An uncommon infection of the penis characterized by superficial erosions. It must be differentiated from syphilis by a darkfield examination and blood serology.
  xerotica obliterans. *See* Atrophies of the Skin. It is to be differentiated from leukoplakia.

Basic dermatologic tray, 233

Bazin's disease. Erythema induratum. *See* Tuberculosis

Beau's lines of nails, *195,* 196

Behçet's syndrome, 70

Bejel. The name given to syphilis as it occurs among the Arabs.

Berger, Dr. Saul, 202

Beriberi, 180

Berlock dermatitis. Similar to the *melanosis of Riehl* and can result from contact with toilet

waters containing oil of bergamot or other essential oils, followed by exposure to sunlight, causing a dermatitis that appears to drip down the neck, like a pendant (berloque). *See also* Dermatitis, berlock
Biologic false-positive serology, 117, 118, 126
Biopsies, 10
Biopsy set-up, 235
Bismuth. Formerly used in the treatment of syphilis because of its antispirochetal effect. Now mainly used in treatment of lichen planus and flat warts in the form of Bismuth Cevitamate (Smith) given intramuscularly, and Bistrimate (Smith) given orally.
Bite(s), brown spider, *203*
in Midwest, 202
chigger, **204**
in Midwest, 202
fire ant, 204
flea, 204
tick, 202
Black dot ringworm. Tinea of the hair caused by *Trichophyton violaceum, T. sulfureum* and *T. crateriforme*. These endothrix fungi do not produce fluorescent hairs under the Wood's light and may occur in adults.
Blank, Dr. Harvey, 204
Blastomycosis, North American, 153
Blister beetle dermatitis. Beetles of the family *Meloidae* contain cantharidin which on contact with the skin causes the formation of a tense, itching, burning bulla.
Blister beetle vesicle, *203*
"B.O.," 6
Bockhart's impetigo. A very superficial bacterial infection of the hair follicle.
Boeck's sarcoid, 110
Boil, 100
Boric acid. A mild antiseptic agent prescribed most often as a 2% solution for wet dressings. It is poisonous to infants who mistake the powder for sugar and eat it.
Botfly dermatitis, 205
Bowen's disease, *212*, 216
Brazilian pemphigus. *See* Fogo selvagem
British Columbia dermatoses, 201
Bromhidrosis. The odor of the body which is associated with sweating, commonly called "B.O." Freshly secreted sweat has no odor, but an odor develops when the sweat becomes contaminated with bacteria.
Bromoderma. A dermatosis, usually pustularlike, due to the ingestion of bromides. *See* Drug eruptions, 55
Bronze diabetes. *See* Hemochromatosis
Brucellosis. The human infection of undulant fever is infrequently accompanied by a nondescript skin eruption. However, after delivering an infected cow, a high percentage of veterinarians experience an itching, red, macular, papular or pustular dermatitis on the contaminated arms and hands that lasts for a few days to 3 weeks without systemic illness.
Buerger's disease, 71, **178**
Bullae, 12
Bullous dermatoses, 159
Burow's solution. A solution of aluminum acetate which in its original formula contained lead. A lead-free Burow's solution for wet dressings can be made by adding Domeboro tablets or powder to water to make a 1:20 or 1:10 solution.
Burton, Dr. Arthur M., 202

Cactus granuloma, 203
Calciferol, 181
Calcinosis. *Localized calcinosis* can occur in many tumors of the skin and following chronic inflammatory lesions. *Metabolic calcinosis* may or may not be associated with an excess of blood calcium and is divided into universal calcinosis and circumscribed calcinosis.
California dermatoses, 202
Callus. A hyperkeratotic plaque of the skin due to chronic pressure and friction.
Cancer(s), internal, and skin lesions, 181
and radiodermatitis, *199*
skin, in Southwest, 202
Candidiasis. *See* Moniliasis, 149
Canities. Gray or white hair.
Canker sore. Another name for Aphtha.
Carbuncle, 101
Carcinoma, epidermoid, 218
See also Epitheliomas, prickle cell
squamous cell, 218
See also Epitheliomas, prickle cell
Caseation necrosis. Histologically, this is a form of tissue death with loss of structural detail leaving pale eosinophilic, amorphous, finely granular material. It is seen especially in tuberculosis, syphilis, granuloma annulare and beryllium granuloma.
Cat scratch disease. Manifested by inflammation at the site of a cat scratch or bite obtained a few days previously. Malaise, headache, low-grade fever, chills, generalized lymphadenopathy and splenomegaly occur. A maculopapular skin rash or erythema nodosumlike eruption occurs occasionally.
Causalgia. A condition characterized by burning pain aggravated by touching the neuralgic site.
Cellulitis, 102
dissecting, of the scalp, 102

Chalazion. A small cyst of the meibomian glands of the eyelid.
Chamomile solution. A solution of whole chamomile flowers used in wet dressings for its mild anti-inflammatory action. The solution can be conveniently made by the addition of a Chamo-Powder (Dome) packet to 1 pint of tap water.
Chancre, monorecidive. A relapsing form of syphilis characterized by the development of a lesion reduplicating the primary sore.
primary syphilis. *See* Syphilis, 112
redux. *See* Chancre, monorecidive
Chancre-type, primary diseases. *See* Primary chancre-type diseases
Chancroid, *19,* 108
Charcot joints. A type of joint destruction in patients with central nervous system syphilis of the paretic type.
Chédiak-Higashi syndrome. A fatal syndrome in children characterized by pigmentary disturbances, photophobia, pyogenic infections, excessive sweating, pale optic fundi, splenomegaly and lymphadenopathy.
Cheilitis. *See* Mucous membrane disorders
Chickenpox, 126
Chigger bites, in California, 202
Chilblains. Also called *pernio.* A cutaneous reaction, either acute or chronic, from exposure to excessive cold.
in California, 202
Chloasma, 167
Chromhidrosis. The excretion of colored sweat, usually brownish, grayish, bluish or yellowish.
Chromoblastomycosis. The signature of this tropical fungus disease caused by the *Hormodendrum* species is a pruritic papule on the leg that very slowly extends to form warty hard plaques.
Chrysarobin. A reducing agent which hastens keratinization when it is applied to the skin. It can be incorporated in petrolatum or chloroform but must be used with great caution and in mild strength such as 0.25% to 3%. Mainly used in treatment of resistant cases of psoriasis and tinea cruris.
Clutton's joints. A symmetric serous synovitis of the knee joints with hydrothrosis due to congenital syphilis.
Coccidioidomycosis. This fungus disease of the arid southwestern part of the United States is caused by *Coccidioides immitis* and originates in the soil. Inhalation of the spores produces an asymptomatic pulmonary infection that may be accompanied by erythema nodosum leg lesions or urticaria. Primary cutaneous coccidioidomycosis and the disseminated form are rare.
in Arizona, 203
in California, 202
Collagen diseases, 171
Colloid degeneration (colloid milium). A rare and chronic degeneration characterized by occurrence of pinhead and slightly larger-sized yellowish nodules on cheeks and forehead.
Condyloma, acuminata, 129
lata, 113
Congenital ectodermal defect. A hereditary group of diseases that present many ectodermal defects such as keratoses of hands, feet, and body, eye cataracts, decrease or absence of sweat and sebaceous glands, changes in nails and hair, and dry skin that may be smooth or keratotic.
Congenital ichthyosiform erythroderma. *See* Ichthyosis.
Congo red test. An intravenous test used to diagnose generalized amyloidosis. An intradermal skin test using Congo red solution will stain localized amyloid nodules red.
Corn. A corn or clavus is a small, sharply circumscribed hyperkeratotic lesion which may be hard with a central horny core or may be soft as commonly seen between the toes. Underlying bony protuberances are causative.
Cowpox, 127
Crabs. *See* Pediculosis, 157
Creeping eruption, 205
Crusts, 12
Cryptococcosis (torulosis). A world-wide disease caused by a yeastlike fungus. *Cryptococcus neoformans.* It characteristically invades the central nervous system via the respiratory tract. Variable skin lesions are uncommon.
Curtis, Dr. George, 202
Cushing's syndrome, 178
Cutis verticis gyrata. A rare abnormality of the scalp where the skin is thrown into waves and folds resembling the cerebral convolutions of the brain.
Cyst(s), dermoid, 209
epidermal, 209
hair. This granulomatous reaction to buried hair occurs in the hands of barbers.
mucous retention, 209
sebaceous, 209
synovial, 209

Dalibour solution. An astringent and mildly antiseptic solution used for the treatment of pyodermas. It contains zinc sulfate, copper sulfate and camphor. It can be made readily by the addition of a Dalidome (Dome) powder packet to 1 pint or more of tap water.
Dandruff, 73. *See also* Seborrheic dermatitis

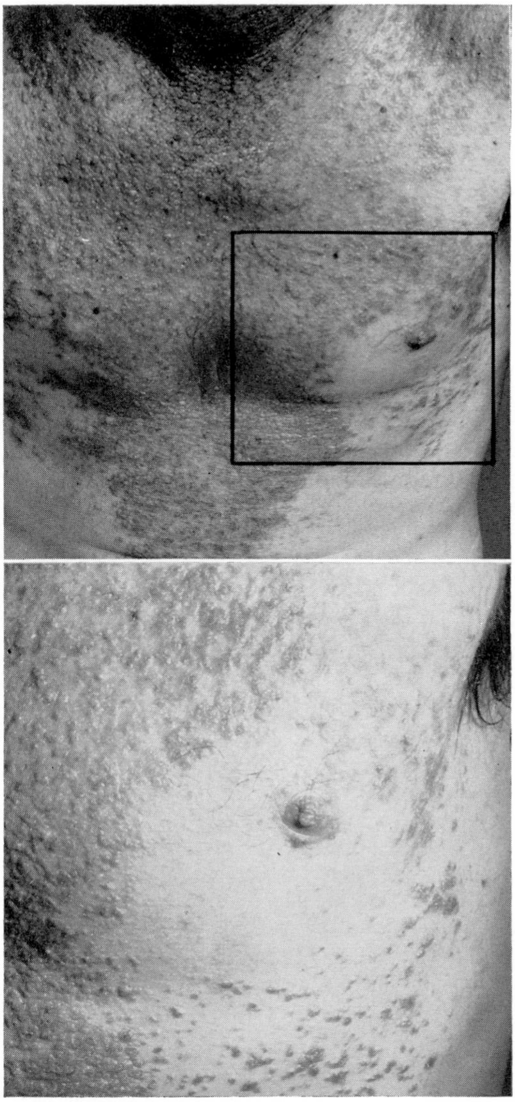

Fig. 135. Darier's disease.

(*K.U.M.C.*)

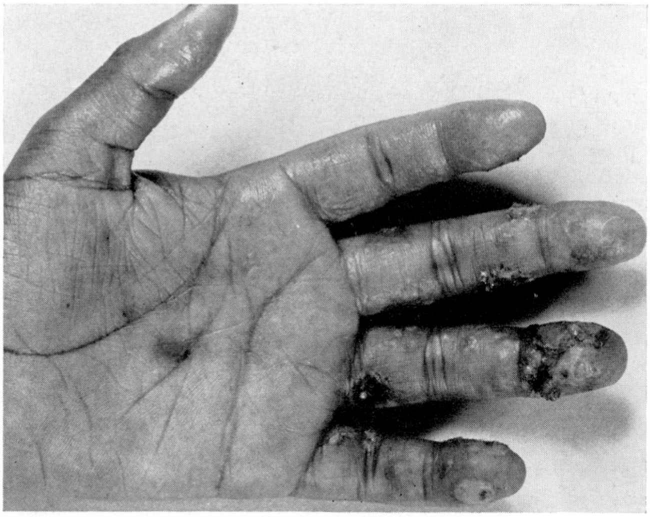

Fig. 136. Dyshidrosis with secondary infection. (Negro)

Diphtheria, cutaneous. The skin ulcer due to *Corynebacterium diphtheriae* has a characteristic rolled firm border and a grayish membrane that progresses to a black eschar with surrounding inflammation, vesicles and anesthesia.

Duke's disease. A mild exanthem occurring in children, usually in the spring or summer months, with an incubation period of from 9 to 21 days. The eruption becomes generalized within a few hours, is bright red in color and is accompanied by a low-grade fever.
Dyshidrosis (Fig. 136). A syndrome characterized by blisters on the palms of hands and feet. If the cause is known, this term should not be used. The common causes of dyshidrosis, or *pompholyx,* are mycotic, contact dermatitis, drugs, and associated as a manifestation of a generalized skin disease.

Dyskeratosis, benign. A histopathologic finding of faulty keratinization of individual epidermal cells with formation of corps ronds and grains. Seen in Darier's disease and occasionally in familial benign chronic pemphigus.
Dyskeratosis congenita. With pigmentation, dystrophia unguis and leukokeratosis oris, this is a rare syndrome characterized by a reticulated pigmentation, particularly of the neck, dystrophy of the nails, and a leukoplakialike condition of the oral mucosa. Increased sweating and thickening of palms and soles may occur.
Dyskeratosis, malignant. A histopathologic finding in Bowen's disease and also in prickle cell epithelioma and senile keratosis where premature and atypical keratinization of individual cells is seen.

Ectodermosis erosiva pluriorificialis. A synonym for Stevens-Johnson form of erythema multiforme.

Ehlers-Danlos Syndrome. Known also as *cutis hyperelastica,* this is a rare congenital anomaly of the skin composed of marked fragility of the skin resulting in the formation of pseudotumors, hyperelasticity of the skin, and abnormal hyperflexibility of the joints.

Epidermodysplasia verruciformis. A rare, apparently hereditary disease manifested by papulosquamous and warty lesions present at birth with no site of predilection. The prognosis for life is poor because of the eventual development of prickle cell epitheliomas from the lesions.

Epidermophytid. A dermatophytid due to *Epidermophyton* infection.
Epidermophytosis. A fungus infection due to *Epidermophyton.*
Epiloia. A triad of mental deficiency, epilepsy and adenoma sebaceum.

Epulis. This term refers to any growth involving the gums.

Erosio interdigitale blastomycetica. A complex term signifying a monilial infection of the webs of the fingers.

Erysipeloid. A chancre-type infection on the hand occurring at the site of accidental inoculation with the organism. *Erysipelothrix rhusiopathiae,* seen in butchers, veterinarians and fishermen. A localized form runs its course in 2 to 4 weeks. A generalized form develops a diffuse eruption with occasional constitutional symptoms such as arthritis. A very rare systemic form exhibits an eruption, joint pains and endocarditis.
Erythema, ab igne. A marmoraceous-appearing redness which follows the local application to the skin of radiant heat such as from a heating pad.

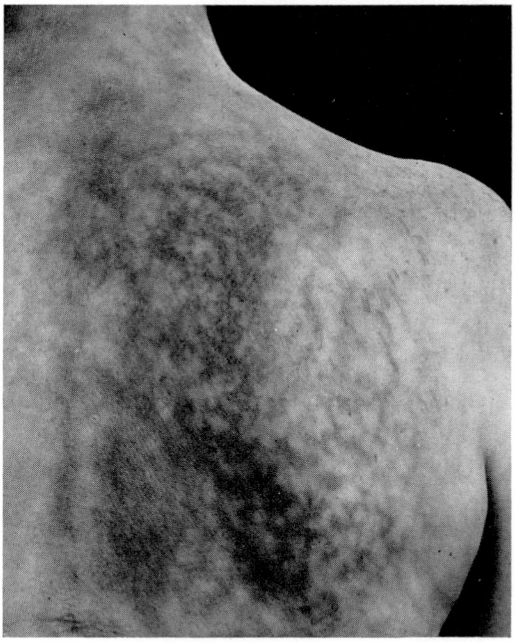

Fig. 137. Erythema ab igne from hot water bottle.

(K.U.M.C.)

Erythema elevatum diutinum. A persistent nodular, symmetrical eruption usually seen in middle-aged males with a rather characteristic histologic picture. This may be a deeper form of *granuloma annulare.*

Erythema of the ninth day. A morbilliform erythema of sudden onset appearing around the 9th day after the initiation of organic arsenic therapy for the treatment of syphilis. It may be accompanied by generalized lymphadenopathy and fever.

Erythema, palmar. Redness of the palms of the hands, which may be due to heredity, pulmonary disease, liver disease, rheumatoid arthritis, or pregnancy.

Erythema perstans. Over a dozen entities have been described which fit into this persistent group of diseases that resemble erythema

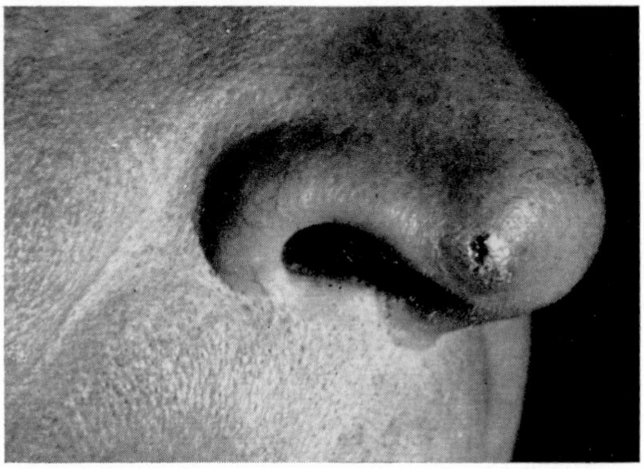

Fig. 138. Folliculitis, perforating, of the nose.

(*Dr. Chester Lessenden*)

Erythema perstans (*Cont.*)
multiforme. The following entities are included in this group:
Erythema annulare centrifugum (Darier); erythema chronicum migrans (Lipschutz), may be due to a tick bite for which Penicillin is effective therapy; *erythema gyratum perstans (Fox); erythema figuratum perstans (Wende);* and *erythema gyratum repens (Gammel).*
Erythrasma, 143
Erythredema. *See* Acrodynia
Erythroderma. *See* Exfoliative dermatitis, 165
Erythrodermia desquamativa. Another term for Leiner's disease.
Erythromelalgia. A rare disorder of hands and feet, most common in males; characterized by burning pain which is activated by exertion or heat and is refractory to treatment.
Erythrose pigmentaire peribuccale. A rare condition of middle-aged women, characterized by diffuse brownish-red pigmentation about the mouth, the chin and the neck with or without a slight burning sensation.
Exanthem subitum. Another term for roseola infantum or sixth disease.
Excoriations, 13
Exfoliative dermatitis, **165,** *169*
nail changes, *195*
primary, 165
secondary, 166

Factitial dermatitis, 181
Fall dermatoses, 22
False-positive serology, 117, 118, 126
Fat necrosis in the newborn. A benign, self-limited localized process over the bony prominences in infants born after a difficult labor.
Favus, 191

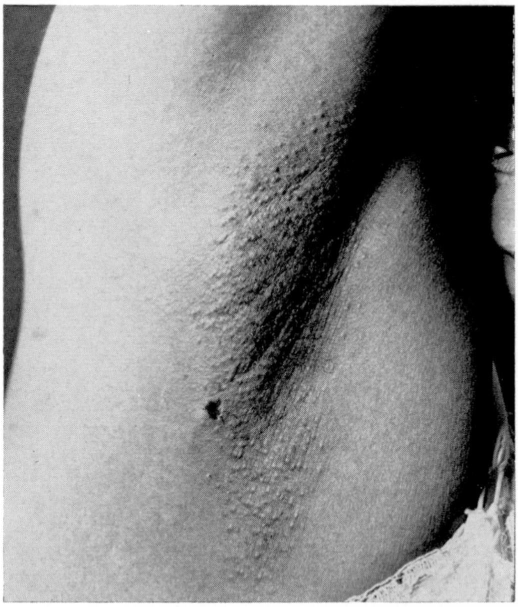

Fig. 139. Fox-Fordyce disease of axilla.

Fever blisters, 121
Fibromas, pedunculated, 221
Fibrosarcoma, 223
Fifth disease, 133
Fissures, 13
Fixed drug eruption, 59
Florida dermatoses, 204
Fogo selvagem. Also known as *Brazilian pemphigus,* this epidemic bullous disease resembles acute pemphigus foliaceus. It is accompanied by high fever, loss of hair and marked secondary infection of the skin. It is fatal in 90% of cases.
Folliculitis, 98
decalvans, 100, 189, **191**
Folliculitis, perforating, of the nose (Fig. 138). A folliculitis of the stiff hairs of the nasal mucocutaneous junction that penetrates deeply through to the external nasal skin. Unless the basic pathology is understood and corrected by plucking the involved stiff hair, the condition cannot be cured. The external papule can simulate a skin cancer.
Foot and mouth disease. A virus disease of animals and occasionally man, characterized by a painful, self-limited vesicular stomatitis.
Formulary, 31-37
Foshay test. A 48-hour intradermal test which, if positive, indicates that the person has or has had *tularemia.*
Fourth disease. Another term for Dukes' disease.

Fox-Fordyce disease (Fig. 139). A rare intensely pruritic, chronic papular dermatosis of the axillae and the pubic area in women. The intense itching is due to the closure of the apocrine gland pore with rupture of the duct and escape of the apocrine sweat into the surrounding epidermis.

Frambesia. *See* Yaws

Freckles (ephelides). Small, brownish macules that develop around puberty and are accentuated by sunlight. They are to be differentiated from lentigines which develop around the age of 2 and are more widespread on the body. *See* 228.

Frostbite. Exposure to cold can cause pathologic changes in the skin which are related to the severity of the exposure but vary with the susceptibility of the individual. Other terms in use that refer to cold injuries under varying conditions include *trench foot, immersion foot, pernio* and *chilblain*. *See* Chilblain.

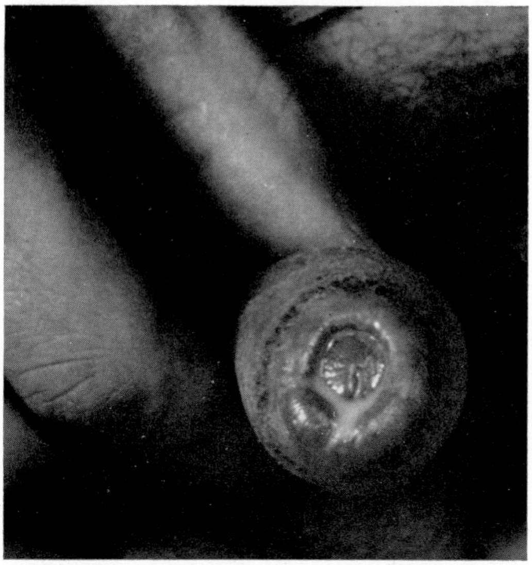

Fig. 140. Fusospirochetal balanitis.

Fusospirochetal balanitis. *See* Balanitis, fusospirochetal (Fig. 140)

Gangosa. A severe ulcerative and mutilating form of yaws affecting the palate, the pharynx and nasal tissues.

General paresis. A psychosis due to syphilitic meningo-encephalitis.

Gentian violet. A pararosaniline dye which destroys gram-positive bacteria and some fungi.

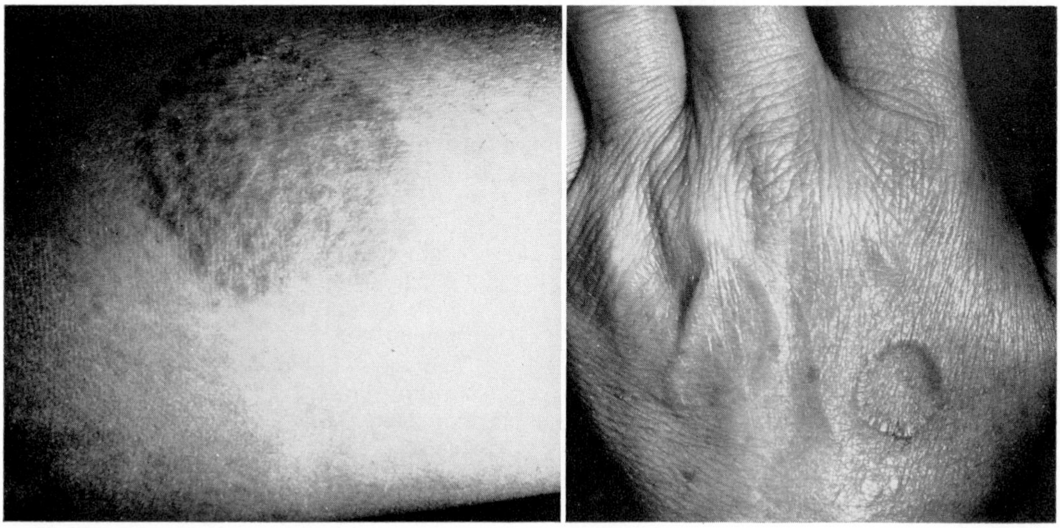

Fig. 141. Granuloma annulare.
(*Left*) On calf of leg of 7-year-old female.
(*Right*) On dorsum of hand. (Dr. Chester Lessenden)

Hemochromatosis. A rare hereditary metabolic disease characterized by a deposit of hemosiderin in the glandular tissues, and hemofuscin in the connective tissues, the spleen and the smooth muscles. *See under* Pigmentary Diseases
Henoch's purpura. A form of nonthrombocytopenic purpura most commonly seen in children characterized by recurrent attacks of purpura accompanied by gastro-intestinal pathology. It is thought to be related to *Schönlein's purpura.*
Hereditary skin diseases. The following list is adapted from Dermatology, by Pillsbury, Shelley, and Kligman (Philadelphia, Saunders, 1956). This and other more comprehensive texts should be consulted for further information on hereditary skin diseases.

A. Neurocutaneous Group
  1. Neurofibromatosis (von Recklinghausen's Disease)
  2. Epiloia, a triad of mental deficiency, epilepsy and skin lesions called adenoma sebaceum.
  3. Encephalotrigeminal angiomatosis (Sturge-Weber syndrome)
B. Pigmentary Group
  1. Incontinentia pigmenti
  2. Albinism
  3. Freckles
C. Vascular Group
  1. Hereditary hemorrhagic telangiectasis (Rendu-Osler-Weber disease)
  2. Congenital lymphedema (Milroy's disease)
D. Diseases of the Corium: Pseudoxanthoma elasticum
E. Diseases with Prominent Epidermal Reactions
  1. Pityriasis rubra pilaris
  2. Benign familial pemphigus
  3. Epidermolysis bullosa, simple and dystrophic forms
  4. Xeroderma pigmentosum
  5. Acanthosis nigricans, benign and malignant forms
  6. Darier's disease (keratosis follicularis)
  7. Ichthyosis of various types
  8. Psoriasis
F. Metabolic Group
  1. Xanthomatosis, primary hypercholesteremic form
  2. Porphyria, congenital and hepatic forms
  3. Gout
G. Tumors
  1. Trichoepithelioma
  2. Keloids

Several nail and hair disorders are hereditary, including male-pattern hair loss and gray hair.

Herpangina. A name applied to a primary form of virus infection of the herpes simplex type that occurs on the mucous membranes of the mouth in children. Fever and malaise accompany this acute infection which lasts approximately 2 weeks. *See* Herpes simplex.

Herxheimer reaction. An acute reaction characterized by fever and aggravation of existing cutaneous lesions following the administration of penicillin or organic arsenic for the treatment of patients with syphilis, particularly the infectious form. In patients with central nervous system syphilis neurologic findings may be aggravated. In patients with cardiovascular syphilis the reaction may be fatal, but some observers doubt the occurrence of this severe form of Herxheimer reaction.

Higoumenakis' sign. Enlargement of the sternoclavicular joint due to osteitis and periostitis of congenital syphilis.

Histoplasmosis. Histoplasmosis is endemic in the Midwestern United States and is caused by *Histoplasma capsulatum,* a soil saprophyte. Inhalation of the spores produces an asymptomatic pulmonary infection that rarely goes on to produce a disseminated organic disease. The secondary skin lesions are multiform, consisting of granulomatous ulcers, purpura, impetiginized lesions, and abscesses.

Hutchinson's teeth. Changes in the teeth of patients with congenital syphilis characterized especially by narrowing of the upper incisors with a central depression of the cutting edge.

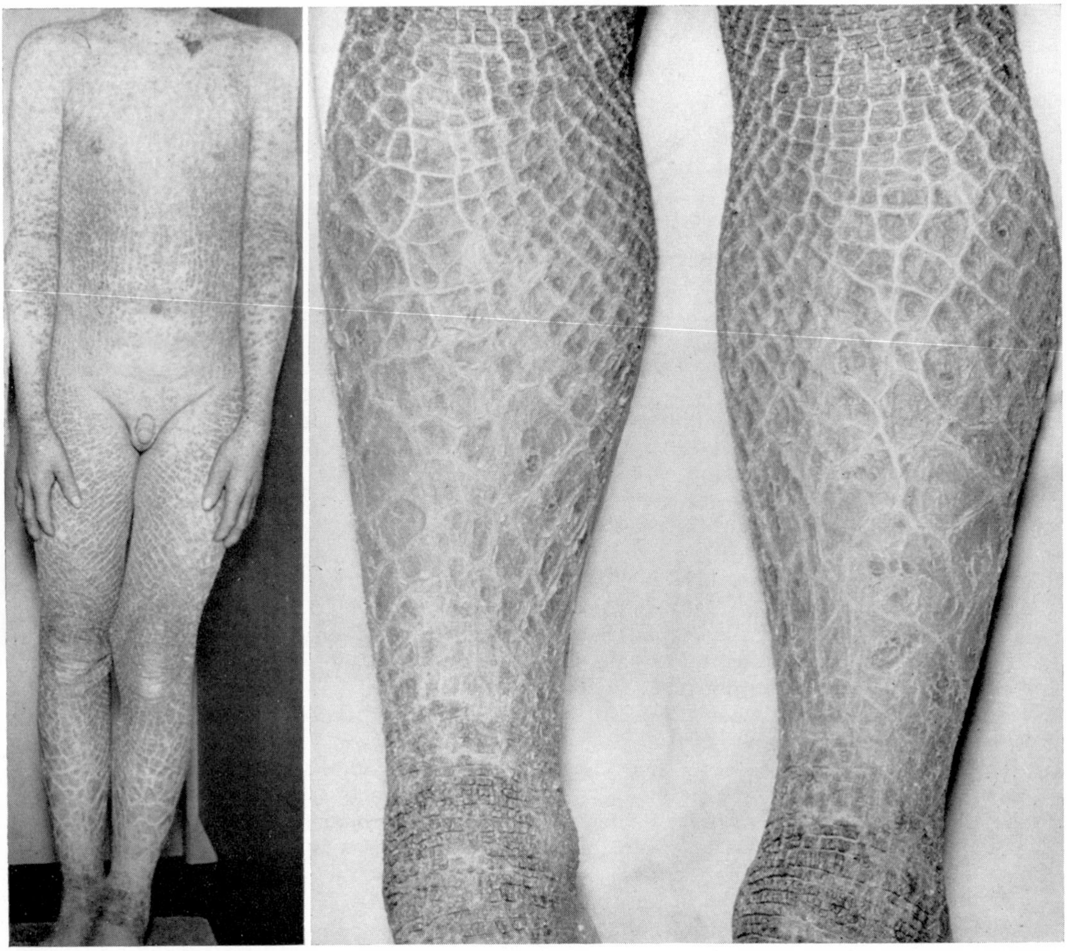

Fig. 142. Ichthyosis, congenital, showing fully body and close-up of legs.
(*Dr. David Morgan, K.C.G.H.*)

Hutchinson's triad. The occurrence in patients with congenital syphilis of ocular keratitis, deafness and dental defects.

Hydroa aestivale. This rare recurrent vesicular dermatoses, occurs in the summer on the exposed areas of the body. It is more common in young males and usually disappears at the age of puberty. The erythema, urticarialike lesions, vesicles and crusted lesions develop following sun exposure and are aggravated by continued exposure. When the vesicle shows a central depression, as in a vaccination, the eruption is called *hydroa vacciniforme*.

vacciniforme. *See* Hydroa aestivale.

Hyperkeratosis. Excessive thickness of the horny layer.

Ichthyosis. Several conditions come under this general heading. (*See also* p. 60.)

Congenital ichthyosis (Fig. 142) is present at birth or shortly thereafter and can be mild or severe. A severe form is known as the Harlequin Fetus where the skin is dry, fissured, unelastic, and usually results in death. Milder cases of ichthyosis are worse in the winter time, due to the low humidity in the home. Usually the flexural aspects of the body are not involved.

Acquired ichthyosis or xerosis occurs rather commonly in elderly patients and is associated with hypothyroidism and vitamin A deficiency.

Ichthyosis hystrix is a rare form of congenital "nevus" characterized by extensive horny, papillary, hyperpigmented elevations of the skin.

Congenital ichthyosiform erythroderma is to be differentiated from ichthyosis. It is a rare ectodermal defect where the skin is generally thickened, red, shiny, and shows a tendency to lichenification over the larger joints. This condition can be differentiated from ichthyosis in that it involves the flexural surfaces of the body, whereas ichthyosis usually does not.

Keratosis palmaris et plantaris (Fig. 143). Hereditary symmetrical thickening of the palms and the soles noticed at an early age, seen alone or associated with ichthyosis or with congenital ectodermal defect.

Mal de Meleda. A hereditary ectodermal defect resembling keratosis palmaris et plantaris due to inbreeding of persons on the Isle of Mljet.

Keratosis punctata. A form of keratosis palmaris et plantaris characterized by the presence of numerous small crateriform pits on the palms and the soles.

Id, dermogram, 17
  reaction, due to tinea, 148
Id Reaction. This phenomenon is characterized by an erythematous, vesicular or eczematous eruption that occurs in disseminated parts of the skin. Most commonly id reactions are seen to follow fungus infections of the feet, varicose ulcers, fungus infections of the scalp, and severe contact dermatitis of the hands. *See* Dermatophytid, Epidermophytid, Monillid and Trichophytid.
Immersion foot. *See* Frostbite
Impetigo, 96
  bullous, 159
  due to chigger bites, 205
  herpetiformis, 159
Incontinentia pigmenti. A rare pigmentary anomaly characterized by hyperpigmented patches that occur in symmetrical whorls on the skin. Some cases are preceded by a bullous and lichenoid eruption which is present at birth, or soon after. The name is derived from the histopathologic findings of melanin in the corium suggesting that the epidermis was incontinent.
Industrial dermatoses, 47
Infantile eczema. *See* Eczema, atopic

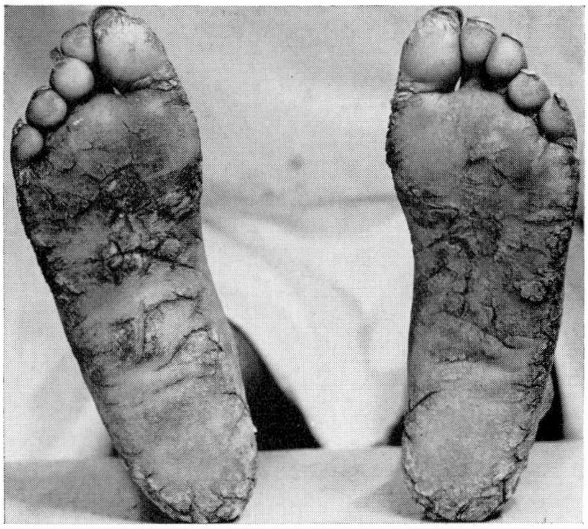

Fig. 143. Keratosis plantaris of patient with pityriasis rubra pilaris.

Infectious mononucleosis, 133
Ingrown beard hairs, 100
Insects, 155
Internal diseases, and skin, 177
Interstitial keratitis. A resistant eye affection occurring in patients with congenital syphilis.
Intertrigo, bacterial, 106
  monilial, 150
Intracutaneous test, 7
Ioderma. A dermatosis due to the ingestion of iodides, usually of a pustular nature. *See also* Drug eruption, 55
Itching, 4

Jarisch-Herxheimer reaction. *See* Herxheimer reaction
Jessner's syndrome. Lymphocytic infiltration of the skin mainly of the face resembling deep chronic discoid lupus erythematosus.
Jungle rot. A "G.I." term for a group of bacterial and mycotic infections of the skin seen in the South Pacific during World War II.
Jüngling's disease. *Osteitis fibrosa cystica* of the small long bones, particularly of the fingers, due to sarcoidosis.
Juxta-articular nodes. These are syphilitic gummatous tumors occurring in the corium or subcutaneous layer of the skin in the region of the joints.

Kaposi, sarcoma of. *See* Tumors of vascular tissue
  varicelliform eruption, 124
Kassowitz-Diday's law. The observation that successive children of a syphilitic mother will become progressively less infected with syphilis or not at all.

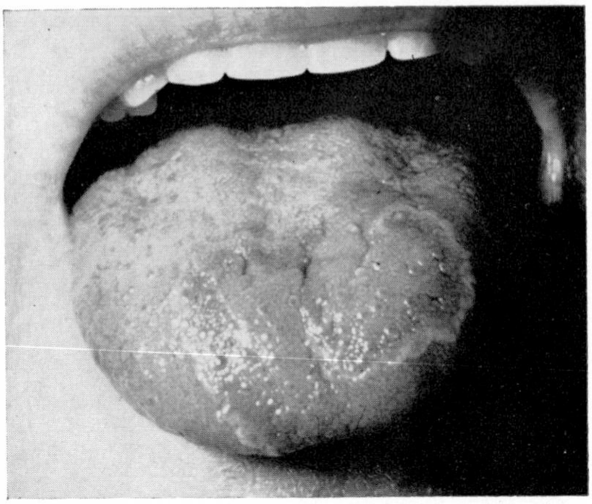

Fig. 144. Geographic tongue.

Mucous membrane disorders (*Cont.*)
ical causes (sucking of lips, pressure sores, burns, actinic or sunlight cheilitis, tobacco, other chemicals, and allergens). (2) *Infectious diseases* from viruses, bacteria, fungi and animal parasites (gangrenous bacterial infections are called *noma. Ludwig's angina* is an acute cellulitis of the floor of the mouth due to bacteria, abscesses and sinuses; may be due to dental infection. *Trench mouth, or Plaut-Vincent's disease,* is an acute ulcerative infection of the mucous membranes caused by a combination of a spirochete and a fusiform bacillus). (3) *Systemic diseases.* (4) *Drugs* (Dilantin sodium causes a hyperplastic gingivitis, bismuth orally and intramuscularly causes a bluish black line at the edge of the dental gum; certain drugs cause hemorrhage and secondary infection of the mucous membranes). (5) *Metabolic diseases.* (6) *Tumors,* local or systemic.

Halitosis, or fetor oris, is a disagreeable odor of the breath.

Periadenitis mucosa necrotica recurrens. Also known as Sutton's disease, this is a painful, recurrent, ulcerating disease of the mucous membranes of the oral cavity.

Black tongue (hairy tongue, lingua nigra). Overgrowth of the papillae of the tongue apparently caused by an imbalance of bacterial flora due to the use of antibiotics and other agents.

Geographic tongue (Fig. 144). A very common eruption on the tongue; of no medical importance. The patient who becomes suddenly aware of this condition needs to be reassured that it is not a malignancy. Clinically, circinate and annular red areas are seen on the top of the tongue that spread and disappear spontaneously.

Moeller's glossitis. A painful, persistent, red eruption on the sides and the tip of the tongue that persists for weeks or months, subsides, and then recurs. The etiology is unknown.

Burning tongue (glossodynia). A rather common complaint, particularly of middle-aged women; usually accompanied by no visible pathology. The etiology is unknown, and therapy is of little value; but the many diseases and local factors that cause painful tongue must be ruled out from a diagnostic viewpoint.

Cheilitis glandularis apostenatosa. A chronic disorder of the lips manifested by swelling and secondary inflammation due to hypertrophy of the mucous glands and their ducts.

Furrowed tongue (grooved tongue, scrotal tongue). A tongue that is usually larger than normal containing deep longitudinal and lateral grooves of congenital origin or due to syphilis.

Glossitis rhombica mediana. A rare disorder characterized by a smooth reddish lesion, usually in the center of the tongue. This term is poor because there is no inflammation, and the reddish plaque may not always be in the center.

Multiple, benign, tumorlike new growths of the skin. *See* Atrophies, anetoderma of Schweninger-Buzzi

Mundt, Dr. Leslie K., 204

Mycology, 135. *See also* Fungus infections *and* Tinea

Mycosis fungoides, 231
See Granuloma fungoides

Myiasis. Infestation of the skin with flies *(Diptera),* usually the larva.

Myxedema, generalized, 179
localized, 179

Nail disorders. In addition to those disorders discussed in Chapter 23, the following are listed.

Anonychia. Total congenital absence of the nail.

Onychatrophia. Simple atrophy of the nails which may be congenital, hereditary, traumatic, or due to any severe local or systemic disease.

Softened nails (hapalonychia). A rare atrophic condition usually concurrent with the aging process.

Spoon nails (koilonychia). Usually a congenital defect but seen with certain systemic diseases and occasionally with Plummer-Vinson syndrome.

Thickening of the nail plates (ony-

Ochronosis (*Cont.*)
the term "alcaptonuria." *See* Pigmentary disorders
Ohio dermatoses, 202
Oid-Oid disease, 206. *See also* Dermatosis, exudative discoid and lichenoid chronic
Onycho-. A prefix from the Greek *onyx* meaning nail.
Onychogryphosis, *193*
Onychomycosis. *See* Tinea of nails, 140
Optic atrophy. Atrophy of the optic nerve due to syphilitic involvement of the central nervous system of the tabetic type. Blindness is the end result.
Orf. A viral infection characterized by a vesicular and pustular eruption of the mouth and the lips of lambs. Sheepherders and veterinarians become inoculated on the hand and develop a primary-chancre type lesion.
Otitis, external, 63

Panniculitis, nodular, 71
Papilloma. An upward proliferation of the papillae which is seen histiologically in nevus verrucosus, senile keratosis, seborrheic keratosis, verruca vulgaris and acanthosis nigricans.
Papillomatoses. Three forms of papillomatoses have been described and all are very rare.
Papules, 12
Papulosquamous diseases, 83-95
Paraffinoma. A foreign body granuloma due to the injection of paraffin into the subcutaneous tissue for cosmetic purposes.
Parakeratosis. An example of imperfect keratinization of the epidermis resulting in the retention of nuclei in the horny layer. In areas of parakeratosis the granular layer is absent.
Parapsoriasis. A term for a group of persistent macular and maculopapular scaly erythrodermas. An acute form with the synonym *pityriasis lichenoides et varioliformis acuta (Habermann)* appears as a reddish macular generalized eruption with mild constitutional signs, including fever and malaise. Vesicles may develop and also papulonecrotic lesions. This form disappears in several months. A chronic form of parapsoriasis, *parapsoriasis guttata,* can resemble guttate psoriasis or seborrheic dermatitis. This condition does not itch and persists for years. Another chronic form of parapsoriasis, *parapsoriasis en plaque,* is characterized by nonpruritic or slightly pruritic scaly brownish patches and plaques. A high percentage of patients that are given this diagnosis terminate with granuloma fungoides.
Parapsoriasis, 87
Parasitology, 155
Paronychia, bacterial, **193,** 150
monilial, 150
Patch tests, 7
Pearls, diagnostic, 12, 19
syphilis, 119-120
therapy, 30
Pediatric (childhood) dermograms, 23
Pediatric (infancy) dermograms, 23
Pediatric skin diseases, 22
Pediculosis, 157
capitis, 158
corporis, 158
pubis, 158
Pellagra, 180
Pemphigoid. A chronic bullous eruption most commonly occurring in elderly adults; usually not fatal. It is differentiated from true pemphigus by the histologic presence of a subepidermal bullae without acantholysis, from erythema multiforme by the chronicity and absence of iris lesions, and from dermatitis herpetiformis by the absence of response to sulfapyridine or Diasone therapy.
Pemphigus, benign mucous membrane (Fig. 145). A disabling but nonfatal bullous eruption of the mucous membranes but most commonly involving the eyes. As the result of scarring, which is characteristic of this disease and separates it from true pemphigus, the eyesight is eventually lost. Over 50% of the cases have skin lesions. Histologically, the bullae are subepidermal and do not show acantholysis.
erythematosus, 161
familial benign chronic, 159
foliaceus, 161
neonatorum, 97, 159
ocular. *See* Pemphigus, benign mucous membrane
Senear-Usher type. *See* Pemphigus erythematosus, 161
vegetans, 161
vulgaris, 161
Periadenitis mucosa necrotica recurrens. *See* Mucous membrane disorders
Periarteritis nodosa, 71, **178**
Perlèche, 151
Pernio. See Chilblain *and* Frostbite
Petechiae, 12
See also Purpura
Peutz-Jehgers syndrome. *See* Pigmentary disorders
Phobias, 182
Phrynoderma, 180

Phthiriasis. Infestation with the crab louse.

Pigmentary disorders. A classification follows:

A. Melanin hyperpigmentation or melanoderma
  1. Chloasma
  2. Incontinentia pigmenti
  3. Secondary to skin diseases
    a. Chronic discoid lupus erythematosus
    b. Tinea versicolor
    c. Stasis dermatitis
    d. Many cases of dermatitis in Negroes and other dark-skinned individuals
    e. Scleroderma
  4. Secondary to external agents
    a. X-radiation
    b. Ultraviolet
    c. Sunlight
    d. Tars
    e. Photosensitizing chemicals as in cosmetics causing development of the clinical entities labeled as Riehl's melanosis, poikiloderma of Civatte, berlock dermatitis and others.
  5. Secondary to internal disorders
    a. Addison's disease
    b. Chronic liver disease
    c. Pregnancy
    d. Hyperthyroidism
    e. Internal carcinoma causing malignant form of acanthosis nigricans
    f. Hormonal influence on benign acanthosis nigricans
    g. Intestinal polyposis causing mucous membrane pigmentation (Peutz-Jehgers syndrome)
    h. Albright's syndrome
    i. Schilder's disease
    j. Fanconi's syndrome
  6. Secondary to drugs such as ACTH, estrogens, progesterone, melanocyte stimulating hormone

B. Nonmelanin pigmentations
  1. Argyria due to silver salt deposits
  2. Arsenical pigmentation due to ingestion of inorganic arsenic as in Fowler's solution and Asiatic pills.
  3. Pigmentation from heavy metals such as bismuth, gold, and mercury.
  4. Tattoos
  5. Black dermographism, the common bluish-black or green stain seen under watches and rings in certain people from the deposit of the metallic particles reacting with chemicals already on the skin.

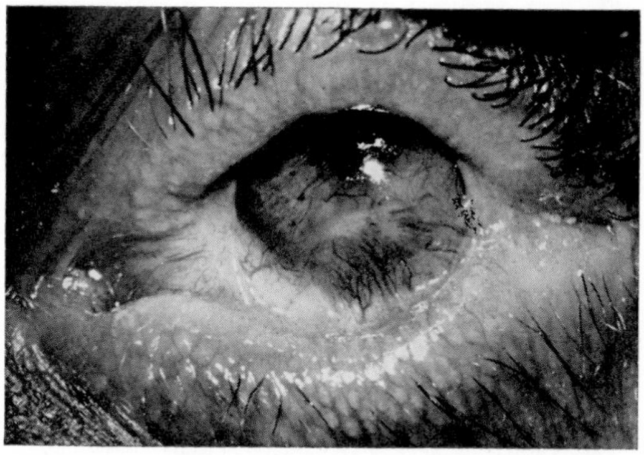

Fig. 145. Pemphigus, benign mucous membrane type of eye.
(Drs. L. Calkins and A. Lemoine)

  6. Hemosiderin granules in hemochromatosis or bronze diabetes.
  7. Bile pigments from jaundice
  8. Yellow pigments following Atabrine and chlorpromazine ingestion
  9. Carotene coloring in carotinosis
  10. Homogentisic acid polymer deposit in ochronosis

C. Hypopigmentation
  1. Albinism
  2. Vitiligo
  3. Leukoderma or acquired hypopigmentation
    a. Secondary to skin diseases such as tinea versicolor, chronic discoid lupus erythematosus, localized scleroderma, psoriasis, secondary syphilis, pinta, etc.
    b. Secondary to chemicals such as mercury compounds and monobenzyl ether of hydroquinone
    c. Secondary to internal disease as hormonal diseases, and in Vogt-Koyanagi syndrome
    d. Associated with pigmented nevi (leukoderma acquisitum centrifugum or Sutton's disease).

Pigmented purpuric eruption. Three rare non-thrombocytopenic purpuric skin conditions are included under this heading: *purpura annularis telangiectodes* (*Majocchi*), *progessive pigmentary dermatosis* (*Schamberg*) and *pigmented purpuric lichenoid dermatitis* (*Gougerot-Blum*). Majocchi's disease commonly begins on the legs but slowly spreads to become generalized. Telangiectatic capillaries become confluent and produce annular or serpiginous lesions. The capillaries break down, causing purpuric lesions. Schamberg's disease is a slowly progressive pigmentary

Pigmented purpuric eruption (*Cont.*)
condition of the lower part of the legs which fades after a period of months. The Gougerot-Blum form is accompanied by severe itching; otherwise, it resembles Schamberg's disease.

Pink disease. *See* Acrodynia

Pinta. Caused by *Treponema carateum;* is similar to syphilis and yaws. Common in Mexico and Central America and characterized by a striking patchy depigmentation of the skin accompanied by other cutaneous and organ changes similar to syphilis. Penicillin therapy is effective.

Pityriasis lichenoides chronica (Juliusberg). A form of guttate parapsoriasis.

Pityriasis lichenoides et varioliformis acutis (Habermann). *See* Parapsoriasis

Pityriasis rubra pilaris. One of the nutmeg-graterlike diseases. It appears mainly in young adults and is characterized by hard, reddish-yellow hyperkeratotic papules situated at the mouths of the hair follicles and the sweat ducts. Vitamin A therapy is helpful. Fatal cases of this rare disease are unusual.

Pityriasis simplex faciei. A common disorder of children seen predominately in the winter as a rather well-localized scaly oval patch on the cheeks. The end result is depigmentation of the area, but the normal pigment returns when the eruption clears up (usually in the summer). I believe this condition to be a mild form of atopic eczema.

Plaut-Vincent's disease. *See* Mucous membrane disorders

Plummer-Vinson syndrome. A syndrome characterized by dysphagia, glossitis, hypochromic anemia and spoon nails in middle-aged women. The associated dryness and atrophy of the mucous membranes of the throat may lead to leukoplakia and squamous cell epithelioma.

Poikiloderma of Civatte. Characterized by a diffuse patch of hyperpigmentation and atrophy occurring in a network of patches on both sides of the neck and the face. Most commonly seen in women of the menopausal age. Probably identical with melanosis of Riehl.

Poikiloderma congenitale. A rare syndrome characterized by telangiectasis, pigmentation, defective teeth and bone cysts. This may be similar to dyskeratosis congenita.

Pompholyx. *See* Dyshidrosis

Porokeratosis. A rare disorder that begins as a small, slightly elevated, wartlike papule that slowly enlarges, leaving an atrophic center with a keratotic ridgelike border. The small individual lesions may coalesce.

Porphyria. A rare metabolic disorder of certain red pigments of the body called porphyrins. Uroporphyrin and coproporphyrin I and III are the most significant porphyrins from the standpoint of disease states. There are 2 types of porphyrin disturbance: the erythropoetic type and the hepatic type. The erythropoetic type manifests itself clinically as *congenital porphyria,* which begins in childhood and is characterized by a reddish discoloration of the teeth and the long bones; the urine, which is red, contains large amounts of uroporphyrin I. The striking skin change is a marked photosensitivity with bullae and a positive Nikolsky test. The hepatic type occurs as acute porphyria and chronic porphyria. *Acute porphyria* is the commonest of the porphyrias. This form occurs most commonly in women from the age of 20 to 40 and often can be related to excessive intake of alcohol, barbiturates, sulfonamides and other drugs. Skin changes are absent or present only as hyperpigmentation. There is no photosensitivity. Neurologic symptoms are the most dominant. *Chronic porphyria* is milder than the acute form and occurs later in adult life and more frequently in males. Photosensitivity with vesiculation and bulla formation is common. This form also is aggravated by certain drugs and alcohol consumption.

Potassium permanganate. An oxidizing antiseptic usually used as a wet dressing in the concentration of 1:10,000.

Prausnitz-Küstner reaction. A demonstration of passive sensitization of the skin of a nonsensitive individual. This is accomplished by the intradermal injection of serum from a sensitive patient into the skin of a nonsensitive individual. After 24 to 48 hours the atopen to be tested is injected intracutaneously into the previously injected site on the nonsensitive individual's skin. Passive transfer of the sensitivity is manifested by the formation of a wheal.

Primary chancre-type diseases.
Anthrax
Blastomycosis, primary cutaneous type
Chancroid
Coccidioidomycosis, primary cutaneous type

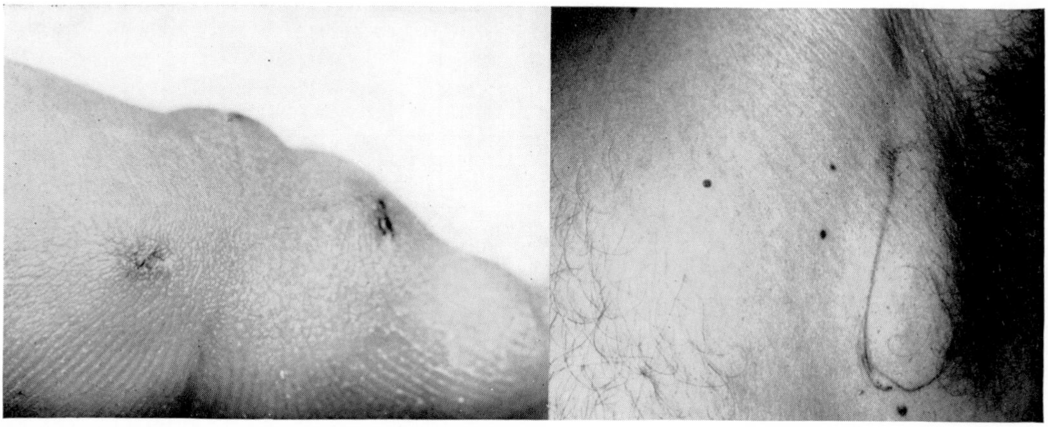

Fig. 146. Primary chancre-type disease.
(*Left*) Tularemic chancre on finger.
(*Right*) Axillary adenopathy of same patient. (Dr. Lawrence Calkins)

Cowpox
Cutaneous diphtheria
Erysipeloid
Furuncle
Milker's nodules
Orf
Sporotrichosis
Syphilis (genital but also extragenital)
Tuberculosis, primary inoculation type
Tularemia (Fig. 146)
Vaccinia
Protozoal dermatoses, 155
Prurigo nodularis. A rare chronic dermatosis, usually of women, consisting of discrete nodular pruritic excoriated papules and tumors scattered over the arms and the legs.
Pruritic dermatoses, 60
Pruritus, ani, 64
essential, 62
generalized, 60
genital, 66
scrotal, 66
senile, 60
vulvar, 66
winter, 60
Pseudochancre redux. A late, gummatous, syphilitic inflammation, occurring at the site of the original chancre.
Pseudoepitheliomatous hyperplasia, 220
Pseudopelade. *See* Alopecia cicatrisata
Pseudoxanthoma elasticum, 183
Psoralens, 169
Psoriasis, *18, 20,* 21, **83,** *84, 85*
and arthritis, 182
dermogram, 14
nails in, *194,* 195
pustular, *20, 21*
of toenails, 140
Psychoses, and skin diseases, 181
Puberty state, 177
Purpura, 12
Purpura (Fig. 147). There are several forms of purpuric lesions. *Petechiae* are small superficial purpuric lesions. *Ecchymoses* are more extensive, round or irregularly shaped purpuric lesions. *Hematomata* are large, deep, fluctuant, tumorlike hemorrhages of the skin. The purpuras can be divided into the thrombocytopenic forms and the nonthrombocytopenic forms.
Purpura, senile. This is a rather common form of nonthrombocytopenic purpura seen on legs, arms and dorsum of hands of elderly patients.
Purpura, thrombocytopenic. May be idiopathic or secondary to various chronic diseases or a drug sensitivity. The platelet count is below normal, the bleeding time is prolonged, and the clotting time is normal, but the clot does not retract normally.
Pustules, 12
Pyoderma(s), 96-111
gangrenosum, 104
See also Bacterial infections

Radiation, 41
Radiodermatitis, 198
Rat-bite fevers. The bite of a rat can cause *sodoku* and *Haverhill fever*. Sodoku, caused by *Spirillum minus,* is manifested by a primary-type chancre and later by an erythematous rash. Haverhill fever, caused by *Streptobacillus moniliformis,* is characterized by joint pains and an erythematous rash.
Raynaud's phenomenon, *174,* 175
Refrigeration, 40

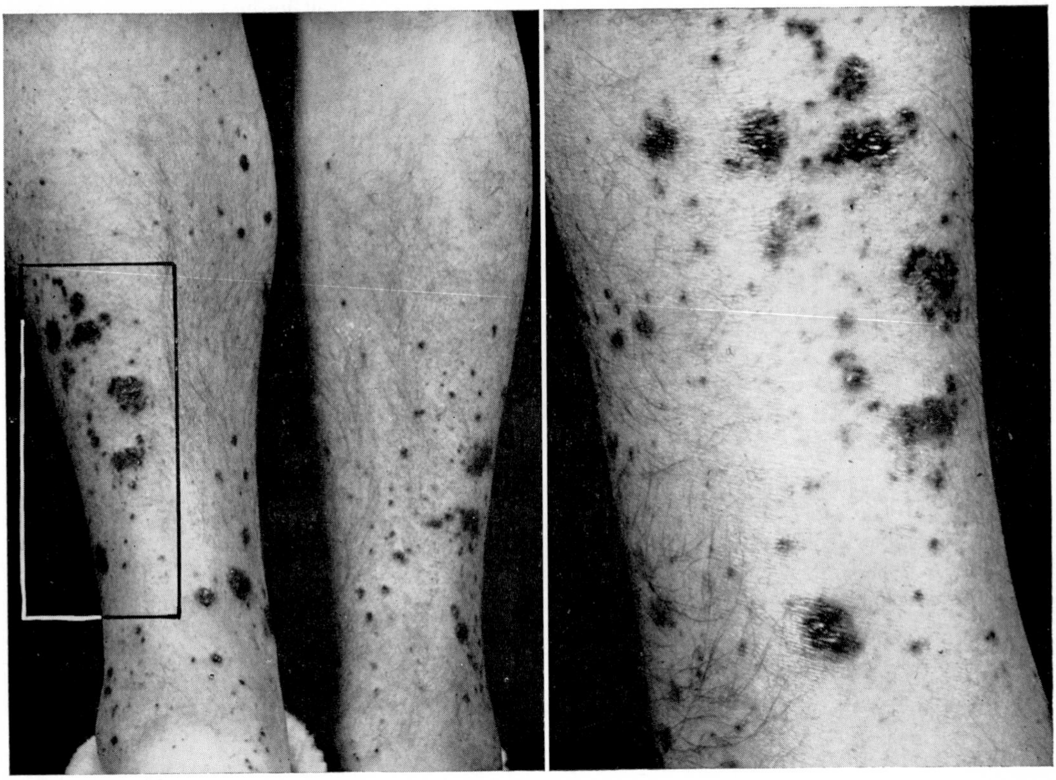

Fig. 147. Purpura of unknown cause on legs.
(K.U.M.C.)

Resorcinol. This agent is similar in its properties and use to salicylic acid.

Rhinosporidiosis. The fungus, *Rhinosporidium seeberi,* causes a raspberrylike papillomatous tumor of the nares of the nose.

Rickettsial diseases. The commonest rickettsial disease in the United States is *Rocky Mountain Spotted Fever* which is spread by ticks of various types. The skin eruption occurs after 3 to 7 days of fever and other toxic signs, and is characterized by purpuric lesions on the extremities, mainly the wrists and the ankles, which then become generalized. The Weil-Felix test using Proteus OX19 and OX2 is positive. The broad spectrum antibiotics are effective.

The typhus group of rickettsial diseases includes *epidemic* or *louse-borne typhus, Brill's disease* and *endemic Murine* or *flea-borne typhus.* Less common forms include *scrub typhus* (tsutsugamuchi disease), *trench fever* and *rickettsialpox.* The last rickettsial disease is produced by a mite bite. The mite ordinarily lives on rodents. Approximately 10 days after the bite a primary lesion develops in the form of a papule that becomes vesicular. After a few days fever and other toxic signs are accompanied by a generalized eruption that resembles chickenpox. The disease subsides without therapy.

Romberg's sign. Swaying of the body when standing with the feet close together and the eyes closed which occurs in patients with central nervous system syphilis of the tabetic type.

Rothmund's syndrome. A rare hereditary syndrome characterized by cataracts, scleroderma and poikilodermalike changes with telangiectasis developing in childhood. This syndrome is thought to be related to *Werner's syndrome,* but the latter manifests itself in the 2nd and the 3rd decade of life.
Rowe elimination diet, 9
Roys, Dr. Harvey, 202
Rubella. *See* Measles, German
Rubeola. *See* Measles

Sabouraud's media, 9
Salicylic acid. Locally, this agent acts as a keratoplastic chemical in strengths up to 3% and keratolytic in strengths over 3%. Its greatest use is in treatment of chronic fungus infection of the feet, and lichenified patches seen with psoriasis or neurodermatitis. It macerates and peels off the thickened horny layer of the skin when used in the stronger strengths.
Sanarelli-Shwartzman phenomenon. A local hemorrhagic and necrotizing inflammatory response seen in rabbits which appears promptly after the intravenous injection of a bacterial filtrate, in a site which 24 hours previously was injected intracutaneously with that bacterial filtrate. A fatal systemic reaction results if the preparatory injection was administered intravenously.
Sarcoid, Darier-Roussy. A deep subcutaneous form of sarcoid resembling erythema induratum.
  Spiegler-Fendt. *See* Tumor, Lymphomas
Sarcoidosis, 110
Scabies, **155,** *156*
Scales, 12
Scarlet fever, 106
Scars, 13
  traumatic, 175
Schick test. An intradermal test using diphtheria toxin which, if positive, as shown by the development of an erythematous wheal, indicates that the person lacks immunity for diphtheria.
Schistosomal dermatitis, 205
Schönlein's purpura. A form of nonthrombocytopenic purpura most commonly seen in children; accompanied by joint symptoms. It is thought to be related to *Henoch's purpura.*
Schüller-Christian syndrome, 180
Schultz-Charlton reaction. A blanching reaction seen when the scarlet fever antitoxin or convalescent serum is injected intradermally into a bright red area of the scarlet fever rash. Neutralization of the streptococcal toxin causes the blanching.
Scleredema. A self-limited rare disease characterized by benign but spreading induration and swelling of the skin and the subcutaneous tissues. It usually follows an acute infection. It resembles *scleroderma* but usually involutes in 3 to 12 months.
Sclerema adiposum. This rare highly fatal disease of newborns is characterized by cadaveric induration first on the lower extremities that extends rapidly to cover the entire body. It is to be differentiated from *fat necrosis of the newborn.*
Scleroderma, 174
  diffuse, 175
  localized, 174
  saber-cut type, 175
Sclerosing hemangioma, 222
Scratch tests, 7
Scurfy scalp. A scalp dermatosis in infants which can be either true dandruff, or the so-called "milk crust" due to the disinclination of the mother to cleanse the presumably delicate scalp of the newborn, or lastly a mixture of dandruff and lack of cleanliness. This old term may also be used by the lay person to designate atopic eczema of the scalp in infants.
Scurvy, 181
Seabather's eruption, 205
Seasonal skin diseases, 22
Sebaceous glands, 5
Seborrheic dermatitis dermogram, 14
  keratosis. *See* Keratosis, seborrheic, 221
Secondary infection, 103
Senear-Usher syndrome. Another term for pemphigus erythematosus.
Senile skin diseases, 24
Serologic tests, 117
Seven-year itch. *See* Scabies, 155
Shingles, 124
Silhouettes, dermatologic. *See* Dermograms
Silica granuloma, 111
Simmond's disease. Also known as hypophyseal cachexia, this disease is characterized by emaciation, amenorrhea, hypogenitalism, hypoglycemia, hypotension and generalized pigmentation. The disease is due to necrosis of the pituitary usually due to postpartum hemorrhage into the gland.
Sixth disease. Another term for roseola infantum.
Sjögren's syndrome. A very rare entity characterized by dryness of all of the mucous membranes and of the skin in middle-aged women. This may be related to *Plummer-Vinson syndrome.*
Skin tags, 221
Smallpox, 126

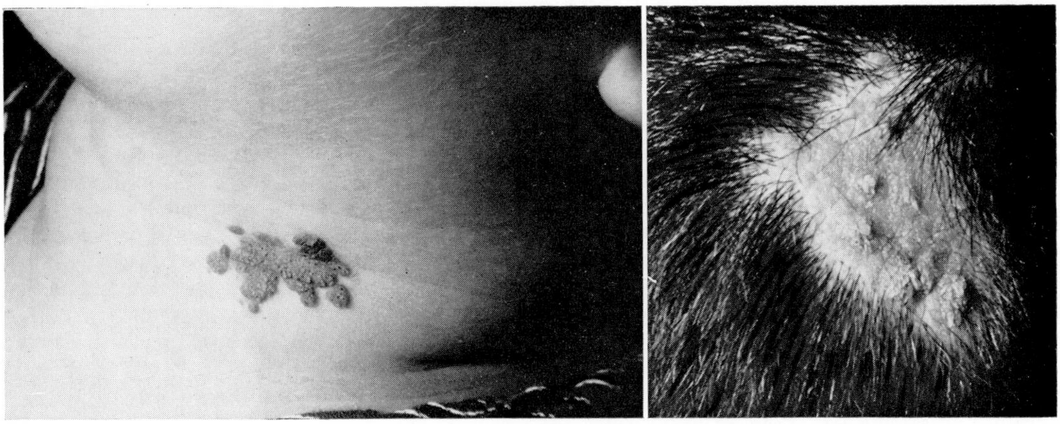

Fig. 148. Tumors. Nevus verrucosus on the neck (left) and on the scalp (right).

of nails, **140**
organisms, 136
pedis. *See* Tinea of foot, 136
of scalp, **144,** *145,* 190, 191
inflammatory type, 147
noninflammatory type, 144
due to *T. tonsurans,* in Southwest, 204
of smooth skin, *142,* **143**
suppurative, 202
therapy, griseofulvin, 149
versicolor, *18,* **90,** *91*
dermogram, 14
Tongue diseases. *See* Mucous membrane disorders
TPI test. (Treponema pallidum-immobilizing antibody test.) *See* Tests, for syphilis
Trench foot. *See* Frostbite
Tricho-. A prefix from the Greek *thrix* meaning hair.
Trichophytid. A dermatophytid due to *Trichophyton.*
Trichophyton test, 7
Trichophytosis. An infection due to *Trichophyton.*
Trichotillomania, **190**
of adults, 181
of children, 182
Triple response of Lewis. A response that occurs following scratching of the skin or injection of histamine and other related compounds which consists of (1) an immediate red flush due to local capillary dilation, (2) wheal formation due to increased capillary permeability, and (3) an erythematous flare due to reflex dilation of arterioles.
Trombidiosis, 204
Tuberculid, rosacealike, of Lewandowsky, 81
Tuberculin skin test, 7
Tuberculosis, 109
Tuberculosis of the skin. (Classification from Dermatology, by Pillsbury, Shelley, and Kligman, Philadelphia, Saunders, 1956)
1. True cutaneous tuberculosis. (Lesions contain tubercle bacilli.)
A. Primary tuberculosis. (No previous infection, individuals tuberculin-negative in initial stages.)
(1) Primary inoculation tuberculosis. Tuberculous chancre. (Exogenous implantation into skin producing the primary complex.)
(2) Miliary tuberculosis of the skin. (Hematogenous dispersion.)
B. Secondary tuberculosis. (Lesions develop in person already sensitive to tuberculin as result of prior tuberculous lesion. Tubercle bacilli difficult or impossible to demonstrate.)
(1) Lupus vulgaris. Inoculation of tubercle bacilli into the skin from external or internal sources.
(2) Tuberculosis verrucosa cutis. Inoculation of tubercle bacilli into the skin from external or internal sources.
(3) Scrofuloderma. Extension to skin from underlying focus in bones or glands.
(4) Tuberculosis cutis orificialis. Mucous membrane lesions and extension onto the skin near mucocutaneous junctions.
2. Tuberculids. (Allergic origin, no tubercle bacilli in lesions)
A. Papular forms.
(1) Lupus miliaris disseminatus faciei. Purely papular.

Tuberculosis of the skin, tuberculids (*Cont.*)
(2) Papulonecrotic tuberculid. Papules with necrosis.
(3) Lichen scrofulosorum. Follicular papules or lichenoid papules.
B. Granulomatous, ulceronodular forms.
(1) Erythema induratum. Nodules or plaques subsequently ulcerating.

Tularemia. The commonest form is the ulceroglandular form with its primary chancre-type lesion and regional and generalized lymphadenopathy. Caused by *Pasteurella tularensis*. Other forms are oculoglandular, glandular and typhoidal.

Tumor, 12

Tumorlike keratosis of Poth. Another term for Keratoacanthoma.

Tumors. The rarer tumors of the skin not discussed in Chapter 26 will be defined here. This complete classification is based on the histology. An asterisk signifies those tumors discussed in Chapter 26.
A. Epidermal tumors
I. Tumors of the surface epidermis
a. Nevoid tumors
1. Nevus verrucosus (Fig. 148). A rather common tumor usually present at birth consisting of single or multiple lesions in various forms that give rise to several clinical designations such as hard nevus, epidermal nevus, nevus unius lateralis, papilloma, ichthyosis hystrix, etc. No nevus cells are present.
2. Cysts
*(a) Epidermal cyst
*(b) Sebaceous cyst
*(c) Milium
*(d) Dermoid cyst
*(e) Mucous retention cyst
b. Precancerous tumors
*1. Senile or actinic keratosis and cutaneous horn
*2. Arsenical keratosis
*3. Leukoplakia
c. Epitheliomas
*1. Basal cell epithelioma
*2. Prickle cell epithelioma
*3. Keratoacanthoma
4. Bowen's disease and Erythroplasia of Queyrat. Bowen's disease is a single red scaly lesion with a sharp but irregular border that grows slowly by peripheral extension. Histologically it is an intraepidermal prickle cell epithelioma. Erythroplasia of Queyrat represents Bowen's disease of the mucous membranes and occurs on the glans penis and rarely on the vulva. The lesion has a bright red velvety surface.
5. Paget's disease. A unilateral scaly red lesion resembling a dermatitis, usually present on the female nipple. The early lesion is an intraepidermal prickle cell epithelioma that also involves the mammary ducts and deeper connective tissue.
*d. Seborrheic keratosis and dermatosis papulosa nigra
*e. Pedunculated fibromas
II. Tumors of the epidermal appendages
a. Nevoid tumors
1. Organic nevi
(a) Sebaceous nevi
(1) Nevus sebaceous (Jadassohn). Seen on the scalp or face as a single lesion present since birth, slightly raised, firm, yellowish, with furrowed surface.
(2) Adenoma sebaceum (Pringle). Part of a triad of epilepsy, mental deficiency and the skin lesions of adenoma sebaceum. The skin lesions occur on the face and consist of yellowish brown papular nodular lesions with telangiectases.
(3) Senile sebaceous nevus. This appears on the face in elderly persons and consists of one or several small yellowish translucent nodules.
(4) Fordyce disease. A rather common condition of pinpoint-sized yellowish lesions of the vermilion border of the lips or the oral mucosa.
2. Adenomas
(a) Sebaceous adenoma. A very rare solitary tumor of the face or scalp, smooth, firm, elevated, often slightly pedunculated and measuring less than 1 cm. in diameter.
(b) Apocrine adenomas
(1) Syringocystadenoma papilliferum. This adenoma of the apocrine ducts appears as a single verrucous plaque, usually seen on the scalp. Basal cell epitheliomatous change does occur.
(2) Hidradenoma papilliferum. This adenoma of the apocrine glands oc-

curs almost exclusively on the labia majora and perineum of women as a single intracutaneous tumor covered by normal epidermis.

(3) Benign epitheliomas

(a) Sebaceous epithelioma. A rare solitary, small nodule or plaque that has no characteristic clinical appearance.

(b) Apocrine epithelioma

(1) Syringoma. This is characterized by the appearance of pinhead sized soft, yellowish nodules at the age of puberty in women developing around the eyelids, chest, abdomen, and the anterior aspects of the thighs.

(2) Cylindroma. These appear as numerous, smooth, rounded tumors of various size on the scalp in adults and resemble bunches of grapes or tomatoes. These tumors may cover the entire scalp like a turban and are then referred to as turban tumors.

(3) Myoepithelioma. This occurs as a rare, moderately large solitary, intracutaneous tumor. Mixed tumors of the salivary gland type clinically and histologically resemble myoepithelioma.

(c) Hair epitheliomas

(1) Trichoepithelioma. Also known as epithelioma adenoides cysticum and multiple benign cystic epithelioma. This begins at the age of puberty frequently on a hereditary basis and is characterized by the presence of numerous, pinhead to pea-size rounded yellowish or pink nodules on the face and occasionally on the upper trunk. Ulceration occurs when these lesions change into a basal cell epithelioma.

(2) Calcifying epithelioma (Malherbe). A rather rare solitary, hard, deep seated nodule of the face or upper extremities. Malignant degeneration does not occur.

b. Carcinomas of sebaceous glands, and eccrine and apocrine sweat glands (rare)

B. Mesodermal tumors.

I. Tumors of fibrous tissue

*a. Histiocytoma and dermatofibroma

b. Xanthogranuloma (Fig. 149) (nevoxanthoendothelioma; juvenile xanthoma). A moderately rare condition characterized by the occurrence of several or many yellowish-brown papules or nodules usually on the extremities of young children that disappears spontaneously over the period of a few months or years.

*c. Keloid

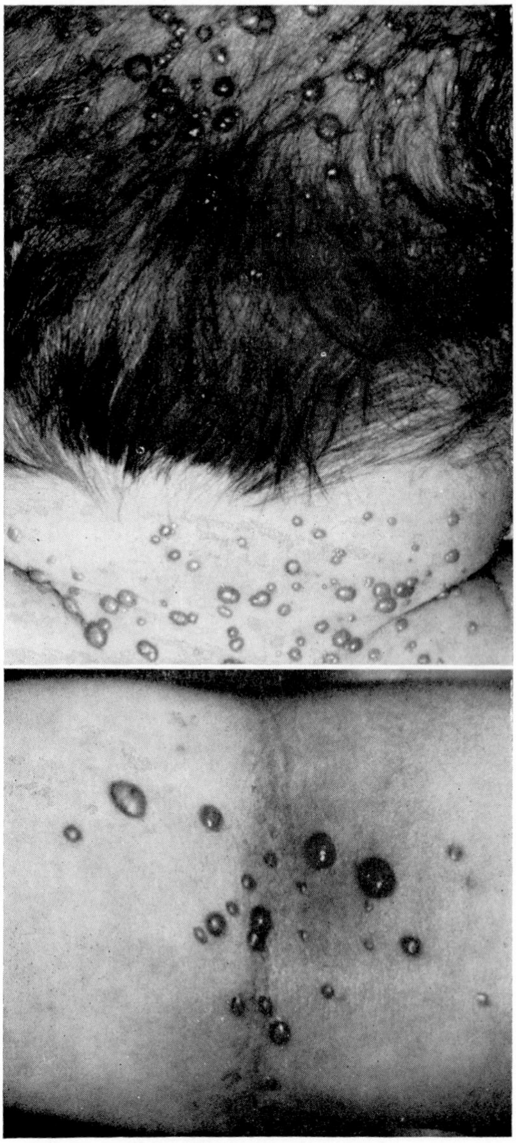

Fig. 149. Tumors. Xanthogranuloma.
(*Top*) Back of head and neck of child.
(*Bottom*) Arm of same child.
(*Dr. David Morgan*)

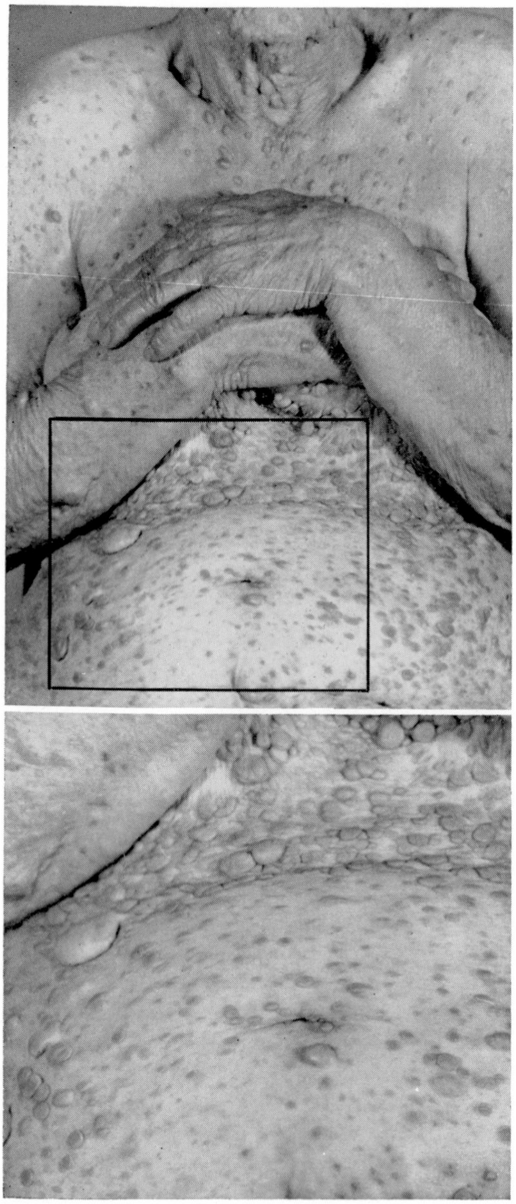

Fig. 150. Tumors. Neurofibromatosis.

Tumors, mesodermal, of fibrous tissue (*Cont.*)

d. Fibrosarcoma

1. True fibrosarcoma. A rare tumor that starts most commonly in the subcutaneous fat, grows rapidly, causes the overlying skin to appear purplish and finally ulcerates.
2. Dermatofibrosarcoma protuberans. A small tumor that grows slowly in the corium and spreads by the development of adjoining reddish or bluish nodules that may coalesce to form a plaque which can eventually ulcerate.

II. Tumors of mucoid tissue

a. Myxoma. Clinically seen as fairly well circumscribed, rather soft intracutaneous tumors with normal overlying epidermis.

b. Myxosarcoma. Subcutaneous tumors which eventually ulcerate the skin.

*c. Synovial cyst of the skin

III. Tumors of fatty tissue

a. Lipoma. A rather common tumor which may be multiple or single, lobulated, of varying size, and in the subcutaneous tissue.

b. Hibernoma. A form of lipoma composed of embryonic type of fat cells.

c. Liposarcoma

d. Malignant hibernoma

IV. Tumors of nerve tissue and mesodermal-nerve sheath cells

a. Neuroma. Rare, single or multiple small reddish or brown nodules that are usually tender as well as painful.

b. Neurofibromatosis (Fig. 150). Also known as von Recklinghausen's disease, this hereditary disease classically consists of pigmented patches, pedunculated skin tumors, and nerve tumors. All of these lesions may not be present in a particular case.

c. Neurolemoma

V. Tumors of vascular tissue

*a. Hemangiomas

b. Granuloma pyogenicum. Also known as proud flesh, this is a rather common end-result of an injury to the skin which may or may not have been apparent. Vascular proliferation with or without infection produces a small red tumor that bleeds easily. It is to be differentiated from a malignant melanoma. Mild electrocoagulation is curative if the known cause is removed.

c. Osler's disease. *See* Rendu-Osler-Weber disease.

d. Lymphangioma. A superficial form, lymphangioma circumscriptum, appears as a group of thin walled vesicles on the skin surface, whereas the deeper variety, lymphangioma cavernosum, causes a poorly defined enlargement of the affected area such as the lip or tongue.

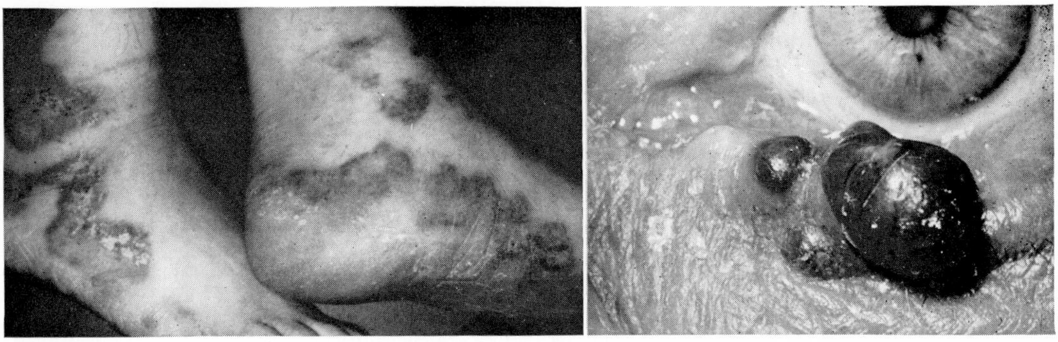

Fig. 151. Tumors. Kaposi's sarcoma.
(*Left*) Of feet (Dr. David Morgan).
(*Right*) Of lower eyelid (Drs. A. Lemoine and L. Calkins).

e. Glomus tumor. A rather unusual small, deep-seated, red or purplish nodule which is tender and may produce severe paroxysmal pains. The solitary lesion is usually seen under a nail plate, on the finger tips or elsewhere on the body.
f. Hemangiopericytoma
g. Kaposi's sarcoma (multiple idiopathic hemorrhagic sarcoma (Fig. 151). Most commonly seen on the feet and ankles as multiple bluish red or dark brown nodules and plaques associated with visceral lesions. Sarcomatous malignant degeneration can occur.
h. Hemangio-endothelioma
i. Postmastectomy lymphangiosarcoma

VI. Tumors of muscular tissue
a. Leiomyoma. Solitary leiomyomas may be found on the extremities and on the scrotum whereas multiple leiomyomas occur on the back and elsewhere as pinhead to pea-size, brown or bluish firm elevated nodules. Both forms are painful and sensitive to pressure, particularly as they enlarge.
b. Granular-cell myoblastoma. From embryonal striated muscle cells, this appears usually as a solitary tumor of the tongue, skin or subcutaneous tissue.

VII. Tumors of osseous tissue
a. Osteoma cutis
1. Primary. The primary form of osteoma cutis develops from embryonal cell rests. These may be single or multiple.
2. Secondary. Secondary bone formation may occur as a form of tissue degeneration in tumors, in scar tissue, in scleroderma lesions, and in various granulomas.

VIII. Tumors of cartilaginous tissue
a. Nodular chondrodermatitis of the ear. A painful, hyperkeratotic nodule usually on the helix of the ear of elderly males.

C. Nevus cell tumors
I. Nevi
*a. Junction (active) nevus
*b. Intradermal (resting) nevus
c. Lentigines. These represent early junction nevi which are to be differentiated from freckles (ephelides). A freckle histologically shows hyperpigmentation of the basal layer but no elongation of the rete pegs and no increase in the number of clear cells and dendritic cells.
d. Mongolian spot. These are seen chiefly in Oriental or Negro babies usually around the buttocks. They disappear spontaneously during childhood.
e. Blue nevus. Clinically, the blue nevus appears as a slate-blue or bluish-black sharply circumscribed, flat or slightly elevated nodule occurring on any area of the body.
*II. Malignant melanoma

D. Lymphomas
I. Monomorphous group. This includes stem-cell lymphoma, reticulum-cell lymphoma, lymphoblastic lymphoma, lymphocytic lymphoma and follicular lymphoma. Lymphomas may have specific skin lesions containing the lymphomatous infiltrate, or nonspe-

Tumors, lymphomas, monomorphous group (*Cont.*)
cific lesions may be seen. These latter consist of macules, papules, purpuric lesions, blisters, eczematous lesions, exfoliative dermatitis, and secondarily infected excoriations that are a part of severe itching. Synonymns for follicular lymphoma include Brill-Symmers disease, giant follicular lymphoblastoma, and the localized variety of Spiegler-Fendt sarcoid. The disseminate variety of Spiegler-Fendt sarcoid is now classified as a reticulum cell lymphoma.
II. Polymorphous group
a. Hodgkin's disease. Specific lesions are very rare but nonspecific dermatoses are rather commonly seen.
*b. Granuloma fungoides
E. Myelosis
I. Leukemia. Refers to circulating abnormal blood cells. May be seen along with lymphomas but it is almost always associated with myelosis, such as myeloid leukemia. Cutaneous lesions are quite uncommon but may be specific or nonspecific.
II. Reticulogranulomas. (Discussed under Xanthomas.)
a. Letterer-Siwe disease
b. Hand-Schuller-Christian disease
c. Eosinophilic granuloma
precancerous, 210
skin, 207-232
age, classification, 208
clinical classification, 208
histologic classification, 207
Tzanck cells. Cells uncovered from the floor of fresh bullae of pemphigus. These cells are altered epithelial cells, rounded and devoid of intercellular attachments.

Ulcer(s), 13
corneal, 121
infected, 104
phagedenic, 104
primary, 104
secondary, 104
stasis leg, 104
Ulcus vulvae acutum. A rare self-limited disease mainly of virgins characterized by shallow ulcerated lesions of the vulva. Thought to be caused by *Bacillus crassus* or a virus.
Ultraviolet therapy, 41
Urticaria, 67
papular, 204
pigmentosa, **182,** 229
Utah dermatoses, 202

Vaccinia, 126
Vaccinoid reaction, 127
Vaginitis, monilial, 151
trichomonal, 151
Varicose vein dermatitis, 71
Varioloid, 126
Vascular supply of skin, 3
Venous stars, 225
Venules, dilated. These occur very commonly in young and middle-aged women on the thighs and the legs. They can be removed easily by inserting an electrosurgical needle along the length of several of the venous arms or perpendicularly at several spots along the vein.
Verrucae, 127-130
Vesicles, 12
Virology, dermatologic, 121-134
Vitamin(s), 58, **180**
A, 180
B, 180
B_1, 180
B_2, 180
B_{12} therapy, 181
C, 181
D, 181
K, 181
Vitiligo, 169
in Arizona, 203
Vleminckx's solution. A solution of sulfur salts used as wet dressing therapy for the treatment of cystic acne. A fresh solution can be made by the addition of a Vlem-dome powder packet (Dome) to 1 pint of hot tap water.
Vogt-Koyanagi syndrome, characterized by nontraumatic bilateral uveitis, premature graying of the hair, alopecia, symmetric vitiligo of hands, wrists and feet, and dysacousia.
von Recklinghausen's disease. *See* Neurofibromatosis *under* Tumors

Warts, 127-130
around nails, 195
common, 127
filiform, 128
flat, 128
moist, 129
plantar, 129
Washington State dermatoses, 202
Weber-Christian disease, 71
Wegener's granulomatosis. This rare fatal syndrome of unknown etiology is characterized by granulomatous tumors of the upper re-

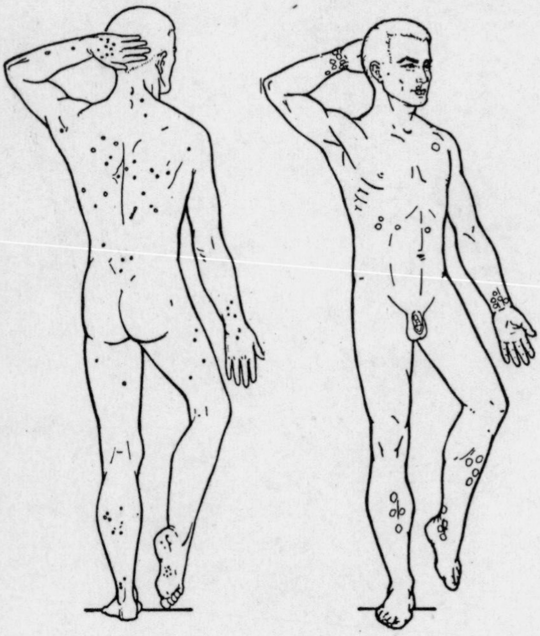

LICHEN PLANUS

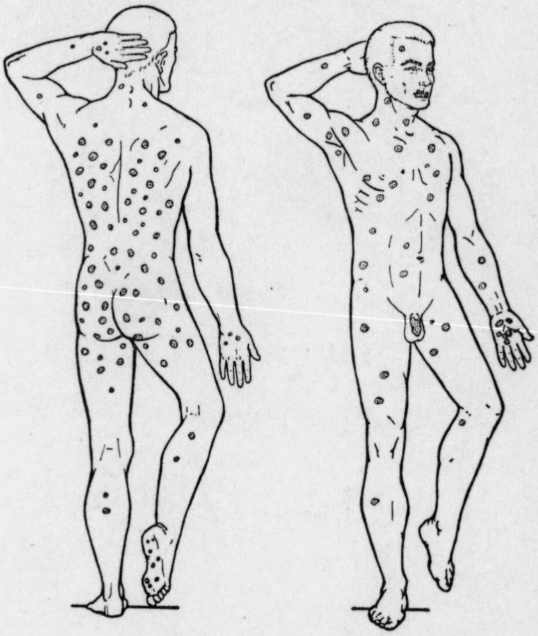

SECONDARY SYPHILIS

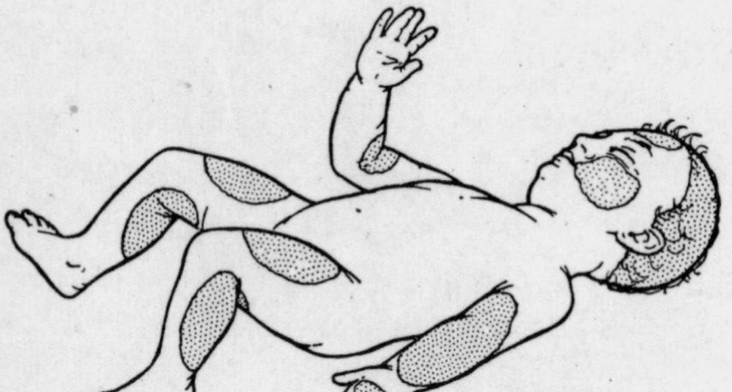

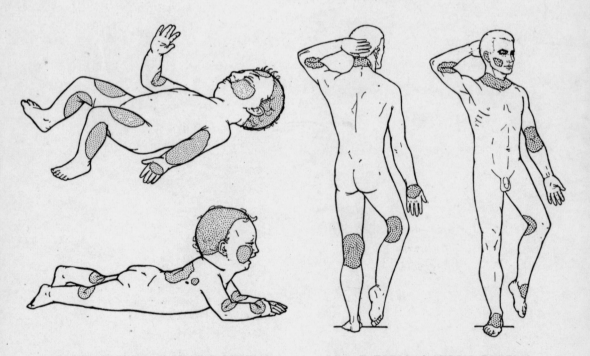

INFANTILE FORM of ATOPIC ECZEMA

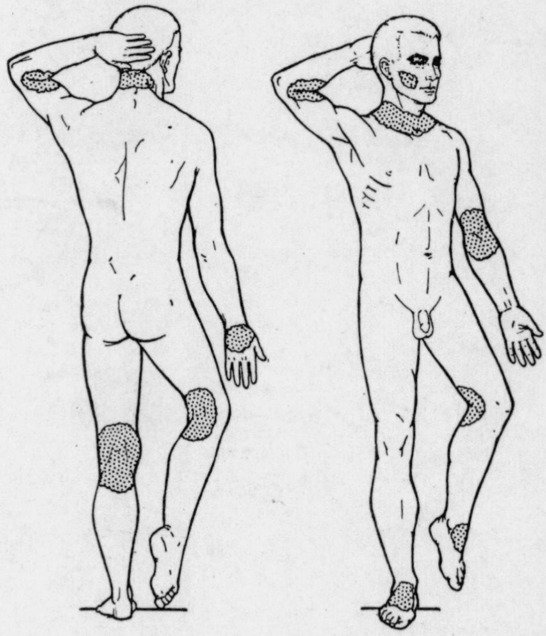

ADULT FORM of ATOPIC ECZEMA